Advances in Experimental Medicine and Biology

Volume 1350

Advances in Experimental Medicine and Biology provides a platform for scientific contributions in the main disciplines of the biomedicine and the life sciences. This series publishes thematic volumes on contemporary research in the areas of microbiology, immunology, neurosciences, biochemistry, biomedical engineering, genetics, physiology, and cancer research. Covering emerging topics and techniques in basic and clinical science, it brings together clinicians and researchers from various fields.

Advances in Experimental Medicine and Biology has been publishing exceptional works in the field for over 40 years, and is indexed in SCOPUS, Medline (PubMed), Journal Citation Reports/Science Edition, Science Citation Index Expanded (SciSearch, Web of Science), EMBASE, BIOSIS, Reaxys, EMBiology, the Chemical Abstracts Service (CAS), and Pathway Studio.

2019 Impact Factor: 2.450 5 Year Impact Factor: 2.324

More information about this series at http://www.springer.com/series/5584

Debabrata Banerjee • Raj K. Tiwari
Editors

Tumor Microenvironment: Cellular, Metabolic and Immunologic Interactions

Springer

Editors
Debabrata Banerjee
Department of Pharmacology
Robert Wood Johnson Medical School
Rutgers, The State University
of New Jersey
Piscataway, NJ, USA

Raj K. Tiwari
Department of Pathology, Microbiology
and Immunology
New York Medical College
Valhalla, NY, USA

ISSN 0065-2598 ISSN 2214-8019 (electronic)
Advances in Experimental Medicine and Biology
ISBN 978-3-030-83281-0 ISBN 978-3-030-83282-7 (eBook)
https://doi.org/10.1007/978-3-030-83282-7

This Springer imprint is published by the registered company Springer Nature Switzerland AG
The registered company address is: Gewerbestrasse 11, 6330 Cham, Switzerland

Preface

Appreciation of the important role of tumor microenvironment in supporting growth and dissemination of tumors has come as a result of increasing knowledge of the complexities of the tumor microenvironment. The field has grown from the early observations on spread of tumors to our current knowledge regarding the wide array of host cells and how they contribute to many aspects of tumor growth and spread.

In 1889, the English surgeon Stephen Paget proposed the "seed and soil" hypothesis, based on his study of autopsy records of hundreds of breast cancer patients, which basically suggested that tumors or "seeds" are dispersed in all directions but can thrive only if they fall on the right "soil." This view was subsequently challenged by James Ewing who suggested that metastasis is determined by purely mechanical means and had little to do with the "soil." Thanks to the pioneering work of Prof. Isaah Fidler and colleagues we now have an improved understanding of cancer metastasis; the soil is now termed the "tumor microenvironment" and is widely accepted as an equal partner in determining metastasis outcome [1–6].

Tumor microenvironment has many different facets, and each are important in their own right in shaping tissue homeostasis if one recognizes that the tumor is an externally growing immunologically tolerized organ constantly trying to adapt itself in the host. Immunologically it survives by invoking the classical tolerance mechanism and physically by interception of survival mechanism be it metabolic or oxidative respiration. In the present series, our aim has been to decipher the immediate cellular milieu and how it shapes tumor phenotype, specifically the metastases phenotype. This cutting-edge analysis is expected to give the highest return in terms of therapeutic intervention and our ability to manage cancer as it can impact metastases directly. It is our contention that if metastasis is preventable, then cancer becomes a manageable chronic disease.

In this context updates on evasion of immune surveillance (Tiwari chapter), metabolic support (Mishra chapter), growth factor and cytokine signaling, provide structural support to the tumor enabling invasive behavior. We have just begun to understand how cell–cell interaction in the TME is not limited to released factors from one cell that then reaches a target cell and produces an effect but can also occur via exosomes which carry a number of molecules that evoke a variety responses in the target cell (Rameshwar chapter). It is well known that hematopoiesis is sustained in the bone marrow (BM) via mechanisms involving the microenvironment which includes several cell types, neurotransmitters from innervated fibers, growth factors, extracellular matrix proteins, as well as extracellular vesicles. Besides its hematopoietic function, the BM microenvironment can also accommodate survival of malignant cells that communicate with cells of the BM microenvironment through exchange of exosomes, a subset of extracellular vesicles that deliver molecular signals between cells. A better understanding of exosomal packaging, cargo, and production can be leveraged therapeutically to impede cancer progression. The crucial role of exosomes in the development and progression of BM-associated cancers, such as hematologic malignancies and marrow-metastatic breast cancer, are presented. Attention is also paid to exosome-based therapeutic strategies and their limitations.

Mishra and Banerjee reflect on tumor stroma metabolic interaction. Tumor microenvironment (TME) contains stromal cell of different types including fibroblasts, immune cells, and endothelial cells having varied influence on the local metabolic activity. Recent advances in the understanding of complex tumor microenvironment have revealed that a multifaceted interaction between tumor cells with their neighboring stroma is essential for tumor growth and metastasis. The tumor stroma presents distinctive features which enhance tumor growth such as recruitment and ultimate activation of bone marrow–derived mesenchymal stem cells to cancer-associated fibroblasts (CAFs). This underscores molecular interactions in the tumor microenvironment and allows reciprocal exchange of nutrients, secretory molecules, and other signals between tumor and stromal cells. The reciprocated molecular interactions between tumor cells and non-malignant stromal cells in the tumor microenvironment not only promote tumor development and progression, but largely control most of the characteristic hallmarks of tumorigenesis and stimulate chemotherapeutic drug resistance. Shared interactions between tumor and stromal cells facilitated either directly by cell-to-cell contact or via the release of secretory molecules including, cytokines, chemokines and extra cellular matrix (ECM) aid in remodeling proteins to activate signaling pathways that encourage cell growth, survival and overall development. The secretory molecules shared among tumor cells and neighboring cells instigate epithelial-mesenchymal transition (EMT), tumor cells migration, invasion, and dissemination to secondary sites. The metabolic activities in the microenvironment are influenced by tumor and stromal factors present in the microenvironment. Metabolic reprogramming allows fulfillment of demands of growing tumor cells. Different stromal components in the tumor microenvironment provide additional nutrients that supplement local nutrient pool. Stromal cells present in the immediate proximity of tumor cells are inevitably most affected by the metabolic alterations caused by neighboring cancerous cells. Stromal fibroblasts present in the tumor microenvironment also known as cancer-associated fibroblasts (CAFs) play a key role in metabolic reprogramming. CAFs are predominantly resident mesenchymal cells in origin that get activated and reprogrammed in response to signals from cancer cells. Tumor cells display heightened glucose uptake and even under normoxic conditions display increased generation of lactate from pyruvate by aerobic glycolysis, also known as the Warburg effect. This adaptation not only allows generation of biosynthetic precursors for added nutritional demands of tumor cells but also directs the metabolic reprogramming of neighboring stromal cells. The lactate generated as a result of metabolic reprogramming of tumor cells and stromal cells play diverse role in the tumor microenvironment. Both tumor and stromal CAFs consume and secrete lactate differently, which makes it an integral modulating factor in tumor microenvironment. Molecular evidences collected over the last several years have prompted deeper examination of tumor stroma interactions. Mishra and Banerjee have covered role of cytokines, chemokines, and lactate in driving tumor-stroma interactions in the microenvironment. Pro-tumorigenic molecular interactions between tumor cells and CAFs mediated via altered signaling pathways, cytokines, chemokines, and lactate in the tumor vicinity are discussed. A better understanding of the complex cancer cell–CAF interactions will help in designing successful therapeutic strategies targeting the stromal rich tumors in the clinic.

Freeman writes on the structural aspects of the tumor microenvironment. Cancers can be described as "rogue organs" because they are composed of multiple cell types and tissues and appear to be independent of control mechanisms operative in normal organs and tissues. The transformed cells can recruit and alter healthy cells from surrounding tissues for their own benefit. It is these interactions that create the tumor microenvironment (TME). The TME describes the cells, factors, and extracellular matrix proteins of the tumor and the area around it. Alterations in the TME can lead to growth and development of the tumor, the death of the tumor, or tumor metastasis, a process by which cancer spreads from its initial site to different sites. Metastasis occurs when cancer cells enter the circulatory system or lymphatic system after breaking away from a tumor. Once the cells reach the circulatory system, they can travel to a different part of the body and form new tumors. Understanding the TME therefore becomes critical to fully understand cancer and develop strategies to control it. Knowledge of the TME can better inform researchers of the ability of potential therapies to reach tumor cells. It can also identify potential targets within the tumor. Instead of directly killing the cancer cells, therapies can target an aspect of the TME which could then halt tumor development or lead to tumor death. In other cases, targeting another aspect of the TME could make it easier for another therapy to kill the cancer cells. The TME can be split simply into cells and the structural matrix and include fibroblasts, structural proteins, immune cells, lymphocytes, bone marrow-derived inflammatory cells, blood vessels, and signaling molecules. From structure scaffolds to providing nutrients for growth, each of these components impacts cancer growth, development, and resistance to therapies. This chapter describes the TME and underscores the importance of cellular and structural elements of the TME.

Gene expression analyses have also brought to light the emerging role of long non-coding RNAs in cellular communication in the TME (Geliebter chapter). The idea of regulating gene expression was prominent in tumor cells and has contributed to a wealth of information in the discovery of all the transcriptional factors and their role in oncogenesis and metastases. Although transcriptional factors have been difficult target, they have been of immense benefit. Recent advances in regulators of gene expression include long noncoding RNAs which may be more amenable to novel therapies that use gene deletion techniques such CRISPR but not limited to one technique. Linking these molecules with cancer differentiation phenotype is a foundational discovery in carcinogenesis that brings gene expression and genotype variation with observed cancer phenotype in the mainstream of cancer biology. This is indeed cutting-edge discovery in our battle to understand the heterogeneity of cancer and devise personalized therapy.

Dr. Maniyar furthers the concept of linking cancer phenotype resulting from genetic lesions with the cellular environment of the tumor microenvironment specifically as dictated by the immune cells. This is an attempt to define the negative and positive regulators of immune activation and checkpoints so as to advance a combinatorial therapy that can target the genetic lesion–based signal transduction pathway together with the checkpoint inhibitor–based immunotherapy. Taking a stock of the immune cells in the tumor microenvironment one characterizes the exhausted effector tumor cells that have now become signals of preexisting immune activation and the various modalities to specifically use the characteristics of these exhausted effectors cells to tailor-made novel combinatorial dual targeted cancer therapies. One directed against the driver mutations and the other to boost immune effector cells. The emphasis in this chapter is also in the need to characterize the expression of checkpoint molecules on the tumor cells itself so that the therapy can be tailored to thwart the tumor's attempt to propagate an immunosuppressive environment. These finding and the concepts put forward in the context of melanoma by Maniyar et al apply to other cancers as well.

A very important piece of the carcinogenesis puzzle is to identify a set of markers that can define the phenotype of the growing tumor preferably in biological fluids. Almost 70 years of research has resulted in tumor-associated markers. Most of these markers reflect our technical advances to compare tumor versus normal in regard to macro molecules, enzymes and proteins, lipids, and cell-surface carbohydrates culminated into genes and regulators of gene expression. Tumor-specific markers remain elusive though tumor-associated markers have contributed to defining subsets of tumors. Cell-cell communication in the evolution of tumorigenic phenotype is a recent discovery, and more significantly, we have been characterizing the template of this communication where secretory exosomes play a significant role. It is the contention of **Jarboe et al** that these exosomes have defined cargo and reflect both the inflammatory cell phenotype and the evolving cancer using anaplastic thyroid cancer as a model system and the deregulated miRNAs in ATC tissues they propose a novel category of biomarker(s) that could define metastatic propensity. The use of these miRNA markers in secreted fluids remains to be analyzed; however, such analysis and categorization of inflammation promoting markers especially in secretory exosomes in serum can provide us important clues on tissue tumor evolution.

The success of immunotherapy, specifically checkpoint inhibitor, is at least partly dependent on the selection of the right target that thwarts the tumor-induced immune suppression. Chakraborty et al promote the contention, using anaplastic thyroid cancer as a model, that there are several tumor-intrinsic and tumor-extrinsic factors that shape the final response. Extrinsic factors include quality of T cell infiltrates, composition of cytokines, and percentage of immune suppressor cells such as MDSCs. All these eventually shape the immune response in a highly individualized manner. High percentage of tumor-associated macrophages and immune suppressive cytokines are well established features of the immune landscape in ATC. In the three-way cell-cell communication, antigen presentation cells, T cells, and tumor cells, the cytokine milieu is of major significance that can be measured in serum as end point markers. These inflammatory markers can provide important clues to ATC evolution, and the characterization of the expression of positive and negative regulators on tumor cell surface leads to additional immunotherapeutic targets as identified by Chakraborty et. al.

The importance of cellular components of the tumor microenvironment in promoting tumor cell growth and dissemination is now well accepted in the field of cancer biology. The interaction between these components and the tumor cells is becoming an area of intense research, and chapters in this series have touched upon various aspects of these interactions. An increased understanding of these interactions will likely result in improved therapeutic strategies to control growth and spread of tumor cells from the primary site. Comprehension of these complex interactions is limited due to studies being conducted in isolated systems under restrictive experimental conditions. We regret that other important aspects of TME such as innervation of tumors and cancer stem cells in the TME could not be included in this volume.

References for general reading on history of Tumor Microenvironment:

1. Langley, R. R., & Fidler, I. J. (2007). Tumor cell-organ microenvironment interactions in the pathogenesis of cancer metastasis. *Endocrine Reviews, 28*, 297–321. [PubMed: 17409287].
2. Fidler, I. J. (2003). The pathogenesis of cancer metastasis: The 'seed and soil' hypothesis revisited. *Nature Reviews. Cancer, 3*, 453–458. [PubMed: 12778135].
3. Talmadge, J. E., Benedict, K., Madsen, J., & Fidler, I. J. (1984). Development of biological diversity and susceptibility to chemotherapy in murine cancer metastases. *Cancer Research, 44*, 3801–3805. [PubMed: 6744297].
4. Paget, S. (1889). The distribution of secondary growths in cancer of the breast. *The Lancet, 133*(3421), 571–573.
5. Fidler, I. J., & Poste, G. (2008). The "seed and soil" hypothesis revisited. *The Lancet Oncology, 9*(8), 808.
6. Ewing, J. (1928). *Metastasis, neoplastic disease: A treatise on tumors*. Philadelphia and London.

Valhalla, NY, USA — Raj K. Tiwari
Piscataway, NJ, USA — Debabrata Banerjee

Contents

About the Editors

Debabrata (Debu) Banerjee, Ph.D., is an Emeritus Professor, Rutgers University having retired as Assistant Dean, School of Graduate Studies and an Associate Professor in the Department of Pharmacology at Rutgers University. He is also an Adjunct Associate Professor at the New York Medical College, positions he has held since 2002. Prior to this, he was an Associate Lab Member at Memorial Sloan-Kettering Cancer Center, New York. Dr. Banerjee obtained a PhD in Biochemistry from Calcutta University and also served as an Adjunct Lecturer for the Department of Biochemistry at Calcutta University. Dr. Banerjee completed his Postdoctoral Fellowship training in the Department of Biology, McGill University, Canada. He has published over 100 peer reviewed research articles in scientific journals. In addition, to his academic appointments, Debu serves as a Member of the Editorial Board for journals Cancers, Cells, PLoS, World Journal of Stem Cells and Current Signal Transduction and Therapy. He is a Reviewer for the journals: Cancer Research, Oncogene, Clinical Cancer Research, Gynecologic Oncology, Journal of Cancer Chemotherapy, British Journal of Cancer, Stem Cells, and Blood. He has extensive experience in preclinical drug development. He has also been awarded 5 patents for his scientific innovations.

Raj K. Tiwari is currently a Professor and Graduate Program Director at New York Medical College's Department of Pathology, Microbiology and Immunology and the Department of Otolaryngology. He was interim Chair of the Department of Microbiology and Immunology for over 3 years. Tiwari received his BS in Chemistry at St. Xavier's College in Calcutta, his Masters in Biochemistry at Calcutta University, and his Ph.D. in Biochemistry at Calcutta University. Tiwari has an internationally recognized profile for his contributions in Cancer Biology on the early observations of the JAK/STAT pathway, use of peptides mimotopes as Cancer Vaccines and more recently on the Cell-Cell communication in the tumor microenvironment. His focus is on a variety of Cancers, Breast, Prostate, Melanoma and Thyroid. He teaches immunology to medical and graduate students and take pride in successfully mentoring a large number of graduate students, clinical fellows and junior faculty.

Inflammatory Components of the Thyroid Cancer Microenvironment: An Avenue for Identification of Novel Biomarkers

Tara Jarboe, Neha Y. Tuli, Sanjukta Chakraborty, Rachana R. Maniyar, Nicole DeSouza, Xiu-Min Li, Augustine Moscatello, Jan Geliebter, and Raj K. Tiwari

1 Tumor Microenvironment of Solid Tumors

1.1 Defining the Tumor Microenvironment

Solid tumors consist of two interdependent compartments – the carcinoma cells and the stroma (Fig. 1). Unlike the normal interstitial connective tissue, the tumor stroma is involved in malignant growth. The cellular constituents of the tumor stroma surrounding and embedded in the tumor make up the tumor microenvironment (TME). The tumor stroma consists of various stromal cells and a structural component known as the extracellular matrix (ECM). The stromal cells secrete macromolecules that make up the ECM. These macromolecules are made of proteoglycans and glycoproteins, such as laminin, fibronectin, and structural proteins, including collagen and elastin. The stromal cells also secrete proteolytic enzymes leading to ECM degradation. This phenomenon along with disruption of the basement membrane becomes a prerequisite for the invasion process. During invasion, the matrix of the stroma is degraded by active proteases secreted into the tissue microenvironment leading to migration of tumor cells along the various components of the ECM [1, 2]. The ECM is responsible for the generation of signals that influence cellular proliferation, growth, migration, invasion, angiogenesis, and differentiation of cancer cells. Also, normal cells undergo apoptosis in the absence of contact with the ECM, proving it to be an important factor for cell survival. The composition of the ECM is modified and remodeled as the tumor progresses. As such,

T. Jarboe · N. Y. Tuli · N. DeSouza · Xiu-Min Li · J. Geliebter · R. K. Tiwari (✉)
Departments of Pathology, Microbiology and Immunology, New York Medical College, Valhalla, NY, USA
e-mail: Raj_Tiwari@nymc.edu

S. Chakraborty
Departments of Pathology, Microbiology and Immunology, New York Medical College, Valhalla, NY, USA

Weill Cornell Medicine, New York, NY, USA

R. R. Maniyar
Departments of Pathology, Microbiology and Immunology, New York Medical College, Valhalla, NY, USA

Memorial Sloan Kettering Cancer Center, New York, NY, USA

A. Moscatello
Department of Otolaryngology, Westchester Medical Center, Valhalla, NY, USA

D. Banerjee, R. K. Tiwari (eds.), *Tumor Microenvironment: Cellular, Metabolic and Immunologic Interactions*, Advances in Experimental Medicine and Biology 1350,
https://doi.org/10.1007/978-3-030-83282-7_1

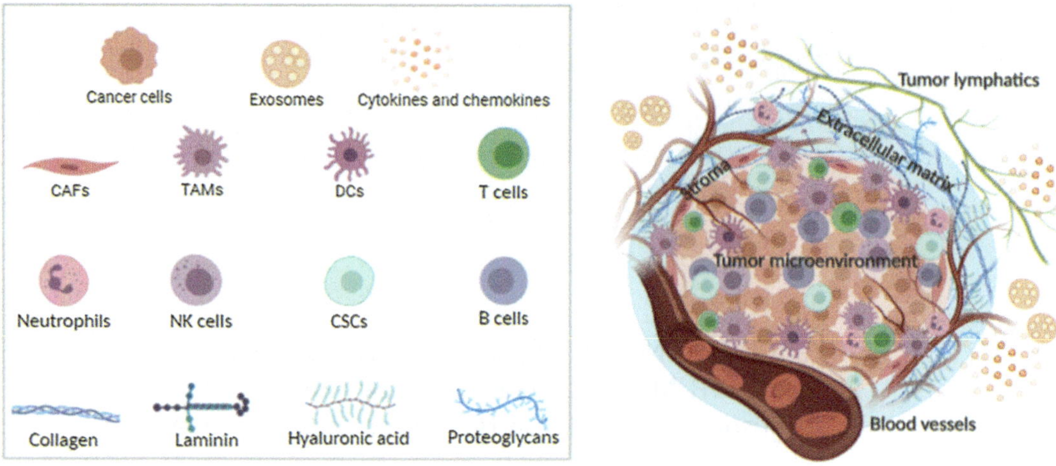

Fig. 1 Tumor Microenvironment of solid tumors and its cellular, structural, and secretory constituents

the malleable ECM microenvironment does not just provide structural support, but also has a profound influence on tumorigenesis [3]. The cellular components of the tumor stroma consist of cancer-associated fibroblasts (CAFs), pericytes, vascular endothelial cells, cancer stem cells and immune cells. The immune cells include dendritic cells, tumor-infiltrating lymphocytes, monocytes, and tumor-associated macrophages (TAMs). These cells, as well as the secretory molecules released by these cells and the tumor cells making up the TME including cytokines, chemokines, growth factors, and exosomes carrying cargo that all remodel the composition of the TME (Fig. 1), will be described in greater detail throughout this chapter. The interactions of these cells and their cellular constituents lead to consistent alterations in the TME network showcasing the dynamic nature of the TME.

1.2 Cellular Constituents of the Tumor Microenvironment

1.2.1 Cancer-Associated Fibroblasts (CAFs)

The main connective tissue cells that reshape the tumor stroma are fibroblasts and myofibroblasts. During the early stages of tumorigenesis, the fibroblasts undergo a change in both activity and phenotype, transforming into cancer-associated fibroblasts (CAFs). These cells produce macromolecules of the ECM, aid in angiogenesis, and synthesize various growth factors and cytokines. The basic fibroblast growth factor is a mitogenic factor for smooth muscle and is involved in various intracellular signaling pathways [4–6]. The interaction between fibroblasts and activated myofibroblasts occurs via direct cell-cell contact or by means of paracrine signaling. Presence of these cells is correlated with increased tumor aggressiveness and poor prognosis [7].

1.2.2 Endothelial Cells (ECs)

Endothelial cells (ECs) form the inner lining of the blood vessels. The associated vasculature is responsible for the delivery of nutrients and oxygen to tissues, organs, as well as developing tumors. Therefore, the formation of new blood vessels (neovascularization) and sprouting of new blood vessels from preexisting ones (angiogenesis) are both essential for the growth and the metastasis of tumors. Numerous pro-angiogenic factors, such as vascular endothelial growth factor (VEGF), platelet-derived growth factor (PDGF), basic fibroblast growth factor (bFGF), and angiopoietins, are secreted into the TME to stimulate angiogenesis; this phenomenon is observed in the thyroid cancer TME. Among these growth factors, VEGF is the key pro-angiogenic factor, and activation of its receptor,

VEGF receptor-2 (VEGFR-2), results in endothelial cell survival, proliferation, and vessel tubule formation. The degree and intensity of angiogenesis depend on the balance between the pro- and anti-angiogenic factors and their regulation [8].

1.2.3 Cancer Stem Cells (CSCs)

This subpopulation of tumor cells actively participates in the initiation and promotion of tumor formation. Cancer stem cells (CSCs) can self-renew, differentiate to diverse cell lineages, and seed new tumors. In vitro and in vivo experiments have shown that CSCs can differentiate into vascular endothelial cells. There is also speculation that CSCs can also differentiate into immune cells, such as tumor-associated macrophages (TAMs), in the TME, furthering the process of tumorigenesis and metastasis [9]. An interesting study done in mammary cancer cells by Mani et al. suggests that epithelial to mesenchymal transition (EMT) generates CSCs from mammary epithelial cancer cells [10].

1.2.4 Immune Cells

Pathological reports have shown that solid tumors are surrounded by abundant immune cell infiltrates. These cells belong to both arms of the immune system – innate and adaptive. These cells include lymphocytes, tumor-associated macrophages (TAMs), and various antigen-presenting cells (APCs). These cellular types are explained in further detail in Sect. 1.3.

1.3 Immune Cells of the Tumor Microenvironment

1.3.1 Natural Killer Cells (NK Cells)

Natural killer (NK) cells belong to the innate immune system and actively take part in initial tumor immune surveillance. The two types of NK cells, immunoregulatory and cytotoxic, are distinguished based on the expression of specific surface molecules – cluster of differentiation 16 (CD16) or 56 (CD56). The relative levels of immunoregulatory versus cytotoxic NK cells impact whether or not the TME has a pro-tumor phenotype, with a desire to polarize these NK cells in the cytotoxic direction to improve prognosis of disease, as described in the context of papillary and anaplastic thyroid cancer (ATC) in Sect. 2.6 [11].

1.3.2 Dendritic Cells

Dendritic cells (DCs) are key immune regulatory components that facilitate a critical connection between the innate and adaptive immune system, and arise from a hematopoietic stem cell lineage. Their main role lies in their antigen presentation ability, characterizing them as antigen-presenting cells (APCs). DCs are classified as one of the more "professional" APCs, a conclusion made on the basis of their efficient migration and T-cell activation. Upon foreign antigen detection, DCs will internalize, process, and project the antigen on its periphery, resulting in naive T-cell recognition and thus activation of an adaptive, and specifically tailored, immune response. DCs will present antigens in the context of major histocompatibility complex (MHC) class II and I in secondary lymphoid organs, a phenomenon termed as "cross-presentation." In the event of pathologic environment establishment, DCs have the ability to recognize certain molecular patterns (pathogen-associated molecular patterns (PAMPs) or danger-associated molecular patterns (DAMPs)) and elicit an immune response through migration and upregulation of costimulatory molecules. Examples of these costimulatory molecules include CD40, CD80, and CD86, which support the generation of a second set of signals that will initiate the adaptive immune response.

Within the tumor microenvironment (TME), there is a plethora of DC infiltrates that represent a variety of maturation stages and DC subsets. These subsets include plasmacytoid DCs (pDC), conventional DCs (cDCs) 1 and 2, and monocyte-derived DCs (mo-DCs). Tumors are said to contain seldom mature DCs, due to the fact that the TME is highly immunosuppressive, a characteristic that favors tumor proliferation [12]. With this being said, there is a correlation between increased levels of mature DCs and a positive prognosis. However, it has been seen that in certain TMEs, DCs have the potential to switch from serving as an immunostimulatory cell that drives potent anti-tumor activity to becoming an immunosuppressive accomplice. Cancer cells secrete immunosuppressive factors that are said to facilitate this pathologic "switch" in DC activity, leading to the formation of tumor-associated DCs (TADCs). TADCs characteristically promote neovascularization, which greatly favors tumor growth and establishment. This population of TADCs exerts their tumor-promoting effects through hindering antigen uptake and presentation, which greatly reduces the generation of an immune response; therefore, subsets of TADCs can serve as a target for the facilitation of therapeutic intervention [13].

1.3.3 Mast Cells

Mast cells are immune cells that elicit their effector function through either one of two processes: piecemeal degranulation and anaphylactic degranulation. The granules of mast cells are loaded with histamine, a potent inflammatory mediator that is released when an immune response is generated. Mast cell activation is typically triggered via IgE Fc region interaction with their FcεRI, making them key players in allergic responses. Mast cells are also prominent factors within the tumor microenvironment (TME) due to their extensive role in inflammation and their ability to induce neovascularization and support angiogenesis. Mast cells are said to support the proliferation of the TME and can contribute to the pathogenic nature and aggression of certain cancer types [14]. Depending on the anatomical location and type of tumor, mast cell involvement contributes to either a good or poor prognosis [15]. Within the TME, mast cells interact with other cellular residents, either through direct contact or through the release of characteristic mediators that have the ability to lead to TME remodeling. Studies have shown a plausible correlation between mast cells and the development of thyroid cancer. This correlation was made on the basis of significant mast cell infiltration within thyroid cancers that were more aggressive and invasive. Mast cell recruitment to the tumor site occurs via chemoattractant responses to vascular endothelial growth factor-A (VEGF-A), a protein released by thyroid cancer cells [16]. Thyroid carcinoma cells were also shown to alter the mast cell transcriptome, which was demonstrated through an IL-6, tumor necrosis factor-α (TNF-α), and colony-stimulating factor mRNA upregulation, which greatly supports the proliferative and inflammatory nature of the TME. Similar to thyroid cancer cells, pancreatic cancer cells also lead to the induction of mast cell migration. Upon mast cell infiltration into the TME, release of their associated cytokines, IL-13 and tryptase, leads to a proliferation of pancreatic cancer cells. Since the presence of mast cells favors tumor proliferation, blocking mast cell migration has led to the suppression of pancreatic cancer cell growth, and has contributed to a prognostic improvement [14].

1.3.4 T Regulatory Cells (Tregs)

CD4+ T helper (Th) cells can be polarized to express two different types of immune responses: the anti-tumorigenic Th1 response and the pro-tumorigenic Th2 response. T regulatory cells (Tregs) are associated with the pro-tumorigenic Th2 response. The polarization of the CD4+ T cells is influenced by the factors present in the TME.

Interestingly, double negative T cells have been more recently observed as previously undiscovered type of lymphocyte infiltration, which was showcased in a study by Imam et al. The double negative T cells do not express either CD8 or CD4 cell surface markers, and their secreted cytokines, particularly interferon-gamma (IFN-γ) and interleukin-17 (IL-17), repress the activation of CD8+ and CD4+ T cells. Thus, these double negative T cells make the TME favorable for persistent chronic inflammation, encouraging the tumor progression [17].

1.3.5 CD8+ Cytotoxic T Cells (CTLs)

Cluster of differentiation 8 (CD8) is a well-defined glycoprotein that spans the membrane of T lymphocytes and is further defined as a co-receptor for the T-cell receptor (TCR). Collectively, these cells are specifically denoted as $CD8^+$ T lymphocytes and are key components of the adaptive immune system. Upon activation through presentation of tumor-associated antigens by antigen-presenting cells (APCs), these cells will differentiate into cytotoxic T lymphocytes (CTLs) and are responsible for eliciting their cytotoxic effects upon stimulation via interaction with major histocompatibility complex I (MHC I) and cognate antigen. This primes the CTLs against tumor cells expressing those specific antigens. Antigen presentation is an immunogenic phenomenon that describes the internalization of antigen followed by presentation on the cell periphery to elicit an immune-specific response through immune cell activation and differentiation. These cells will receive their antigen-specific signal, followed by subsequent activation via costimulatory signals and cytokines delivered by the APC to promote their targeted and specific effector functions. Activated $CD8^+$ T cells will secrete two key cytokines that contain potent anti-tumor effects: tumor necrosis factor-alpha (TNF-α) and interferon-gamma (IFN-γ). These cells can also release two protein classes stored within their cytoplasmic granules, known as perforins and granzymes, which are pore-forming and pro-apoptotic proteins, respectively. These proteins work in concert to elicit an immune response on a foreign target. In addition to their released cytotoxic mediators, CTLs also will express chemokine receptors that will allow the cell to gain access to peripheral tissues [18]. Activation through tumor antigen recognition and presentation leads to the generation of an adaptive immune response, involving the activation of CTLs, and their subsequent recruitment and infiltration (tumor-infiltrating lymphocytes, TILs) into the area in which the tumor environment is being established. CTLs are a key component of discussion when referring to the tumor microenvironment (TME). TILs and inflammation together serve as a key feature of cancer [19]. Despite the high degree of heterogeneity of the TME, a major portion of the cellular composition is attributed to T-cell residents. $CD8^+$ T-cell analysis within cancer patients has led to a better understanding of tumor immunology and antigen-specific immunotherapy. Activated T cells express a programmed cell death-1 (PD-1) receptor on its periphery, whereas its corresponding ligands, PD-L1 and PD-L2, are expressed by dendritic cells and macrophages. When activated CTLs bearing PD-1 receptors migrate to the TME, the receptor/ligand interactions promote resistance to endogenous anti-tumor activity that is typically exemplified by CTLs. Within the TME, PD-L1 is said to be overexpressed on the resident tumor cells, which greatly favors their further establishment and immune evasion through inhibition of CTLs. For example, in breast cancer (BC), instances of poorer prognosis have been shown in patients that express high levels of PD-1^+ TILs, which coincides with their inhibition. Furthermore, in BC patients, their sites of malignant tissue had significantly less IL-2 and IFN-γ, which corresponds to the progressive loss/inhibition of cytotoxic activity, a phenomenon termed "T-cell exhaustion" [20].

To determine the impact that blocking PD-1 has on the establishment of CTLs within the TME, there is a stage-specific requirement that will determine whether or not the abrogated expression of the receptor will lead to a rise in CTL cytotoxicity or favor immune evasion. Results have shown that anti-PD-1 monoclonal antibody therapy can serve as a revitalization tool for exhausted T cells and has led to an increased production of IFN-γ, thus confirming successful activation of CTL activity [21]. This PD-1 blockade, however, is only successful when it occurs in a stage-specific manner. Blocking of PD-1 must occur after the CD8 T lymphocyte is exposed to the presented antigen. If anti-PD-1 is administered prior to antigen exposure, the CD8 T lymphocyte will become anergic, and linker for activation of T cells (LAT) and Akt will lack phosphorylation: an implication of failed cellular activation [21]. CTLs that express high levels of PD-1 have been correlated with an increased expression of T-cell immunoglobulin and mucin domain-3 (TIM-3) and lymphocyte activation gene 3 (LAG3), two inhibitory checkpoint molecules [22]. TIM-3 has specifically been identified as a marker for anti-PD-1 resistance, which makes this inhibitory molecule a key target for future study regarding cancer immunotherapy [22].

1.3.6 Tumor-Associated Macrophages (TAMs)

Macrophages are key components of the innate immune system; they serve as the first responders to inflammation or pathogens and foreign antigens. Common myeloid progenitor cells give rise to blood monocytes that eventually differentiate into macrophages [23]. These cells of monocyte-macrophage lineage are very important for the maintenance of homeostasis in body tissues. Macrophages have multiple subtypes and possess the plasticity to switch between these subtypes. Based on the signals within the tissue microenvironment, macrophages can either be activated classically to an M1 phenotype or alternatively to an M2 phenotype. Cytokines secreted by Th1 cells, such as IFN-γ and tumor necrosis factor-alpha (TNF-α), or the bacterial moiety lipopolysaccharide (LPS), have the ability to activate macrophages to the M1 phenotype. On the other hand, M2 macrophages are subdivided into M2a, M2b, and M2c subtypes based on their activation stimulus. Th2 cytokines, such as IL-13 and IL-4, activate monocytes to the M2a macrophage phenotype. M2b macrophages are stimulated by LPS, toll-like receptors (TLRs), and IL-1 receptor antagonists. Lastly, M2c macrophages are induced by transforming growth factor beta (TGF-β), IL-10, or glucocorticoids [24]. The diversified phenotype of macrophages, based on their polarization, exhibits differential expression of cytokines, chemokines, and surface proteins. M1 macrophages are pro-inflammatory and produce inflammatory cytokines such as IL-6, IL-1, and TNF-α, which aid in the generation of an anti-tumor immune response. In contrast, M2 macrophages exert pro-tumorigenic, anti-inflammatory, and pro-vasculogenic actions. These actions are exerted via immunosuppressive cytokines, including IL-4, IL-13, and IL-10, as well as immune complexes and apoptotic cells.

Solid tumors, such as thyroid cancer, are composed of a highly heterogeneous mass of mutant cells embedded in the stroma, with these macrophages being a vital and prominent component. Hence, these macrophages are termed as tumor-associated macrophages or TAMs. A vast number of studies have shown that these TAMs exhibit the same characteristics of the immunosuppressive M2 macrophages in the TME and aid in tumor development and promotion, not just by cytokine secretion, but also by angiogenesis, increased survival, and metastasis of tumor cells [25, 26].

Studies done in mouse mammary carcinoma, murine fibrosarcoma, and B16 melanoma reveal high expression of immunosuppressive cytokines by TAMs isolated from such cancers. This is fortified by the presence of certain M2 markers, which include, but are not limited to, arginase-1, FIZZ1, and YM1 [27]. However, more studies are presenting newer evidence suggesting that the polarization of macrophages depends on the stage of the tumor. Tumorigenic M1 macrophages at sites of chronic inflammation contribute in the early stages of tumor progression [28], whereas M2 macrophages support angiogenesis, tumor growth, and tissue repairs in established tumors [26, 29, 30]. Epidemiological and clinical studies have shown the correlation between various infections causing chronic inflammation and an increased risk of cancer. Detailed investigation of this link between inflammation and cancer suggests that macrophages play a vital role in tumor onset at sites of chronic inflammation [31, 32].

Studies conducted in breast cancer suggest that the density of TAMs positively correlates with the angiogenic potential of the tumor, where increased density is associated with poor prognosis [33]. A meta-analysis study done on more than a thousand patients with solid tumors suggested that the plasticity and duplicity of TAMs can serve as a critical indicator for prognosis. The presence of immunosuppressive M2 macrophages correlates with poor prognosis of disease, in contrast to the anti-tumor M1 macrophages which improve the prognosis of the patients, therefore suggesting an anti-tumor role. Thus, there are varying and contradictory reports on the role of TAMs in cancer prognosis. A macrophage balance based on the TME signals will indicate the prognosis of the solid tumor [34].

The most important question remaining is that if these M1 macrophages are pro-inflammatory, how are they involved in tumorigenesis? It is believed that these pro-inflammatory M1 macrophages, through their persistent secretion of cytokines and reactive oxygen species (ROS), cause extensive surrounding tissue and DNA damage, generating mutations and altered p53 activity. This event predisposes the tissue cells to undergo premalignant, neoplastic transformation and tumor initiation [28, 29, 35]. Moreover, in vivo studies support this M1 macrophage activity by demonstrating how inflammatory cytokines like TNF-α, IL-1β, and IL-6 enhance tumorigenesis by sending out pro-survival signals to the proliferating neoplastic cells [36, 37]. Thus, it is the M1 phenotype that is present in tumor initiation and causes neoplastic transformation, a phenotypic transition, whereas M2 macrophages reside in the established tumors [27, 38]. "Mixed phenotype" macrophages also exist in established tumors. In vivo studies conducted to ascertain the TAM population in tumors suggest the presence of TAMs expressing M1 and M2 markers. Pro-inflammatory M1 macrophages express inducible nitric oxide synthase (iNOS), which is utilized to metabolize arginine to nitric oxide (NO) or reactive nitrogen species (RNS). In contrast, M2 immunosuppressive macrophages express arginase and metabolize arginine to urea and L-ornithine. This difference in arginine metabolism is one of the major indicators of the M1 vs M2 phenotype. However, TAMs of certain solid tumors express both arginase and iNOS, suggesting the presence of both phenotypes in the TME.

A study by Auffray et al. shows that macrophage phenotype can switch from M1 to M2, and vice versa, based on tissue environment [39]. This heterogeneity and plasticity of the macrophages modulates with the signals present in the TME. As the cancer progresses, the phenotype of the macrophage changes in accordance with the secretory factors of the tumor environment. At any given time point during tumorigenesis and advancement, there will be diversity of macrophages present at various stages of M1, M2, or intermediate transition.

2 Specificity of the Thyroid Tumor Microenvironment

2.1 Anatomy of the Thyroid Gland

The thyroid is a highly vascular, butterfly-shaped gland, located in the anterior neck, overlaying the trachea. The thyroid gland weighs approximately 15–25 grams in adults. It is the largest endocrine gland, consisting of two pear-shaped lateral lobes connected by the isthmus. The thyroid gland is surrounded by a dense fibrous capsule of connective tissue. This capsule also encloses four small parathyroid glands which are located posterior to the thyroid gland. Externally, the capsule is enveloped by *pretracheal fascia* (false capsule of deep cervical fascia) encompassing the vessels entering and leaving the gland. Overall, the thyroid gland has a rich blood supply of 5 mL/g/min, which includes the dense network of connecting vessels. The lymphatic vessels drain into the lymph nodes as well as directly into the veins. The gland receives its vasomotor innervations from cervical sympathetic ganglia [40–43]. The adult thyroid consists of about three million spherical-shaped follicles. These follicles are lined by a single epithelial cell layer and serve as the major functional units [41, 44]. Each follicle is composed of a colloid filled central cavity containing thyroglobulin (Tg) glycoprotein and is surrounded by a single layer of thyroid follicular cells. In addition, there are small numbers of parafollicular cells (C cells, parenchymatous cells) in the space surrounding the follicles. The primary function of C cells is to secrete calcitonin, a hormone that reduces blood calcium [45].

2.2 Thyroid Cancer

Thyroid cancer is the most prevalent endocrine malignancy, comprising more than 95% of all such malignancies in the United States [46–48]. It is the most rapidly rising cancer in the United States, with its incidence having tripled in the last 30 years [49]. Pathologically, thyroid cancer can be classified into four morphological types – papillary, follicular, anaplastic (undifferentiated), and medullary thyroid cancer. Papillary thyroid cancer (PTC) and follicular thyroid cancer (FTC) are the differentiated thyroid cancer (DTC) types and are derived from thyroid epithelial cells. PTC and FTC represent 90–95% of all thyroid cancers. Interestingly, PTC alone makes up 75–85% of all thyroid cancers [50]. Medullary thyroid cancer (MTC) is derived from parafollicular C cells and makes up 5–10% of cases. The rarest and most fatal thyroid cancer is anaplastic (undifferentiated) thyroid carcinoma.

2.3 Heterogeneity of Thyroid Cancer Cells

The dynamic heterogeneity of tumors encompasses the transient presence of various cell populations, signaling cascades, and metabolism associated with tumorigenesis, which eventually becomes an established feature of the tumor microenvironment (TME). Clonal evolution occurs as a result of somatic mutations in a population of cells which gradually accumulate over a period of time, leading to tumor initiation. These clonal cells further propagate, gaining branch mutations, which give rise to subclonal populations of cells under the influence of various factors present in the TME. Such clonal and subclonal alterations lead to the formation of intratumoral genetic heterogeneity with genetically distinct clones existing within the same tumor. Such a phenomenon of evolutionary divergence of cellular variants is present in all solid tumors, including advanced thyroid cancer [51]. The heterogeneous genetic and epigenetic alterations in cancer cells offer a selective advantage to the cells in the TME for the promotion of growth and metastasis. Studies of breast cancer cells have denoted that only a few cancer cells are needed with such accrued genetic variants to drive the progression of cancers with individualized genotypes [52].

Thyroid cancer consists of a heterogeneous group of neoplasms as well, which are classified histologically based on the cells of origin. The exact etiology of thyroid cancer remains unclear to date, but it is considered to have a multifactorial etiopathogenesis. External environment factors such as radiation and dietary iodine can influence the incidence of thyroid cancer. Case studies have shown that patients with preexisting thyroid diseases such as goiter or autoimmune disorders – Hashimoto's thyroiditis and Graves' disease – have a constitutional predisposition to thyroid cancer in the future. Most thyroid cancers are sporadic in nature, with genetic and epigenetic modifications that are promoted by external factors as mentioned above [53]. Only about 5% of cases have familial cancer incidence, elucidating the role of molecular pathogenesis in thyroid cancer. Based on the tumorigenesis model of a number of other cancers, it has been proposed that thyroid cancers arise from the sequential accretion of genetic and epigenetic alterations.

The multistep tumorigenesis model suggests that the accumulation of multiple genetic alterations in the genome of thyrocytes leads to the generation of thyroid cancer. The damage in the genome can occur in the oncogenes or tumor suppressor genes, promoting neoplastic conversion. A complete analysis of the papillary thyroid cancer (PTC) genomic landscape was done by the TCGA Network (The Cancer Genome Atlas Network) recently, which suggested a low occurrence of overall somatic gene alterations in well-differentiated thyroid cancer. Unlike other cancers, only a handful of recurrent mutations are present in PTC. This means that PTC and follicular thyroid cancer (FTC) can be derived from activating mutations in RAS (13%) and/or BRAF (60%) genes or rearrangements of fusion proteins associated with receptor tyrosine kinases such as RET/PTC, NTRK1/3, and ALK [54]. Although the abovementioned genetic alterations are found in PTC, thyrocytes give rise to FTC due to point mutations in RAS gene or a rearrangement of PAX8/PPARγ genes. Interestingly, as with breast, ovarian, and pancreatic cancers, it was observed that the original somatic mutations were present in the metastases. Moreover, the secondary metastatic lesions contained additional genetic lesions, offering a greater genetic instability in tumorigenesis [55]. This multistep tumorigenesis model also suggests that poorly differentiated and undifferentiated thyroid cancer, such as anaplastic thyroid cancer (ATC), arises due to progression in acquisition of these small numbers of genetic mutations during dedifferentiation.

This provides two options for ATC formation; it arises either de novo or by dedifferentiation from preexisting well-differentiated thyroid cancer (WDTC), including PTC and FTC. The evidence points toward the latter with the existence of WDTC in ATC specimens, as well as the presence of BRAF and RAS gene mutations in differentiated and undifferentiated thyroid cancer. Cellular heterogeneity is also consequential to tumor progression. It incorporates both different kinds of cells and similar cells that possess different metabolic phenotype – aiding in cancer proliferation. Breast and ovarian cancers have a large population of associated fibroblasts in the TME, which not only are key for cancer progression but can also be used to predict the prognosis. Cellular heterogeneity is also important in thyroid cancer; however, the infiltration of the stromal and immune cells varies based on the aggressiveness of the tumor. Among the well-differentiated thyroid cancers, FTC is mostly considered homogeneous, whereas PTC has a large number of cancer-associated fibroblasts. In contrast, ATC has a higher infiltration of TAMs in the TME. The immune cell infiltrates are associated with poor outcomes in patients; however, the mechanism behind it is still being explored [52].

This heterogeneity of thyroid cancer with an accumulation of very few mutations offers a uniqueness to thyroid cancer. Standard treatment modalities and targeted therapies have made WDTC, especially PTC, curable. However, the same cannot be said about malignant/metastatic PTC, PDTC, or undifferentiated ATC. This propensity of ATC to develop metastasis still needs to be explored.

2.4 Anaplastic Thyroid Cancer

Anaplastic thyroid carcinoma (ATC) is an aggressive, undifferentiated cancer responsible for less than 1.7% of all thyroid cancer cases in the United States. Although rare, it remains one of the most fatal forms of the disease, representing an end stage of thyroid tumor progression. The median survival of patients with ATC is 5 months and the 1-year survival rate is less than 20% [56]. ATC is categorized as stage IV cancer with subgroups based on the involvement of adjacent neck structures or distant sites. Patients with intrathyroidal undifferentiated tumors are stage IVA, extrathyroidal extensions are stage IVB, whereas distant metastases are stage IVC. At the time of diagnosis, almost 90% of patients are in stage IVB and about 20% have distant metastases. ATC has a rapid onset; hence, patients usually present with symptoms suggestive of tracheal, esophageal, and nerve compression due to the rapidly growing neck mass [56, 57].

The undifferentiated phenotype of ATC may arise due to dedifferentiation of preexisting well-differentiated thyroid carcinomas, such as incompletely treated papillary thyroid cancer (PTC) and follicular thyroid cancer (FTC). There is also evidence that about 80% of ATC patients have a long-standing goiter. Histologically, ATC completely loses the thyroid differentiation features and the normal thyroid cellular architecture. Instead, tumors are highly invasive with mitotic figures, multinucleated giant cells, large atypical nuclei, and widespread necrosis present [57–59].

Compared to other types of thyroid cancer, ATC frequently metastasizes, is more aggressive, and is largely incurable, which emphasizes the importance in understanding the molecular and cellular mechanisms contributing toward the disease progression.

2.5 Amplified Metastatic Propensity of Anaplastic Thyroid Cancer

The genetic burden carried by papillary thyroid cancer (PTC) is lower than that of aggressive thyroid cancers, such as anaplastic thyroid cancer (ATC). Despite the presence of a number of mutually exclusive genetic alterations, clinically, PTC is indolent in nature, therefore making it an easy target for available drugs. In contrast, ATC has unfavorable clinical outcomes accompanied by fast growing tumors, metastasis, and invasion of distant sites.

In addition to these pathological manifestations, ATC also exhibits resistance to current therapies, thus leading to poor prognosis of the disease. The fundamentals behind the aggressive nature of ATC have not been elucidated completely.

The metastatic ability of ATC is a fascinating property that is worth investigating to understand the pathogenesis of the disease. The metastatic cascade is said to be associated with the multistep tumorigenesis process. The gain of mutations, aside from the initial driver mutations, aids in progressive dedifferentiation of the cancer cells. The dedifferentiated cells have the ability to undergo epithelial to mesenchymal transition and invade the local structure at the primary site and travel to distant secondary sites.

Very limited information is available regarding the genomic basis of ATC. Aside from the mutations present in PTC, there is an additional accumulation of diverse mutations in TP53, PIK3CA, and the β-catenin encoding gene, specifically during the dedifferentiation process, thus contributing toward the aggressive nature of ATC. TP53 is the most common mutation found in ATC, followed by RAS, BRAF, β-catenin, and PIK3CA. A number of studies have suggested this claim concerning the gain of additional epigenetic and genetic alterations rather than a single genetic event in transforming the differentiated cancer cells into undifferentiated cells. This information is made possible due to the availability of whole exome sequencing and ultradeep sequencing of ATC specimens [54]. Moreover, next-generation sequencing (NGS) of PDTC and ATC has revealed that these tumors may have a unique genetic background that is distinct from the DTCs they originate from [60, 61]. However, it is important to note that most of the abovementioned mutations are pan-mutations commonly found in a number of other cancers.

Although a number of driver mutations (such as BRAF and RAS, as well as additional secondary mutations) that cause nuclear instability and dedifferentiation have been assessed with respect to ATC, it is quite evident that genetic lesions alone cannot define the ATC phenotype. The fact that ATC is still unresponsive to the current targeted therapies against driver mutations and possesses a very high metastatic propensity suggests that there are other factors influencing its pathogenesis. Multiple cancer studies have shown that targeting a single driver mutation will ultimately result in evolution of clones that propagate using alternate pathways. The signals for such evolution can be intrinsically derived from the cancer cells, or can come from other host factors such as the tumor microenvironment (TME), leading to thyroid cancer progression.

2.6 Thyroid Cancer and Inflammation

Several genetic and epigenetic factors affect the irreversible initiation of carcinoma. However, the advancement of tumorigenesis requires a promoting agent that induces proliferation of cancer cells. Chronic inflammation is regarded as a promoting agent for several types of cancer. Persistent infection causing chronic inflammation leads to recruitment of immune cells that secrete pro-inflammatory factors in the tissue microenvironment, causing DNA damage in the proliferating cells. These can permanently alter the genetic makeup of the proliferating cells, by way of point mutations, deletions, or rearrangements, triggering tumor promotion. The axiom of chronic inflammation and cancer is illustrated by bacterial or viral infections leading to associated malignancies, such as *H. pylori*, causing gastric ulcers, and hepatitis B virus, causing hepatocellular carcinoma [29]. Inflammation is an important process linked to tumor development and progression in thyroid cancer as well. It enhances cell proliferation by providing an environment rich in growth factors. It is suggested that inflammation is to be referred to as the seventh hallmark of solid tumors [62].

2.7 Dynamic Nature of the Thyroid Tumor Microenvironment

In the last two decades, several studies have demonstrated the importance of stromal cells in thyroid cancer progression [63, 64].

Papillary thyroid cancer (PTC) stroma consists of the ECM, along with a variety of stromal cells, namely, fibroblasts (and myofibroblasts), inflammatory cells, and blood vessels [65]. The thyroid cancer cells interact with the stromal cells, changing the behavior and coevolving with these stromal cells, whereby the tumor cells build a supportive environment for their own proliferation and propagation. Hence, there is a well-defined reciprocal relationship between the cancer cells and stromal cells in the thyroid cancer tumor microenvironment (TME).

Studies have shown that angiogenesis in the thyroid TME is in fact initiated due to paracrine signaling from the secretory factors of thyroid cancer cells and endothelial cells. This interaction may be influenced by the role of estrogen in promotion of metastatic thyroid cancer. It was observed that estrogen-stimulated VEGF secretion in turn promotes angiogenesis and tumor growth [66, 67]. Moreover, the new blood vessels formed in the tumor are branched and leaky, encouraging a more metastatic environment for thyroid cancer [68].

There is a heterogeneous population of cancer cells in the thyroid TME. This heterogeneity may contribute to the presence of cancer stem cells (CSCs) in the thyroid TME. Thyroid cancer follows the dynamic cancer stem cell (CSC) model, where the cells interconvert between CSCs and non-CSC cells. Such interconversion can be spontaneous or induced by certain processes such as EMT [69–71]. Most interestingly, thyroid CSCs are invasive and highly resistant to conventional treatment modalities, resulting in relapse [72].

Evidence has shown the existence of a mixed population of lymphocytes and macrophages in and around primary thyroid tumors. Thus, there exists a crucial relationship between thyroid cancer cells and immune cells. An association between the differentiated thyroid carcinoma and inflammatory microenvironment has been strongly recommended over the last decade [73].

2.8 Immune Cell Remodeling of the Thyroid Tumor Microenvironment

How does the interplay between thyroid cancer cells and immune cells impact the composition of the thyroid tumor microenvironment (TME), specifically? In terms of natural killer cells, when comparing infiltration of NK cells in papillary thyroid cancer (PTC) patients versus patients with goiters or healthy individuals, greater infiltration of $CD56_{high}$ $CD16_{low}$ NK cells is observed in the PTC patients. The percentage of immunoregulatory NK cells present is inversely correlated to the stage of disease. Although not a major presence, NK cytotoxic cells $CD56_{low}$ $CD16_{high}$ are also present in PTC, which is positively correlated with disease stage. In accordance with PTC trends, anaplastic thyroid cancer is accompanied by a lesser extent of cytotoxic NK cell infiltration, supporting tumor promotion [74, 75]. Thus, the thyroid TME has a mixture of different NK cells, and based on the predominant cell type, the phenotype of thyroid cancer can undergo alteration.

Another immune cell that bridges the gap between the innate and adaptive arms of the immune system is a type of professional antigen-presenting DCs. There exists a mutual relationship between thyroid cancer cells and DCs. PTC cells recruit DCs toward the tumor, and in return, DCs engulf the tumor-associated antigen to prime the host immune response. DC infiltration is observed more in PTC compared to follicular thyroid cancer (FTC) or adenomas. In contrast, DC infiltration is almost absent in poorly differentiated thyroid cancer, such as anaplastic thyroid cancer (ATC) [76, 77]. This might be due to T cells eliminating PTC better than the aggressive thyroid carcinomas, or with a decreased ability for the DCs to find, package, and present tumor-associated antigens from poorly differentiated cancers.

Thyroid cancer cells interact with mast cells in an opposite manner to their interaction with DCs. PTC attracts the mast cells at the tumor cell axis, and in return mast cells secrete cytokines promoting tumor growth, vascularization, and proliferation. Hence, PTC and FTC had a higher density of mast cells compared to adenomas or healthy thyroids [16, 78]. Mast cells also secrete interleukin-8 (IL-8) into the thyroid TME, which induces EMT in thyroid cancer cells, promoting the invasiveness of the cancer [79].

Within the adaptive immune system, thyroid cancer research involving the polarization of CD4+ T cells into Th1, Th2, and Treg cells has gained interest in the last decade. Many studies conducted on PTC samples have shown higher loads of infiltration of FoxP3+ Tregs. There is a direct correlation between the percentage of Treg cell infiltration in PTC and the aggressiveness of the disease. The higher the infiltration, the poorer the prognosis [80–82].

CD8+ cytotoxic T lymphocytes are conventionally believed to be anti-tumorigenic when present in abundance in the TME. However, different studies offer contradictory roles of CTLs in thyroid cancers. An immune-histological study was conducted in differentiated thyroid cancer (DTC) patients with chronic lymphocytic thyroiditis that associated an increase in CD8+ T-cell infiltration with improved disease-free survival. On the other hand, DTC patients with CD8+ T cells and increased Cox-2 expression also had higher relapse rates. Moreover, $BRAF^{V600E}$-mutated PTC tumors showed a low CD8+/Foxp3+ ratio signifying the presence of immunosuppressive environment in BRAF-mutated tumors, thereby promoting the PTC microenvironment. Hence, low CD8+ T-cell recruitment to the tumor site may be the cause of proliferating thyroid cancer [83, 84]. It can be ascertained that the relationship between T cells and thyroid TME is very different from that observed in thyroid autoimmune disease (Hashimoto's thyroiditis) as the lymphocytes in the latter disease actually eliminate the target cells. The double negative T cells are considered the dominant T cells in thyroid cancer, and they downregulate the expression of CD8+ and CD4+ T cells. Such immunoediting in the thyroid cancer microenvironment may lead to better survival of the developing thyroid tumor.

In addition to the important immunomodulatory roles of NK cells, DCs, and T cells as described above, one of the largest players in immune remodeling in thyroid cancer is tumor-associated macrophages. With TAM infiltration being an important facet of thyroid cancer, many studies have investigated its role in clinicopathological aspects of the disease. Qing and colleagues provided documented evidence that high levels of TAMs are associated with papillary thyroid carcinoma lymph node metastasis [85]. In addition, the presence of TAMs in the thyroid cancer microenvironment is correlated with larger tumor size, increased dedifferentiation, and decreased survival rates. Poorly differentiated thyroid cancer had higher density of TAMs, which was correlated with capsular invasions and extrathyroidal extensions [86, 87]. Ryder et al. also showed that conditional activation of BRAF in adult mice thyroids induced PTC along with TAM infiltration. The thyroid cancer cells secrete chemokines and cytokines that act as chemoattractants for the TAMs. Most of these TAMs belong to the immunosuppressive M2 phenotype, where their depletion reduces tumor growth [88]. Thus, several in vivo and human tissue studies indicate the presence of TAMs positively leading to tumor progression. Interestingly, the role of macrophages in differentiated thyroid cancer (DTC) differs from poorly differentiated thyroid cancer (PDTC) [89]. There is a strong association between the density of TAMs present in thyroid TME and its advanced histological grade. More than 50% of ATC tissues consist of TAMs with a peculiar microglial-like morphology. There is a very dense network of TAMs interlinked with cancer cells in ATC [90]. Intrinsic and extrinsic signals from the TME modulate the functions of TAMs to support the metastatic processes. Poorly differentiated and undifferentiated thyroid cancers had higher density of TAMs infiltrating the tumor, resulting in an increased aggressiveness of the tumor.

Although tissue-associated macrophages with various functional states are found to coexist in the same tumor [91], the preponderance of macrophage polarization and their role in thyroid tumor progression is still understudied. In addition, it is believed that crosstalk between TAMs and epithelial cells (ECs) facilitates induction of epithelial to mesenchymal transition (EMT), which is directly associated with cancer progression. Thus, thyroid cancer represents a complex bionetwork where cell-cell and cell-matrix interactions provide mutual influences resulting in cancer promotion, invasion, and metastasis. Thyroid cancer cells express mutated proteins that are recognized as non-self, activating the host immune system for their elimination. One aspect of the immune system is to recruit inflammatory cells to the tumor site to protect the host tissues. However, there is another side to this tumor-immune cell interaction. Tumor cells have their own secretory profile that recruits and activates immune cells. The immune cell secretory mediators are in turn utilized by the tumor cells to promote their own proliferation, migration, and invasion [92]. This to-and-fro interaction between cancer and immune cells is mediated through several secretory cytokines, chemokines, and exosomes, which form the secretome for the thyroid TME. The secretome majorly influences thyroid cancer growth, promotion, and advancement. Thus, it becomes important to understand the functionality of the soluble mediators of thyroid cancer-immune network.

2.9 Immune Surveillance in the Thyroid Tumor Microenvironment

The foremost immune response that occurs in a tumor microenvironment (TME) is the elimination of the cancer cells by a process called cancer immune surveillance. This mechanism was also explored in thyroid cancer relating the presence of T cells, B cells, and macrophages, as well as the absence of dendritic cells (DCs) with a better or worse prognosis in DTC patients, respectively [89]. However, some aggressive cancer cells escape elimination and proliferate in a less immunogenic environment, maintaining an equilibrium stage, and then eventually escaping from the immune surveillance. To hide from the host immune response, cancer cells recruit immune suppressive cells such as regulatory T cells (Tregs) and MDSC which secrete anti-inflammatory cytokines [80]. This makes the TME conducive for the growth and proliferation of the cancer cells. Contrary to previously mentioned reports, some researchers demonstrated that leukocytic infiltration of thyroid TME as well as tumor-associated lymph nodes, in fact, leads to thyroid cancer progression [81, 85]. The tumor-associated lymphocytes in well-differentiated thyroid cancers majorly consist of a mixture of T cells and macrophages, either inside or surrounding the thyroid cancer, which are pro-tumorigenic. The extensive leukocytic infiltration also correlates with the increase in tumor invasion, lymph node metastasis, and decrease in patient survival rates [93, 94]. This suggests that aggressive form of papillary thyroid cancer (PTC) as well as anaplastic thyroid cancer (ATC) might take up several immune escape mechanisms including, but not limited to, concomitant recruitment of immune suppressive and pro-tumorigenic immune cells in the thyroid TME.

2.10 Evolution of the Metastatic Phenotype Via Macrophages

It is believed that triggering epithelial to mesenchymal transition (EMT) in thyroid tumor cells depends on an assortment of external signals [95, 96]. These signals are present in the tumor microenvironment (TME) in the form of various secretory mediators such as cytokines, chemokines, or secretory molecules – exosomes. The *inflammatory* microenvironment plays an important role in thyroid cancer occurrence and advancement. Patients with preexisting chronic inflammatory conditions tend to get advanced thyroid cancer, denoting a link between the inflammatory microenvironment and increased migratory capacity of the thyroid cancer cells. Deciphering the secretome pattern of inflammatory cells in the thyroid TME aids in bettering understanding that link [97, 98], specifically the effect of macrophage secretory components on the thyroid cancer phenotype. Based on macrophage polarization, the secretory mediators in the TME change. To understand the initiation and progression of thyroid cancer, it is important to assess the role of major secretory players which induce EMT. Moreover, the regulators of EMT do not just initiate the tumor progression, but rather influence the increase in cell survival and resistance to apoptosis/senescence, deeming the current therapies inadequate to treat aggressive invasive thyroid cancer. In the future, innovative therapeutic strategies could be explored that will target EMT regulators to curb advanced thyroid cancer, especially anaplastic thyroid cancer (ATC).

2.11 Interacting Molecules of the Thyroid Tumor Microenvironment

2.11.1 Cytokines and Chemokines

Cytokines are immune molecules secreted by the cells of the innate and adaptive immune system in the presence of cellular stress. Apart from the immune cells, tissue cells, like thyroid follicular cells, also secrete these immune mediators. In thyroid cancer, cytokines and chemokines are released from cancer cells, which act as a chemoattractant for inflammatory cells at the tumor site. As discussed above, preexisting inflammation is an important predisposing factor for thyroid cancer. The presence of persistent inflammation leads to excessive production of cytokines and chemokines, which causes tissue destruction and DNA damage in proliferating cells, thus contributing to the pathogenesis of thyroid cancer.

TAMs infiltrating thyroid cancer form a major component of the thyroid cancer immune stromal network. M2 TAMs are present in a significantly higher density in papillary thyroid cancer (PTC) patients. These M2 polarized macrophages are immunosuppressive in nature and release anti-inflammatory IL-4, IL-13, and IL-10. These cytokines have a dual role; they exert a stimulatory effect on the tumor cells while suppressing the activation of cytotoxic T cells, thus promoting thyroid cancer survival and progression [99]. Moreover, PTC patients with concomitant Graves' disease exhibited higher levels of IL-10 and IL-4, suggesting contribution of anti-tumor immunity [100].

Pro-inflammatory cytokines produced in the thyroid tumor microenvironment (TME) consist of IL-1, IL-6, IL-8, TNF-α, TGFβ, and MCP-1 (monocyte chemotactic protein-1). In vitro studies done in WDTC and anaplastic thyroid cancer (ATC) cell lines denote that these pro-inflammatory cytokines are secreted by thyroid cancer cells. Numerous studies have been performed to understand the role of these cytokines in PTC proliferation. Oncogenes upregulate the expression of these cytokines in PTC. Studies have shown that PTC with RET/PTC, RAS, and/or BRAF mutations have higher expression of these cytokines signifying the correlation of inflammation, oncogene activation, and tumor invasion [101–103]. IL-1 induces thyroid tumor growth and proliferation by activating pro-metastatic genes, angiogenesis, and other pro-inflammatory cytokines. Higher levels of IL-1β are found in the serum of PTC patients when compared to thyroiditis patients, suggesting its contribution in tumor pathogenesis [104]. IL-6 is another important interleukin for thyroid cancer survival and proliferation. It increases the migration and invasive properties of thyroid cancer cells by inducing EMT and stemness [79, 99].

Like IL-1, TNF-α is an acute response pro-inflammatory cytokine that activates several immune cells. It has multiple roles in cancer progression; it can induce apoptosis or necrosis, or cause increased angiogenesis, migration, and invasion of cancer cells. TNF-α is secreted by the TAMs in thyroid tumor environment, and its action depends on the particular downstream signaling in addition to its interaction with other cytokines [99, 105]. TNF-α is an important inflammatory stimulus with higher serum concentrations in several cancers. However, its role for thyroid cancer progression needs further investigation. TGFβ is another cytokine with a plethora of functions in cancer promotion. TGFβ promotes Tregs and hence induces a pro-tumorigenic response by suppressing cytotoxic T cells. Murine studies have shown that TAMs as well as thyrocytes produce TGFβ, which induces EMT in thyrocytes. Moreover, there was a higher expression of TGFβ in PTC tissue samples, suggesting its role in enhancing the invasion of thyroid cancer. Hence, the presence of TGFβ is associated with higher aggressiveness of the cancer [106, 107].

Oncogenic activation of MAPK pathways leads to release of a number of chemokines, such as CXCL1, CXCL8, CXCL9, CXCL10, and CXCL11. In vitro studies have revealed that PTC and ATC cell lines normally release huge quantities of IL-8 into the TME, which is enhanced by IL-1 or TNF-α stimulus. This IL-8 can induce EMT and stemness in thyroid cancer cells. Activation of the RET/PTC1 oncogene exogenously induced expression of IL-8 in normal human thyrocytes. PTC human tissues also displayed higher expression of IL-8 and CCL20 when compared to thyroiditis or normal tissues. A study suggests that this expression pattern may be due to a higher number of TAMs secreting IL-8 in PTC, thereby responsible for invasion and metastasis [79, 93, 103, 108]. Among all the chemokines present in thyroid TME, CXCL8 and its role in cancer survival and metastasis has been explored the most.

Although various cytokines and chemokines might be present in the thyroid TME, the focus in this chapter will be on the pro-inflammatory cytokines. Since these soluble mediators of inflammation are secreted by cancer cells and the stromal cells, it is safe to accept that there exists a mutual link between these TME components.

2.11.2 Exosomes

The various factors secreted in the thyroid tumor microenvironment (TME) consist not only of the soluble mediators – cytokines and chemokines – but other secretory mediators from inflammatory cells. An example of these additional secretary mediators comes in the form of small vesicles known as exosomes. Exosomes secreted by the tumor cells and inflammatory stromal cells, especially TAMs, offer a physical means of communication and transfer of regulatory molecules in the thyroid TME. Recent research has uncovered the important role exosomes play in the TME. Exosomes, once considered as "garbage bags," are "cup"-shaped nanovesicles 30–100 nm in diameter and 1.13–1.19 g/mL in density. Although earlier considered as a means to remove unwanted materials from the cell, recently exosomes have gained much spotlight due to their role in the immune response. Exosomes contain functional proteins and nucleic acids, including microRNAs (miRNAs), messenger RNAs (mRNA), and DNA fragments, as their cargo [109, 110]. Exosomes are secreted actively by normal, tumor, and stromal cells through exocytosis pathways. They act as a shuttle for intercellular communication and crosstalk [111]. Tumor cells secrete a large number of exosomes, which provide a physical means to transfer intracellular molecules into the tumor stroma, where the inflammatory cells reside [112]. Thus, exosomes represent a novel link between cancer and inflammatory cells in the TME, especially in thyroid cancer.

Based on the cargo of these vesicles, they can either be degraded by the lysosome or released in the extracellular environment as exosomes. Exactly how the cargo gets sorted into the exosomes is not yet fully understood, but endosomal sorting complex required for transport (ESCRT)-dependent and ESCRT-independent methods are involved. The outer surface of exosomes consists of a complex lipid bilayer with integral membrane proteins, whereas the interior consists of sorted cargo [113]. The secretion or release of exosomes into the extracellular compartment occurs through MVBs/exosomal fusion with the cellular plasma membrane. Some of the components of this endocytic and exocytic machinery consist of Rab GTPases, cytoskeleton regulatory proteins, annexin, myosin, and fusion proteins such as SNAREs (SNAP (soluble NSF attachment protein) receptor) [109, 114]. Once secreted, the exosomes can travel to distant sites where they fuse with the target cell releasing their contents into the recipient cells. The regulatory signals thus pass on from the parent cell to secondary cells by way of exosomes.

Over 4000 different proteins have been isolated and purified from exosomes of patient samples as well as in vitro cell lines. The protein cargo of the exosomes contains many endosomal network-associated proteins. Some of these proteins are as follows: proteins involved in exosome biogenesis, membrane trafficking, and fusion, such as Rab proteins, GTPases, tumor suppressor gene 101, and annexin; heat shock proteins (Hsp70, Hsp60, and Hsp90); cytoskeletal proteins such as myosin, actin, and tubulin; adhesion proteins such as tetraspanins (namely, CD9, CD63, CD81, and CD82); and certain signal transducers, lipid-related proteins, metabolic enzymes, and MHC [115].

The complex lipid bilayer surrounding the exosomal core is enriched in a number of lipids, such as phospholipids, including phosphatidylserine (PS), phosphatidylcholine (PC), phosphatidylethanolamine (PE), and phosphatidylinositol (PI), sphingolipids (sphingomyelin and ceramide), diglycerides, and cholesterol. The exosomes are stable in the biological fluids and cell culture media because of the rigidity offered by the lipid bilayer. The presence of PS on the outer membrane of exosomes aids in the recognition and internalization of exosomes by the recipient cell. Exosomes also function as lipid carriers, aiding in shuttling immunosuppressive lipids in the TME, and thus aiding cancer progression [115, 116]. The exosomal lipid content differs from the parent cells' as the exosomes contain lipids not just from the plasma membrane of the origin cells, but also from the Golgi apparatus. Thus, exosomes undergo selective protein and lipid sorting [117].

The nucleic acid content of the exosomes consists of various RNAs, such as mRNA, ribosomal RNA, long noncoding RNA (lncRNA), miRNA, and some DNA. The microRNAs, which are small noncoding RNA, form the major composition of the nucleic acids and are very important in the cellular regulation at posttranscriptional levels. The miRNAs can bind to the complementary sequences in the 3′-untranslated regions of the mRNA resulting in translational regulation affecting the protein expression. As the exosome shuttles from the parent cell to the secondary recipient cell, the cargo, including the miRNAs, gets transported. These miRNAs are responsible for a number of regulatory functions related to cellular growth, differentiation, and apoptosis.

ExoCarta is an assimilation of data on exosomal cargo, identifying more than 1600 mRNA, around 800 miRNAs, and over 4000 proteins in exosomes from different species and tissues. The protein and nucleic acid contents within the exosomes represent the cell from which it originated. However, different cell types, physiological conditions, or pathological entities cause variation in the exosomal content, making the exosomal cargo specific for that particular disease state. The major function of exosomes is the transport of biological molecules containing genetic and epigenetic information to target cells. Thus, it becomes important to study exosomes with respect to the TME, since various cells in the tumor secrete and uptake exosomes, which eventually regulates the cancer development [109].

Recently, interest has been generated regarding the role of exosomes in the immune response, especially the tumor immune response. This line of thought was instigated decades ago when it was first observed that APCs utilize exosomes enriched with MHC immunomodulatory molecules for antigen presentation. Studies have shown that dendritic cell and B-cell exosomes generate a strong immunogenic response by direct or indirect T-cell activation. Immature dendritic cells secrete exosomes that are taken up by neighboring mature dendritic cells releasing the antigen-MHC complex. This effectively increases the DC response against the specific processed antigen by the DCs who have not yet encountered a pathogen [114, 118, 119]. A study by Skokos and colleagues displayed that the administration of mast cell-derived antigen-containing exosomes into naïve mice led to the maturation of immature dendritic cells against that particular antigen to elicit specific immune response [120]. One way the exosomes elicit an immune response is by carrying bioactive cytokines as cargo, along with certain inflammasome components and IL-1β. Dendritic cell exosomes contain high quantities of TNF-α, which suggests the role of exosomes in activating the innate and adaptive branches of the immune system. This effect is further amplified by the nucleic acid cargo of exosomes that are released at the site of the responsive recipient cell [121, 122]. Another important aspect of exosome functionality is their role as carriers of surface molecules and genetic information. Due to inter- and intracellular shuttling of exosomes, surface protein from one cell can be induced into the recipient transformed or untransformed cells. The proteins contained within the exosomes include oncoproteins such as MET and KRAS, which are important for tumor formation and proliferation. Horizontal transfer of these oncoproteins to neighboring and/or distant normal cells enhances the potential for tumor propagation by transforming normal cells to neoplastic cells. Exosomes, as a multimolecular messenger, mediate cell-cell communication in autocrine, paracrine, and endocrine manners. Exosomal cargo has the ability to initiate signaling responses in tumorigenic cells, thus aiding and encouraging tumor survival and advancement.

In thyroid cancer, tumor cells and the stromal inflammatory cells, together, command the composition of the extracellular milieu. The inter- and intracellular communications occur in an autocrine and paracrine manner, involving soluble mediators such as growth factors, cytokines, chemokines, and exosomes. These interactions of cancer cell mediators can regulate TME to further maintain EMT and continue dissemination of the tumor to secondary sites [123, 124]. Thus, exosomes play an important role in modulating the TME in favor of disease progression [125]. Although miRNAs secreted by tumor-derived exosomes have been explored in a number of diseases, including breast, colon, lung, pancreatic, as well as other cancers, the search for exosomes and miRNAs in thyroid cancer is in nascent stages.

Circulating miRNAs from the serum of papillary thyroid cancer (PTC) and follicular thyroid cancer (FTC) have been studied in the past to understand their role in thyroid tumor progression. miR-146b-5p, miR-221-3p, and miR-222-3p are consistently found to be overexpressed in well-differentiated thyroid cancer as well as anaplastic thyroid cancer (ATC) [126]. Moreover, there is overexpression of circulating miRNAs, such as let-7e, miR-151, and miR-222 in the serum of papillary thyroid cancer (PTC) patients [127]. It was only recently shown that these miRNAs have been identified to be present in the PTC-derived exosomes [128]. Yu et al. further explored the role of miRNAs as biomarkers for the differential diagnosis of various thyroid cancers. They found that the expression of miR-124-3p, miR-9-3p, and miR-5691 was significantly upregulated in PTC patients, whereas there was a downregulation of miR-4701 and miR-196b-5p. When the expression patterns were compared between benign nodules and PTC patients, miR-124-3p and miR-9-3p were found to be overexpressed in PTC patients, suggesting a distinct potential signature of PTC. Contrastingly, miR-196b-5p was expressed higher in benign nodules compared to PTC [129]. Another study by Li et al. showed that serum of PTC patients had that higher expression of circulating miR-25-3p and miR-451a when compared to benign nodules, suggesting their role in PTC differential diagnosis [130]. In order to distinguish PTC and FTC patients based on the plasma exosomal content, Samsonov et al. carried out a study in 60 patients with different thyroid nodal pathologies. They demonstrated a higher expression of miR-126, miR-145, and miR-31 in PTC-derived exosomes and an upregulation of miR-21 in FTC-derived exosomes. Interestingly, reciprocal and inversely related expression patterns of miR-21-5p (miR-221-3p) and miR-181a-5p were observed in PTC and FTC, respectively [131]. Such comparative analysis provides us with factors that are useful for distinguishing PTC and FTC by noninvasive methods.

A number of in vitro and patient sample-derived studies have focused on the expression pattern of the miR-146 family, making it an important effector in thyroid cancer. The miR-146 family, consistently overexpressed in differentiated thyroid cancer and ATC, has been isolated from patient serum and tumor-derived exosomes. The family consists of two genes: miR-146a and miR-146b. Both are under the regulation of transcription factor NFκB which in turn is activated to increase the invasiveness of the tumor by inducing EMT. Overall concomitant activation of signaling pathways (NFκB and Wnt pathways) and transcription of miR-146 family genes promote the aggressiveness of thyroid cancer, making it an important target for future therapies [132, 133].

ATC is characterized by the aggressive nature of the undifferentiated cancer cells to grow rapidly and cause metastasis. Loss of tumor suppressor genes, accumulations of genetic alteration, and impairment of important signaling pathways (MAPK and PI3K signaling pathways) contribute toward the pathogenesis of the anaplastic phenotype. Recent studies attribute this dysregulation to expression of miRNAs secreted into the TME by the anaplastic cancer cells and surrounding stromal cells. MicroRNAs, such as miR-146b, miR-221, and miR-222, are upregulated in ATC as well as differentiated thyroid cancer such as PTC and FTC. However, certain distinct expressions of miRNAs are associated only with ATC. Investigation of ATC samples from ten patients by Visone et al. revealed downregulation of certain miRNAs with tumor suppressor properties by influencing p53 transcription. These miRNAs include miR-30d, miR-125b, miR-26a, and miR-30a-5p. Complementary to this study, downregulation of let-7 and miR-200 families, and an upregulation of miR-221, miR-222, miR-17-92, and miR-125a-3p, was observed. Out of these, miR-200 and miR-30 family miRNAs are known to be involved in EMT regulation. The miR-30 family also blocks autophagy by repressing Beclin1 protein and preventing formation of autophagosomes. This is important as autophagy is known to cause resistance in ATC to chemotherapy. Thus, overexpressing miR-30 in ATC is a way to increase the sensitivity of the cancer cells to chemotherapeutic drugs [132, 134–136]. miR-17-92 clusters consist of seven different miRNAs. This cluster is associated with the BRAFV600E mutation and is present in PTC as well as ATC. Since the presence of this cluster has been associated with the aggressiveness of ATC and various other cancers, blockage of miRNAs associated with this cluster inhibited the growth of ATC by inducing apoptosis [132, 137]. A meta-analysis of various studies conducted in 2015 suggested that there are variation and discrepancies in the miRNA expression pattern of ATC. One possible reason for such discrepancy is the drastic change in the miRNA expression profiles of the tumor cell as it transforms from differentiated to undifferentiated thyroid carcinomas [133].

Moreover, most of the abovementioned studies were performed with the circulating miRNAs. Since the composition of totally circulating miRNAs differs from the tumor-derived exosomal miRNAs, it is important to evaluate the miRNA content of ATC-secreted exosomes and compare it to other thyroid cancers.

3 Cellular Communication in the Tumor Microenvironment

Although it is known that EMT is important for tumor cell progression and metastasis, and macrophages aid in tumor cell metastasis by inducing EMT in epithelial cells, the exact role of macrophages in thyroid cancer progression and induction of EMT in thyroid cancer cells remained understudied for quite some time. Tiwari et al. evaluated the crosstalk between macrophages and thyroid cancer cells using an in vitro model system and human thyroid cancer tissues, and reported that EMT is induced in thyroid cancer cells by pro-inflammatory macrophage secretory components. This was indicated by the enhanced expression of mesenchymal markers, and phenotypic changes, such as increased scattering and elongation of cancer cells. In addition, the migratory properties of the thyroid cancer cells under the influence of macrophages are also enhanced. They also analyzed the secretory components of macrophages, including cytokines and exosomes isolated from conditioned media, that cause phenotypic switching in thyroid cancer cells. These secretory elements activate macrophages at the tumor site, thus aiding thyroid cancer dissemination by induction of EMT in thyroid cancer cells, especially ATC. This establishes the EMT process as a basis for the metastatic propensity of ATC. Moreover, ATC cells secrete cytokines and exosomal miRNAs which aid in recruitment and activation of inflammatory cells, ripening the TME for EMT.

Hence, this mutual interaction between the inflammatory and cancer cells not only helps to decipher "EMT-associated tumor secretome" [97] but also specifies novel markers of thyroid cancer dissemination which can be targeted to suppress the metastatic potential. Overall, this indicates that the mutual interaction and cross-talk between cancer and inflammatory cells modulate the thyroid cancer phenotype – with crosstalk ultimately taking place between the tumor cells, the antigen-presenting cells, and the T cells.

M1 polarized pro-inflammatory macrophage secretory factors induce epithelial to mesenchymal transition in thyroid cancer cells as evidenced by repressed cell adhesion molecules, such as E-cadherin and β-catenin; increased expression of transcription factors such as NFκB, Twist, and Slug more prominently in ATC than PTC; a halt in proliferation; enhanced migration of thyroid cancer cells; and a change in morphology by acquiring mesenchymal phenotype as observed with cells becoming elongated and scattered indicating gain of mobility.

Reciprocal interaction between ATC cells and pro-inflammatory macrophages through chemotactic and secretory mediators (cytokines and exosomal miRNA) defines metastatic phenotype that is defined by pro-inflammatory cytokines/chemokines such as TNF-α, TGFβ, IL-6, IL-8 and IL-1, as well as chemotactic factors like MCP-1/2, MIP-1, and eotaxin-2, along with reactive oxygen species, present within the thyroid TME causing alteration in thyroid cancer cell phenotype; activated macrophage-secreted exosomes induce EMT in thyroid cancer cells – modulation of EM markers, change in morphology to mesenchymal phenotype, and decrease in proliferation; ATC cell-secreted exosomes activate tumor-associated macrophages; ATC cell-secreted exosomes contain a distinct group of tumor suppressive miRNAs that are downregulated.

Macrophage plasticity provides a conducive pro-inflammatory environment in thyroid cancer for phenotypic transition as observed in the human tissues by the presence of a mixed population of TAMs, present in ATC and malignant PTC, with a higher infiltration and greater interaction with tumor cells in ATC; pro-inflammatory M1 polarized macrophages infiltrate anaplastic as well as malignant PTC, which provides a niche for inducing epithelial to mesenchymal transition and promoting metastasis.

4 Future Directions

There are several other requisite features to any solid tumor including thyroid cancer. Hanahan and Weinberg have listed these unique traits of tumor cells which enable them to have sustained growth and metastasis. These well-known "hallmarks of cancer" include sustained proliferation, evasion of apoptosis and suppression, growth promotion, angiogenesis, invasion, and metastasis capabilities. Tumor formation is a multistep process resulting from the simultaneous occurrence of the above processes. In most cases, the initiation of the tumorigenesis is believed to be due to the acquisition of genetic mutations. The genetic alteration leads to transformation of a benign cell to malignant cells, leading to aggressive cancer formation (Hanahan & Weinberg, 2011). As such, looking at how these processes are impacted by alterations within the TME by its interacting components can shape future studies within this field.

4.1 Novel Targets of Therapeutic Intervention

The thyroid tumor microenvironment secretome offers early markers and putative targets for thyroid cancer metastasis and dissemination. The thyroid TME is composed of thyroid cancer cells in addition to stromal cells consisting of macrophages, fibroblast, mast cells, PMNs, and stem cells. Chronic inflammation is a key initiator of thyroid cancer. This was determined by a strong association found between the presence of preexisting inflammatory benign thyroid disease and the incidence of cancer in later years. Moreover, histopathological analysis of thyroid cancer has shown a dense infiltration of innate and adaptive immune cells surrounding, as well as within, thyroid cancer. This clearly indicates the presence of infiltrating lymphocytes and macrophages in thyroid tumors.

The spectrum of infiltrating stromal and immune cells in anaplastic thyroid cancer (ATC) differs from that in DTC. There is a higher number of T cells in papillary thyroid cancer (PTC) and a greater infiltration of TAMs in ATC. In either case, lymphocytic infiltration of thyroid cancer has been associated with poor disease outcomes. Studies conducted in breast, ovarian, and hepatocellular carcinoma have examined the role of TAMs in tumor proliferation and progression. TAMs release certain chemokines and cytokines which cause corresponding changes in the cell. These macrophages are usually in the form of inactive blood monocytes. They become activated in the presence of specific signals from the surrounding microenvironment. Under normal conditions, during the activation, monocytes are differentiated into either M1 (pro-inflammatory) or M2 (anti-inflammatory) phenotype, depending on the type of signals. Macrophages in general have a complex transcriptome, and they are polarized to specific subtypes based on the specific function they have to perform. In the case of the TME, they are needed to accomplish the vital task of supporting the tumor [101, 138, 139]. Given the relationship between inflammation and thyroid cancer, further investigations into the interaction between M1 polarized pro-inflammatory macrophages and thyroid cancer cells, especially the more resilient ATC, and methodologies by which to remodel the macrophage polarization or the level of inflammation within the TME will have major treatment relevance.

TAMs infiltrate the tumor site and get activated by the secretory factors present in the TME. The activation and polarization of macrophages to a pro-inflammatory phenotype lends further support to thyroid cancer cells for proliferation and dissemination. The Tiwari lab has demonstrated that the secretory mediators of ATC cell lines, consisting of chemotactic factors and pro-inflammatory cytokines, recruit and activate the THP-1 monocytes to macrophages. Thus, cell-cell communication takes place between the anaplastic cancer cells and macrophages, which stimulates the macrophages to perform pro-inflammatory functions. However, such cellular interactions are not unidirectional. There exists reciprocal communication between the cancer and stromal cells in the TME as witnessed in a number of cancers [140, 141].

This crosstalk is facilitated by a number of secretory factors, including soluble mediators – cytokines/chemokines, growth factors, and exosomes with their miRNA cargo. Through examination of the secretome of the thyroid TME, and exploration of the mediators of cell-cell communication, the Tiwari lab found that M1 polarized macrophages expressed higher amount of IL-6 and iNOS. Additionally, the secretory profile of these activated macrophages was distinct from the un-activated monocytes. These activated M1 macrophages secreted chemotactic and pro-inflammatory cytokines such as IL-6, MIP-1α/β, TNF-α, IL-1β, ICAM-1, GMCSF, IL-8, IL-16, TGF-β1, RANTES, and MCP-1/2, further demonstrating M1 polarization. Similarly, cytokine profiles of thyroid cancer cells revealed certain distinct secretory profiles of each histological type of thyroid cancer. PTC cell lines secreted high amounts of IL-6, IL-8, and TIMP-2. IL-6 is secreted by the PTC in the range of 1530–1560 pg/ml. Follicular cancer cell lines secreted IL-6 (about 1240 pg/ml), IL-8, MIP-1α, RANTES, TIMP2, and very high quantities of TGFβ (about 800 pg/ml). Anaplastic cancer cell lines on the other hand secreted high levels of chemotactic and pro-inflammatory cytokines consisting of IL-1α, TGFβ (about 750 pg/ml), MIP-1α/β, eotaxin 2, MCP-1, and PDGF-BB. Most of these cytokines are usually in an undetectable range in healthy individuals. Only in cases of inflammation, injury, or disease does the cytokine levels modulate in accordance with the cellular responses. Hence, the detection of cytokines above normal physiological levels suggests some pathology offering clinicians and researchers the means to monitor disease occurrence and progression. The physiological level of IL-6 is less than 10 pg/ml, while TNF-α and TGFβ are less than 100 pg/ml, so if these pro-inflammatory mediators are extremely high in thyroid cancer patients, they could be important tools in diagnosis and prognosis.

The Tiwari lab also observed the secretion of a number of other pro-inflammatory cytokines by tumor cells to attract and recruit pro-tumorigenic immune cells (Table 1). The secretory profile we obtained from the thyroid cancer cells and the macrophages clearly suggests the presence of pro-inflammatory chemokines and cytokines in the TME. All of these cytokines have major implications for regulating the signaling cascade in cancer cells to promote tumorigenesis. The distinct cytokine profiles of papillary cancer and ATC denote the variation in the cellular makeup of each histological type of thyroid cancer. Thus, one way that the cells communicate with each other is through soluble mediators such as cytokines.

Other means of cellular crosstalk include reactive oxygen species and exosomes. Oxidative stress generates reactive oxygen species, which cause recruitment of infiltrating immune cells, as well as damage the cellular DNA. The latter results in initiation of a repair mechanism which leads to further accumulation of genetic mutations and activation of oncogenic pathways, promoting tumorigenesis.

Exosomes are being developed as cancer therapy targets and drug delivery systems. We have seen that exosomes and the cargo within play a critical role in tumor progression. Hence, to target this aspect, strategies are under development to control the release of exosomes from the tumor cells. This is thought to curb the signals that promote tumor formation. Moreover, dendritic cell exosomes, also known as dexosomes, are being developed as immunotherapeutic agents, whereby dexosomes are pulsed with tumor-derived peptides to activate the cytotoxic T-cell response against cancer. Lastly, due to good biodistribution, biocompatibility, and biostability, exosomes are being considered as drug carriers to deliver short interfering RNA (siRNA) and active drugs like paclitaxel to the target cells [109, 117, 154].

Thus, exosomes and their cargo regulating EMT have huge implications in finding putative therapeutic targets for cancer progression and metastasis. Exosomes are considered to be diagnostic and prognostic biomarkers due to the uniqueness of their cargo, particularly miRNA (depending on the pathology). Differences have been noted in the cargo profile of exosomes obtained from serum of healthy versus cancer patient, further emphasizing the use of exosomes as a prognostic marker. Higher levels of miR-195, miR-145, and let-7a in various cancers, followed by decrease in their expression postoperatively, suggest their role as prognostic marker. Additionally, the stability offered by the lipid bilayer makes the exosomes resistant to degradation under non-physiological conditions. This makes exosomes an easy tool for disease screening or using it as a noninvasive biomarker obtained from bodily fluids [155].

The Tiwari lab observed that anaplastic cancer cells under the influence of activated macrophage conditioned media generated higher levels of ROS. This suggests an unexplored role of reactive oxygen species generated from TAMs in

Table 1 Functions of various pro-inflammatory cytokines profiled in conditioned media

Cytokine/Chemokine	Significance	References
RANTES (CCL5)	Chemoattractant for tumor infiltrating macrophages	[142–145]
	Higher affinity to bind with CCL5 receptors tumor cells	
	Tumor growth, proliferation, migration, and invasion	
MIP-1α and β	Chemoattractant for tumor infiltrating lymphocytes	[146–148]
	Pathogenesis of inflammatory disease	
1 L-1β	Important in the induction of inflammation	[149–151]
	Induces invasive capabilities of malignant cells	
1 L-8	Chemoattractant and activator of lymphocytes and neutrophils	[150, 152, 153]
	Mitogenic, angiogenic, and increases metastasis of tumor cells	
	Transdifferentiations of epithelial cells	

enhancing the proliferative and malignant propensity of ATC cells. Conversely, THP-1 monocytes, as well as macrophages, treated with anaplastic cancer cell conditioned media generated higher levels of ROS. Such a reciprocal induction of ROS accumulation between ATC cells and TAMs, which has never been observed earlier, elucidates that ATC cells generate ROS which aids in tumor progression and recruitment of macrophages. This effect of ROS along with the secreted chemotactic cytokines by ATC indicates an additive effect in recruiting the macrophages at the tumor site. Previous work by our group has characterized the miRNA content of activated THP-1 cells using the immunopathology pathway miRNA PCR arrays. The Tiwari lab went one step further and characterized the miRNA content of the exosomes secreted by the thyroid cancer cells.

Researchers are now concentrating on the miRNA functionality for diagnosis and treatment modalities. However, most of the studies performed are focused on the circulating miRNA. The exploration of exosomal miRNA is still in its budding stage. Exosomes can be isolated from bodily fluids in a noninvasive way, and hence can become a very important diagnostic marker based on their content. The exosomal cargo predominantly consists of miRNAs, which are highly conserved noncoding RNA that regulate the posttranscriptional or translational protein expression. Distinct expression of miRNA from ATC-secreted exosomes when compared to PTC- or FTC-secreted exosomes can be observed. Comparative analysis indicated that eight miRNAs were downregulated in FTC-secreted exosomes compared to papillary. On the other hand, ten miRNAs were downregulated in anaplastic 8505C-secreted exosomes compared to papillary BCPAP, whereas three miRNAs were downregulated and four miRNAs upregulated in anaplastic 8505C-secreted exosomes in comparison to follicular CGTHW1. The specific miRNA, miR-30, inhibits the TGFβ1-induced EMT by downregulating transcription factor Snail [156], and interestingly an upregulation of this miRNA was observed in 8505C compared to CGTHW1-secreted exosomes. Another definite miRNA, miR-155, enhances cellular proliferation [128, 157], which was positively correlated in 8505C-secreted exosomes expressing higher levels of this miRNA compared to CGTHW1-secreted exosomes. Increased expression of miR-30c and miR-155 in 8505C-secreted exosomes suggests their imperative role in enhanced growth and dissemination of ATC.

An important miRNA that is considered a cancer biomarker is miR-21-5p. It is associated with an increase in cellular proliferation in aggressive cancer [158–160]. However, contrary to published studies, we observed a downregulation of exosomal miR-21-5p in CGTHW1 and 8505C in comparison to BCPAP. Another miRNA, miR-138, which is known to suppress cancer metastasis and invasion [161, 162], was downregulated in CGTHW1 and 8505C when compared to BCPAP-secreted exosomes. The specific microRNA, miR-26, is associated with different biological processes pertaining to gene regulation. miR-26 is supposed to possess tumor suppressive activity [163], and its downregulation is associated with resistance to chemotherapy drugs [158]. Downregulation of this miRNA as observed in 8505C opposes apoptosis and induces tumorigenesis in ATC.

Another such miR-125-5p functions as oncomiR in a few cancers and as a tumor suppressor in a number of solid tumors including thyroid cancer. An earlier study by Visone and group indicated that an overexpression of this miRNA led to inhibition of cellular growth [136]. Moreover, miR-125b is associated with repression of migration and invasion of ATC by targeting PIK3CD via PI3K/Akt/mTOR pathway [164]. This suggests a tumor suppressive action of miR-125b. The chemosensitivity to cisplatin is enhanced in osteosarcoma with overexpression of miR-125b, indicating that downregulation of this miRNA may be associated with resistance to chemotherapeutics, as observed in aggressive and malignant cancers. This tumor suppressive miRNA was downregulated in our ATC cell line 8505C-secreted exosomes in comparison to BCPAP.

Another set of tumor suppressive miRNAs consist of miR-148a and miR-152-3p, belonging to the miR-148/152 family. Among the miRNAs from this family, miR-152 is known to act as tumor suppressor by targeting PIK3CA [165], whereas miR-148a is associated with inhibition of cancer stemness and self-renewal ability of the cancer cells [166, 167]. Both these miRNAs are downregulated in 8505C-secreted exosomes compared to other thyroid cancer cell-secreted exosomes. Downregulation of this family of miRNAs promotes tumor growth and proliferation in anaplastic cancer cells. Previous studies have shown that downregulation of miR-191 in medulloblastoma, acute myelogenous leukemia, and melanoma is associated with poor prognosis. Overexpression of miR-191 in thyroid follicular adenoma and carcinoma is associated with decreased cellular proliferation and migration by targeting CDK6. Earlier studies have shown a downregulation of this miRNA in FTC but not in PTC or ATC [168]. We observed a downregulation of miR-191 in anaplastic cancer cell line-secreted exosomes compared to papillary cancer cell line-secreted exosomes. Thus, our group has identified a distinct set of tumor suppressive miRNAs consisting of miR-125b, miR-138, miR-148a, miR-152, miR-191, and miR-26b, which are downregulated in ATC cell-secreted exosomes. This distinct miRNA profile of thyroid cancer is proposed to influence the metastatic proclivity/tendency of the cancer as observed here in ATC. A number of these miRNAs, such as miR-146a, miR-21-5p, and miR-138-5p, were upregulated in activated macrophage-derived exosomes. Moreover, miR-146a and miR-132-3p also promote the activation of monocytes [169].

Different biological functions are associated with the miRNAs. The cells in TME secrete exosomes that are shuttled from primary to secondary recipient cells. They carry within them these functional miRNAs, which are transcribed and translated to biologically relevant proteins that regulate cellular processes. This implies that cellular crosstalk is mediated by soluble mediators and exosomes, ultimately promoting tumorigenesis. Previous studies have focused on circulating or tissue miRNAs associated with thyroid cancers, generally in PTC. However, the exploration of miRNA cargo of exosomes secreted from ATC cells is still in its nascent stage. Previous studies have revealed the profile and functionality (to some extent) of the deregulated miRNAs in ATC tissues [132, 170]. The three major families of miRNAs downregulated in ATC are miR-200 family, miR-30 family, and let-7 family. In our comparative analysis between the various thyroid cancer-secreted exosomal miRNAs, we did not observe any variation in expression profile of miR-200 family or let-7 family. Common miRNAs upregulated in ATC tissues consist of miR-146, miR-221/222, and cluster miR-17-92 [132, 136, 170]. These miRNAs were not observed to be upregulated in ATC-secreted exosomes compared to other thyroid cancers. Thus, we can say that the profile of miRNAs obtained from ATC-secreted exosomes can be different from that obtained from the tissue.

The pro-tumorigenic functions of the exosome-derived miRNAs, through the regulation of genes in the recipient cells, have recently started to gain research interest. The role of exosomes as a drug delivery system, and for diagnostic purposes, has further added to their clinical relevance. However, only a handful of studies have examined the miRNA profile of circulating tumor-derived exosomes in FTC or PTC [131]. Exosomal miRNA cargo is understudied in ATC. In this study, we have come across a group of miRNA present in the exosomes secreted by ATC cells that have tumor suppressive effects. The fact that these miRNAs are downregulated suggests a profile of a huge set of genes that are regulated by these miRNAs, contributing to the metastatic phenotype in ATC.

The studies here are a clear indication that phenotype is regulated by epigenetic phenomenon of which miRNAs constitute a major cargo. We have defined the ATC phenotype based on miRNAs – miR-125b, miR-138, miR-148a, miR-152, miR-191, and miR-26b – that play a functional role in suppressing the ATC phenotype. Their downregulation paves the way for procurement of metastatic ATC phenotype, and as such, can be considered as "tumor suppressors." Their biological function and specificity to ATC, however, remains to be determined. The other mode to establish whether PTC to ATC phenotype is linked is to examine the presence and gradual disappearance of these markers in the serum of patients. The steady disappearance of these miRNA from the serum designates them as a transition biomarker for early detection of ATC phenotype, and should be pursued further.

References

1. Egeblad, M., Rasch, M. G., & Weaver, V. M. (2010). Dynamic interplay between the collagen scaffold and tumor evolution. *Current Opinion in Cell Biology, 22*, 697–706.
2. Friedl, P., & Zallen, J. A. (2010). Dynamics of cell–cell and cell–matrix interactions in morphogenesis, regeneration and cancer. *Current Opinion in Cell Biology, 22*, 557–559.
3. Xing, M. (2013). Molecular pathogenesis and mechanisms of thyroid cancer. *Nature Reviews Cancer, 13*, 184–199.
4. Krizman, D. B., Pathak, S., Samaan, N. A., & Hickey, R. C. (1987). Genetic instability in fibroblasts of patients with thyroid cancers (TC). *International Journal of Cancer, 39*, 179–181.
5. Eggo, M. C., Hopkins, J. M., Franklyn, J. A., Johnson, G. D., Sanders, D. S., & Sheppard, M. C. (1995). Expression of fibroblast growth factors in thyroid cancer. *The Journal of Clinical Endocrinology & Metabolism, 80*, 1006–1011.
6. Jolly, L. A., Novitskiy, S., Owens, P., Massoll, N., Cheng, N., Fang, W., Moses, H. L., & Franco, A. T. (2016). Fibroblast-mediated collagen remodeling within the tumor microenvironment facilitates progression of thyroid cancers driven by Braf V600E and Pten loss. *Cancer Research, 76*, 1804–1813.
7. Surowiak, P., Murawa, D., Materna, V., Maciejczyk, A., Pudelko, M., Ciesla, S., Breborowicz, J., Murawa, P., Zabel, M., Dietel, M., & Lage, H. (2007). Occurrence of stromal myofibroblasts in the invasive ductal breast cancer tissue is an unfavourable prognostic factor. *Anticancer Research, 27*, 2917–2924.
8. Hida, K., Ohga, N., Akiyama, K., Maishi, N., & Hida, Y. (2013). Heterogeneity of tumor endothelial cells. *Cancer Science, 104*, 1391–1395.
9. Huang, Z., Wu, T., Liu, A. Y., Ouyang, G., Huang, Z., Wu, T., Yi Liu, A., & Ouyang, G. (2015). Differentiation and transdifferentiation potentials of cancer stem cells. *Oncotarget, 6*, 39550–39563.
10. Mani, S. A., Guo, W., Liao, M.-J., Eaton, E. N., Ayyanan, A., Zhou, A. Y., Brooks, M., Reinhard, F., Zhang, C. C., Shipitsin, M., Campbell, L. L., Polyak, K., Brisken, C., Yang, J., & Weinberg, R. A. (2008). The epithelial-mesenchymal transition generates cells with properties of stem cells. *Cell, 133*, 704–715.
11. NK cells – need to find.
12. Hargadon, K. M., Bishop, J. D., Brandt, J. P., Hand, Z. C., Ararso, Y. T., & Forrest, O. A. (2015). Melanoma-derived factors alter the maturation and activation of differentiated tissue-resident dendritic cells. *Immunology and Cell Biology, 94*(1), 24–38.
13. Laoui, D., Keirsse, J., Morias, Y., et al. (2016). The tumor microenvironment harbours ontogenically distinct dendritic cell populations with opposing effects on tumor immunity. *Nature Communications, 7*, 13720.
14. Ma, Y., Hwang, R., Logsdon, C., & Ullrich, S. (2013). Dynamic mast cell-stromal cell interactions promote growth of pancreatic cancer. *Microenvironment and Immunology, 73*(13), 3927–3937.
15. Komi, D., & Redegeld, F. (2019). Role of mast cells in shaping the tumor microenvironment. *Clinical Reviews in Allergy and Immunology, 58*, 313–325.
16. Melillo, R. M., Guarino, V., Avilla, E., Galdiero, M. R., Liotti, F., Prevete, N., Rossi, F. W., Basolo, F., Ugolini, C., de Paulis, A., Santoro, M., & Marone, G. (2010). Mast cells have a protumorigenic role in human thyroid cancer. *Oncogene, 29*, 6203–6215.
17. Imam, S., Paparodis, R., Sharma, D., & Jaume, J. C. (2014). Lymphocytic profiling in thyroid cancer provides clues for failure of tumor immunity. *Endocrine-Related Cancer, 21*, 505–516.
18. Hashimoto, M., Kamphorst, A. O., Im, S. J., Kissick, H. T., Pillai, R. N., Ramalingam, S. S., Araki, K., & Ahmed, R. (2018). CD8 T cell exhaustion in chronic infection and cancer: Opportunities for interventions. *Annual Review of Medicine, 69*(1), 301–318.
19. Perica, K., Varela, J. C., Oelke, M., & Schneck, J. (2015). Adoptive T cell immunotherapy for cancer. *Rambam Maimonides Medical Journal, 6*(1), e0004.
20. Song, Q., Shi, F., Adair, M., Chang, H., Guan, X., Zhao, Y., Li, Y., Wu, G., & Wu, J. (2019). Cell counts, rather than proportion, of CD8/PD-1 tumor-infiltrating lymphocytes in a tumor microenvironment associated with pathological characteristics of chinese invasive ductal breast cancer. *Journal of Immunology Research*, 1–8.
21. Verma, V., Shrimali, R. K., Ahmad, S., et al. (2019). PD-1 blockade in subprime CD8 cells induces dysfunctional PD-1^{+}-CD38^{hi} cells and anti-PD-1 resistances. *Nature Immunology, 20*, 1231–1243.
22. He, Y., Cao, J., Zhao, C., Li, X., Zhou, C., & Hirsch, F. R. (2018). TIM-3, a promising target for cancer immunotherapy. *OncoTargets and Therapy, 11*, 7005–7009.
23. Hao, N.-B., Lü, M.-H., Fan, Y.-H., Cao, Y.-L., Zhang, Z.-R., & Yang, S.-M. (2012). Macrophages in tumor microenvironments and the progression of tumors. *Clinical and Developmental Immunology, 2012*, 1–11.
24. Sica, A., & Mantovani, A. (2012). Macrophage plasticity and polarization: In vivo veritas. *The Journal of Clinical Investigation, 122*, 787–795.

25. Rőszer, T., & szer T & s. (2015). Understanding the mysterious M2 macrophage through activation markers and effector mechanisms. *Mediators of Inflammation, 2015*, 816460.
26. Mantovani, A., Sozzani, S., Locati, M., Allavena, P., & Sica, A. (2002). Macrophage polarization: Tumor-associated macrophages as a paradigm for polarized M2 mononuclear phagocytes. *Trends in Immunology, 23*, 549–555.
27. Biswas, S. K., Sica, A., & Lewis, C. E. (2008). Plasticity of macrophage function during tumor progression: Regulation by distinct molecular mechanisms. *The Journal of Immunology, 180*, 2011–2017.
28. Balkwill, F., Charles, K. A., & Mantovani, A. (2005). Smoldering and polarized inflammation in the initiation and promotion of malignant disease. *Cancer Cell, 7*, 211–217.
29. Coussens, L. M., & Werb, Z. (2002). Inflammation and cancer. *Nature, 420*, 860–867.
30. Lewis, C. E., & Pollard, J. W. (2006). Distinct role of macrophages in different tumor microenvironments. *Cancer Research, 66*, 605–612.
31. Gordon, S., & Taylor, P. R. (2005). Monocyte and macrophage heterogeneity. *Nature Reviews Immunology, 5*, 953–964.
32. Szebeni, G. J., Vizler, C., Kitajka, K., & Puskas, L. G. (2017). Inflammation and cancer: Extra- and intracellular determinants of tumor-associated macrophages as tumor promoters. *Mediators of Inflammation, 2017*, 9294018.
33. Leek, R. D., Lewis, C. E., Whitehouse, R., Greenall, M., Clarke, J., & Harris, A. L. (1996). Association of macrophage infiltration with angiogenesis and prognosis in invasive breast carcinoma. *Cancer Research, 56*, 4625–4629.
34. Zhang, Q., Liu, L., Gong, C., Shi, H., Zeng, Y., Wang, X., Zhao, Y., & Wei, Y. (2012). Prognostic significance of tumor-associated macrophages in solid tumor: A meta-analysis of the literature M. O. Hoque, ed. *PLoS One, 7*, e50946.
35. Coussens, L. M., & Werb, Z. (2001). Inflammatory cells and cancer. *Journal of Experimental Medicine, 193*.
36. Pikarsky, E., Porat, R. M., Stein, I., Abramovitch, R., Amit, S., Kasem, S., Gutkovich-Pyest, E., Urieli-Shoval, S., Galun, E., & Ben-Neriah, Y. (2004). NF-κB functions as a tumour promoter in inflammation-associated cancer. *Nature, 431*, 461–466.
37. Greten, F. R., Eckmann, L., Greten, T. F., Park, J. M., Li, Z.-W., Egan, L. J., Kagnoff, M. F., & Karin, M. (2004). IKKbeta links inflammation and tumorigenesis in a mouse model of colitis-associated cancer. *Cell, 118*, 285–296.
38. Chanmee, T., Ontong, P., Konno, K., & Itano, N. (2014). Tumor-associated macrophages as major players in the tumor microenvironment. *Cancers, 6*, 1670–1690.
39. Auffray, C., Fogg, D., Garfa, M., Elain, G., Join-Lambert, O., Kayal, S., Sarnacki, S., Cumano, A., Lauvau, G., & Geissmann, F. (2007). Monitoring of blood vessels and tissues by a population of monocytes with patrolling behavior. *Science, 317*, 666–670.
40. Standring, S., & Berkovitz, B. (2005). Thyroid gland. In S. Standring, H. Ellis, J. C. Healey, D. Johnson, & A. Williams (Eds.), *Gray's anatomy* (pp. 560–564). Churchill Livingstone.
41. Wondisford, F. E., & Radovick, S. (2009). *Clinical management of thyroid disease*. Saunders/Elsevier.
42. Bizhanova, A., & Kopp, P. (2009). The sodium-iodide symporter NIS and Pendrin in iodide homeostasis of the thyroid. *Endocrinology, 150*, 1084–1090.
43. Fancy, T., Gallagher, D., III, & Hornig, J. D. (2010). Surgical anatomy of the thyroid and parathyroid glands. *Otolaryngologic Clinics of NA, 43*, 221–227.
44. Khatawkar, A. V., & Awati, S. M. (2015). Thyroid gland – historical aspects, embryology, anatomy and physiology. *International Archives of Integrated Medicine., 2*, 165–171.
45. Hazard, J. B. (1977). The C cells (parafollicular cells) of the thyroid gland and medullary thyroid carcinoma. A review. *The American Journal of Pathology, 88*, 213–250.
46. Parkin, D. M., Bray, F., Ferlay, J., & Pisani, P. (2005). Global cancer statistics, 2002. *CA: A Cancer Journal for Clinicians, 55*, 74–108.
47. Jemal, A., Siegel, R., Ward, E., Hao, Y., Xu, J., & Thun, M. J. (2009). Cancer statistics, 2009. *CA: A Cancer Journal for Clinicians, 59*, 225–249.
48. Aschebrook-Kilfoy, B., Schechter, R. B., Shih, Y.-C. T., Kaplan, E. L., Chiu, B. C.-H., Angelos, P., & Grogan, R. H. (2013). The clinical and economic burden of a sustained increase in thyroid cancer incidence. *Cancer Epidemiology Biomarkers & Prevention, 22*, 1252–1259.
49. American Cancer Society. (2020). Cancer facts and figures 2020, Atlanta.
50. Gimm, O., & Dralle, H. (2001). Differentiated thyroid carcinoma. In R. Holzheimer & J. Mannick (Eds.), *Surgical treatment: Evidence-based and problem-oriented*. Zuckschwerdt: W. Zuckschwerdt Verlag GmbH.
51. Morris, L. G. T., Riaz, N., Desrichard, A., Şenbabaoğlu, Y., Hakimi, A. A., Makarov, V., Reis-Filho, J. S., Chan, T. A., Morris, L. G. T., Riaz, N., Desrichard, A., Şenbabaoğlu, Y., Hakimi, A. A., Makarov, V., Reis-Filho, J. S., & Chan, T. A. (2016). Pan-cancer analysis of intratumor heterogeneity as a prognostic determinant of survival. *Oncotarget, 7*, 10051–10063.
52. Strickaert, A., Saiselet, M., Dom, G., De Deken, X., Dumont, J. E., Feron, O., Sonveaux, P., & Maenhaut, C. (2016). Cancer heterogeneity is not compatible with one unique cancer cell metabolic map. *Oncogene*, 1–6.
53. Makazlieva, T., Vaskova, O., & Majstorov, V. (2016). Etiopathogenesis of differentiated thyroid carcino-

mas. *Open Access Macedonian Journal of Medical Sciences, 4*, 517–522.
54. Landa, I., Ibrahimpasic, T., Boucai, L., Sinha, R., Knauf, J. A., Shah, R. H., Dogan, S., Ricarte-Filho, J. C., Krishnamoorthy, G. P., Xu, B., Schultz, N., Berger, M. F., Sander, C., Taylor, B. S., Ghossein, R., Ganly, I., & Fagin, J. A. (2016). Genomic and transcriptomic hallmarks of poorly differentiated and anaplastic thyroid cancers. *Journal of Clinical Investigation, 126*, 1052–1066.
55. Le Pennec, S., Konopka, T., Gacquer, D., Fimereli, D., Tarabichi, M., Tomás, G., Savagner, F., Decaussin-Petrucci, M., Trésallet, C., Andry, G., Larsimont, D., Detours, V., & Maenhaut, C. (2015). Intratumor heterogeneity and clonal evolution in an aggressive papillary thyroid cancer and matched metastases. *Endocrine-Related Cancer., 22*, 205–216.
56. O'Neill, J. P., & Shaha, A. R. (2013). Anaplastic thyroid cancer. *Oral Oncology., 49*, 702–706.
57. Smallridge, R. C., & Copland, J. A. (2010). Anaplastic thyroid carcinoma: Pathogenesis and emerging therapies. *Clinical Oncology (Royal College of Radiologists (Great Britain)), 22*, 486–497.
58. Quiros, R. M., Ding, H. G., Gattuso, P., Prinz, R. A., & Xu, X. (2005). Evidence that one subset of anaplastic thyroid carcinomas are derived from papillary carcinomas due to BRAF andp53 mutations. *Cancer, 103*, 2261–2268.
59. Haghpanah, V., Fallah, P., Naderi, M., Tavakoli, R., Soleimani, M., & Larijani, B. (2016). Cancer stem-like cell behavior in anaplastic thyroid cancer: A challenging dilemma. *Life Sciences, 146*, 34–39.
60. Xu, B., & Ghossein, R. (2016). Genomic landscape of poorly differentiated and anaplastic thyroid carcinoma. *Endocrine Pathology., 27*, 205–212.
61. Sykorova, V., Dvorakova, S., Vcelak, J., Vaclavikova, E., Halkova, T., Kodetova, D., Lastuvka, P., Betka, J., Vlcek, P., Reboun, M., Katra, R., & Bendlova, B. (2015). Search for new genetic biomarkers in poorly differentiated and anaplastic thyroid carcinomas using next generation sequencing. *Anticancer Research, 35*, 2029–2036.
62. Colotta, F., Allavena, P., Sica, A., Garlanda, C., & Mantovani, A. (2009). Cancer-related inflammation, the seventh hallmark of cancer: Links to genetic instability. *Carcinogenesis, 30*, 1073–1081.
63. Daoud, S. A., Esmail, R. S. E. N., Hareedy, A. A., & Khalil, A. (2015). Stromal modulation and its role in the diagnosis of papillary patterned thyroid lesions. *Asian Pacific Journal of Cancer Prevention: APJCP., 16*, 3307–3312.
64. San Martin, R., Barron, D. A., Tuxhorn, J. A., Ressler, S. J., Hayward, S. W., Shen, X., Laucirica, R., Wheeler, T. M., Gutierrez, C., Ayala, G. E., Ittmann, M., & Rowley, D. R. (2014). Recruitment of CD34(+) fibroblasts in tumor-associated reactive stroma: The reactive microvasculature hypothesis. *The American Journal of Pathology., 184*, 1860–1870.
65. Radu, T. G., Ciurea, M. E., Mogoantă, S. Ş., Busuioc, C. J., Grosu, F., Ţenovici, M., Petrescu, I. O., & Vladu, I. M. (2016). Papillary thyroid cancer stroma – Histological and immunohistochemical study. *Romanian Journal of Morphology and Embryology., 57*, 801–809.
66. Rajoria, S., Suriano, R., Wilson, Y. L., George, A. L., Geliebter, J., Schantz, S. P., & Tiwari, R. K. (2011). Estradiol-mediated tumor neo-vascularization. *Oncology Letters., 2*, 453–457.
67. Kamat, A., Rajoria, S., George, A., Suriano, R., Shanmugam, A., Megwalu, U., Prakash, P. B., Tiwari, R., & Schantz, S. (2011). Estrogen-mediated angiogenesis in thyroid tumor microenvironment is mediated through VEGF signaling pathways. *Archives of Otolaryngology–Head & Neck Surgery., 137*, 1146.
68. Balkwill, F. R., Capasso, M., & Hagemann, T. (2012). The tumor microenvironment at a glance. *Journal of Cell Science., 125*, 5591–5596.
69. Ma, R., Bonnefond, S., Morshed, S. A., Latif, R., & Davies, T. F. (2014). Stemness is derived from thyroid cancer cells. *Frontiers in Endocrinology., 5*, 114.
70. Shimamura, M., Nagayama, Y., Matsuse, M., Yamashita, S., & Mitsutake, N. (2014). Analysis of multiple markers for cancer stem-like cells in human thyroid carcinoma cell lines. *Endocrine Journal., 61*, 481–490.
71. Nagayama, Y., Shimamura, M., & Mitsutake, N. (2016). Cancer stem cells in the thyroid. *Frontiers in Endocrinology., 7*, 20.
72. Vicari, L., Colarossi, C., Giuffrida, D., De Maria, R., & Memeo, L. (2016). Cancer stem cells as a potential therapeutic target in thyroid carcinoma. *Oncology Letters., 12*, 2254–2260.
73. Yano, Y., Shibuya, H., Kitagawa, W., Nagahama, M., Sugino, K., Ito, K., & Ito, K. (2007). Recent outcome of graves' disease patients with papillary thyroid cancer. *European Journal of Endocrinology., 157*, 325–329.
74. Gogali, F., Paterakis, G., Rassidakis, G. Z., Liakou, C. I., & Liapi, C. (2013). CD3-CD16-CD56bright Immunoregulatory NK cells are increased in the tumor microenvironment and inversely correlate with advanced stages in patients with papillary thyroid cancer. *Thyroid: Official Journal of the American Thyroid Association., 23*, 7–9.
75. Wennerberg, E., Pfefferle, A., Ekblad, L., Yoshimoto, Y., Kremer, V., Kaminskyy, V. O., Juhlin, C. C., Höög, A., Bodin, I., Svjatoha, V., Larsson, C., Zedenius, J., Wennerberg, J., & Lundqvist, A. (2014). Human anaplastic thyroid carcinoma cells are sensitive to NK cell-mediated lysis via ULBP2/5/6 and chemoattract NK cells. *Clinical Cancer Research., 20*, 5733–5744.
76. Tsuge, K., Takeda, H., Kawada, S., Maeda, K., & Yamakawa, M. (2005). Characterization of dendritic cells in differentiated thyroid cancer. *The Journal of Pathology., 205*, 565–576.

77. Ugolini, C., Basolo, F., Proietti, A., Vitti, P., Elisei, R., Miccoli, P., & Toniolo, A. (2007). Lymphocyte and immature dendritic cell infiltrates in differentiated, poorly differentiated, and undifferentiated thyroid carcinoma. *Thyroid, 17*, 389–393.
78. Proietti, A., Ugolini, C., Melillo, R. M., Crisman, G., Elisei, R., Santoro, M., Minuto, M., Vitti, P., Miccoli, P., & Basolo, F. (2011). Higher Intratumoral expression of CD1a, Tryptase, and CD68 in a follicular variant of papillary thyroid carcinoma compared to adenomas: Correlation with clinical and pathological parameters. *Thyroid, 21*, 1209–1215.
79. Visciano, C., Liotti, F., Prevete, N., & Cali' G, Franco R, Collina F, de Paulis A, Marone G, Santoro M & Melillo RM. (2015). Mast cells induce epithelial-to-mesenchymal transition and stem cell features in human thyroid cancer cells through an IL-8–Akt–slug pathway. *Oncogene, 34*, 5175–5186.
80. French, J. D., Weber, Z. J., Fretwell, D. L., Said, S., Klopper, J. P., & Haugen, B. R. (2010). Tumor- associated lymphocytes and increased FoxP3 + regulatory T cell frequency correlate with more aggressive papillary thyroid cancer. *The Journal of Clinical Endocrinology & Metabolism., 95*, 2325–2333.
81. French, J. D., Kotnis, G. R., Said, S., Raeburn, C. D., McIntyre, R. C., Klopper, J. P., & Haugen, B. R. (2012). Programmed Death-1 + T cells and regulatory T cells are enriched in tumor- involved lymph nodes and associated with aggressive features in papillary thyroid cancer. *The Journal of Clinical Endocrinology & Metabolism., 97*, E934–E943.
82. Gogali, F., Paterakis, G., Rassidakis, G. Z., Kaltsas, G., Liakou, C. I., Gousis, P., Neonakis, E., Manoussakis, M. N., & Liapi, C. (2012). Phenotypical analysis of lymphocytes with suppressive and regulatory properties (Tregs) and NK cells in the papillary carcinoma of thyroid. *The Journal of Clinical Endocrinology & Metabolism., 97*, 1474–1482.
83. Angell, T. E., Lechner, M. G., Jang, J. K., Correa, A. J., LoPresti, J. S., & Epstein, A. L. (2014). BRAF V600E in papillary thyroid carcinoma is associated with increased programmed death ligand 1 expression and suppressive immune cell infiltration. *Thyroid: Official Journal of the American Thyroid Association., 24*, 1385–1393.
84. Cunha, L. L., Marcello, M. A., Nonogaki, S., Morari, E. C., Soares, F. A., Vassallo, J., & Ward, L. S. (2015). CD8+ tumour-infiltrating lymphocytes and COX2 expression may predict relapse in differentiated thyroid cancer. *Clinical Endocrinology., 83*, 246–253.
85. Qing, W., Fang, W.-Y., Ye, L., Shen, L.-Y., Zhang, X.-F., Fei, X.-C., Chen, X., Wang, W.-Q., Li, X.-Y., Xiao, J.-C., & Ning, G. (2012). Density of tumor-associated macrophages correlates with lymph node metastasis in papillary thyroid carcinoma. *Thyroid, 22*, 905–910.
86. Jung, K. Y., Cho, S. W., Kim, Y. A., Kim, D., Oh, B.-C., Park, D. J., & Park, Y. J. (2015). Cancers with higher density of tumor-associated macrophages were associated with poor survival rates. *Journal of Pathology and Translational Medicine., 49*, 318–324.
87. Ryder, M., Ghossein, R. A., Ricarte-Filho, J. C. M., Knauf, J. A., & Fagin, J. A. (2008). Increased density of tumor-associated macrophages is associated with decreased survival in advanced thyroid cancer. *Endocrine-Related Cancer., 15*, 1069–1074.
88. Ryder, M., Gild, M., Hohl, T. M., Pamer, E., Knauf, J., Ghossein, R., Joyce, J. A., & Fagin, J. A. (2013). Genetic and pharmacological targeting of CSF-1/ CSF-1R inhibits tumor-associated macrophages and impairs BRAF-induced thyroid cancer progression M. Ludgate, ed. *PLoS One, 8*, e54302.
89. Cunha, L. L., Morari, E. C., Guihen, A. C. T., Razolli, D., Gerhard, R., Nonogaki, S., Soares, F. A., Vassallo, J., & Ward, L. S. (2012). Infiltration of a mixture of immune cells may be related to good prognosis in patients with differentiated thyroid carcinoma. *Clinical Endocrinology, 77*, 918–925.
90. Caillou, B., Talbot, M., Weyemi, U., Pioche-Durieu, C., Al Ghuzlan, A., Bidart, J. M., Chouaib, S., Schlumberger, M., & Dupuy, C. (2011). Tumor-associated macrophages (TAMs) form an interconnected cellular supportive network in anaplastic thyroid carcinoma I. Agoulnik, ed. *PLoS One, 6*, e22567.
91. Movahedi, K., Laoui, D., Gysemans, C., Baeten, M., Stangé, G., Van Bossche, J., Den Mack, M., Pipeleers, D., In't Veld, P., De Baetselier, P., & Van Ginderachter, J. A. (2010). Different tumor microenvironments contain functionally distinct subsets of macrophages derived from Ly6C(high) monocytes. *Cancer Research, 70*, 5728–5739.
92. Wahl, L. M., & Kleinman, H. K. (1998). Tumor-associated macrophages as targets for cancer therapy. *Journal of the National Cancer Institute., 90*, 1583–1584.
93. Galdiero, M. R., Varricchi, G., & Marone, G. (2016). The immune network in thyroid cancer. *OncoImmunology., 5*, e1168556.
94. Modi, J., Patel, A., Terrell, R., Tuttle, R. M., & Francis, G. L. (2003). Papillary thyroid carcinomas from young adults and children contain a mixture of lymphocytes. *The Journal of Clinical Endocrinology & Metabolism., 88*, 4418–4425.
95. Sabbah, M., Emami, S., Redeuilh, G., Julien, S., Prévost, G., Zimber, A., Ouelaa, R., Bracke, M., De Wever, O., & Gespach, C. (2008). Molecular signature and therapeutic perspective of the epithelial-to-mesenchymal transitions in epithelial cancers. *Drug Resistance Updates., 11*, 123–151.
96. Moustakas, A., & Heldin, C.-H. (2007). Signaling networks guiding epithelial-mesenchymal transitions during embryogenesis and cancer progression. *Cancer Science., 98*, 1512–1520.
97. Mathias, R. A., Wang, B., Ji, H., Kapp, E. A., Moritz, R. L., Zhu, H.-J., & Simpson, R. J. (2009). Secretome-based proteomic profiling of Ras-

transformed MDCK cells reveals extracellular modulators of epithelial-mesenchymal transition. *Journal of Proteome Research, 8*, 2827–2837.
98. Palena, C., Hamilton, D. H., & Fernando, R. I. (2012). Influence of IL-8 on the epithelial-mesenchymal transition and the tumor microenvironment. *Future Oncology (London, England), 8*, 713–722.
99. Cunha, L. L., Marcello, M. A., & Ward, L. S. (2014). The role of the inflammatory microenvironment in thyroid carcinogenesis. *Endocrine-Related Cancer., 21*, R85–R103.
100. Vella, V., Mineo, R., Frasca, F., Mazzon, E., Pandini, G., Vigneri, R., & Belfiore, A. (2004). Interleukin-4 stimulates papillary thyroid cancer cell survival: Implications in patients with thyroid cancer and concomitant graves' disease. *The Journal of Clinical Endocrinology & Metabolism., 89*, 2880–2889.
101. Guarino, V., Castellone, M. D., Avilla, E., & Melillo, R. M. (2010). Thyroid cancer and inflammation. *Molecular and Cellular Endocrinology., 321*, 94–102.
102. Muzza, M., Degl'Innocenti, D., Colombo, C., Perrino, M., Ravasi, E., Rossi, S., Cirello, V., Beck-Peccoz, P., Borrello, M. G., & Fugazzola, L. (2010). The tight relationship between papillary thyroid cancer, autoimmunity and inflammation: Clinical and molecular studies. *Clinical Endocrinology., 72*, 702–708.
103. Borrello, M. G., Alberti, L., Fischer, A., Degl'innocenti, D., Ferrario, C., Gariboldi, M., Marchesi, F., Allavena, P., Greco, A., Collini, P., Pilotti, S., Cassinelli, G., Bressan, P., Fugazzola, L., Mantovani, A., & Pierotti, M. A. (2005). Induction of a proinflammatory program in normal human thyrocytes by the RET/PTC1 oncogene. *Proceedings of the National Academy of Sciences of the United States of America., 102*, 14825–14830.
104. Kammoun-Krichen, M., Bougacha-Elleuch, N., Mnif, M., Bougacha, F., Charffedine, I., Rebuffat, S., Rebai, A., Glasson, E., Abid, M., Ayadi, F., Péraldi-Roux, S., & Ayadi, H. (2012). Il-?? A potential factor for discriminating between thyroid carcinoma and atrophic thyroiditis. *European Cytokine Network., 23*, 101–106.
105. Lippitz, B. E. (2013). Cytokine patterns in patients with cancer: A systematic review. *The Lancet Oncology., 14*, e218–e228.
106. Eloy, C., Santos, J., Cameselle-Teijeiro, J., Soares, P., & Sobrinho-Simões, M. (2012). TGFbeta/Smad pathway and BRAF mutation play different roles in circumscribed and infiltrative papillary thyroid carcinoma. *Virchows Archiv, 460*, 587–600.
107. Flavell, R. A., Sanjabi, S., Wrzesinski, S. H., & Licona-Limón, P. (2010). The polarization of immune cells in the tumour environment by TGFβ. *Nature Reviews Immunology., 10*, 554–567.
108. Rotondi, M., Coperchini, F., & Chiovato, L. (2013). CXCL8 in thyroid disease: From basic notions to potential applications in clinical practice. *Cytokine & Growth Factor Reviews., 24*, 539–546.
109. Zhang, X., Yuan, X., Shi, H., Wu, L., Qian, H., & Xu, W. (2015). Exosomes in cancer: Small particle, big player. *Journal of Hematology & Oncology., 8*, 83.
110. Wang, Z., Chen, J.-Q., Liu, J.-L., & Tian, L. (2016). Exosomes in tumor microenvironment: Novel transporters and biomarkers. *Journal of Translational Medicine, 14*, 297.
111. Théry, C., Zitvogel, L., & Amigorena, S. (2002). Exosomes: Composition, biogenesis and function. *Nature Reviews Immunology*, Published Online: 01 August 2002, *2*, 569. https://doi.org/10.1038/nri855
112. Atretkhany, K. S. N., Drutskaya, M. S., Nedospasov, S. A., Grivennikov, S. I., & Kuprash, D. V. (2016). Chemokines, cytokines and exosomes help tumors to shape inflammatory microenvironment. *Pharmacology and Therapeutics., 168*, 98–112.
113. Tickner, J. A., Urquhart, A. J., Stephenson, S.-A., Richard, D. J., & O'Byrne, K. J. (2014). Functions and therapeutic roles of exosomes in cancer. *Frontiers in Oncology., 4*, 127.
114. Pant, S., Hilton, H., & Burczynski, M. E. (2012). The multifaceted exosome: Biogenesis, role in normal and aberrant cellular function, and frontiers for pharmacological and biomarker opportunities. *Biochemical Pharmacology, 83*, 1484–1494.
115. Roma-Rodrigues, C., Fernandes, A. R., & Baptista, P. V. (2014). Exosome in tumour microenvironment: Overview of the crosstalk between normal and cancer cells. *BioMed Research International, 2014*, 179486.
116. Record, M., Carayon, K., Poirot, M., & Silvente-Poirot, S. (2014). Exosomes as new vesicular lipid transporters involved in cell–cell communication and various pathophysiologies. *Biochimica et Biophysica Acta (BBA) – Molecular and Cell Biology of Lipids., 1841*, 108–120.
117. Barile, L., & Vassalli, G. (2017). Exosomes: Therapy delivery tools and biomarkers of diseases. *Pharmacology & Therapeutics*.
118. VanNiel, G., Mallegol, J., Bevilacqua, C., Candalh, C., Brugière, S., Tomaskovic-Crook, E., Heath, J. K., Cerf-Bensussan, N., & Heyman, M. (2003). Intestinal epithelial exosomes carry MHC class II/peptides able to inform the immune system in mice. *Gut, 52*, 1690–1697.
119. Sprent, J. (2005). Direct stimulation of naïve T cells by antigen-presenting cell vesicles. *Blood cells, Molecules & Diseases., 35*, 17–20.
120. Skokos, D., Botros, H. G., Demeure, C., Morin, J., Peronet, R., Birkenmeier, G., Boudaly, S., & Mécheri, S. (2003). Mast cell-derived exosomes induce phenotypic and functional maturation of dendritic cells and elicit specific immune responses in vivo. *Journal of Immunology (Baltimore, Md. : 1950), 170*, 3037–3045.
121. Qu, Y., Franchi, L., Nunez, G., & Dubyak, G. R. (2007). Nonclassical IL-1 beta secretion stimulated by P2X7 receptors is dependent on inflammasome activation and correlated with exosome release

in murine macrophages. *Journal of Immunology (Baltimore, Md.: 1950), 179*, 1913–1925.
122. Obregon, C., Rothen-Rutishauser, B., Gerber, P., Gehr, P., & Nicod, L. P. (2009). Active uptake of dendritic cell-derived exovesicles by epithelial cells induces the release of inflammatory mediators through a TNF-α-mediated pathway. *The American Journal of Pathology., 175*, 696–705.
123. Atay, S., & Godwin, A. K. (2014). Tumor-derived exosomes: A message delivery system for tumor progression. *Communicative and Integrative Biology., 7*, e28231.
124. Bergmann, C., Strauss, L., Wieckowski, E., Czystowska, M., Albers, A., Wang, Y., Zeidler, R., Lang, S., & Whiteside, T. L. (2009). Tumor-derived microvesicles in sera of patients with head and neck cancer and their role in tumor progression. *Head & Neck., 31*, 371–380.
125. Huber, V., Filipazzi, P., Iero, M., Fais, S., & Rivoltini, L. (2008). More insights into the immunosuppressive potential of tumor exosomes. *Journal of Translational Medicine, 6*, 63.
126. Lee, J. C., Zhao, J. T., Clifton-Bligh, R. J., Gill, A., Gundara, J. S., Ip, J. C., Glover, A., Sywak, M. S., Delbridge, L. W., Robinson, B. G., & Sidhu, S. B. (2013). MicroRNA-222 and MicroRNA-146b are tissue and circulating biomarkers of recurrent papillary thyroid cancer. *Cancer, 119*, 4358–4365.
127. Yu, S., Liu, Y., Wang, J., Guo, Z., Zhang, Q., Yu, F., Zhang, Y., Huang, K., Li, Y., Song, E., Zheng, X., & Xiao, H. (2012). Circulating MicroRNA profiles as potential biomarkers for diagnosis of papillary thyroid carcinoma. *The Journal of Clinical Endocrinology & Metabolism., 97*, 2084–2092.
128. Lee, Y. S., Lim, Y. S., Lee, J.-C., Wang, S.-G., Park, H.-Y., Kim, S. Y., & Lee, B.-J. (2015). Differential expression levels of plasma-derived miR-146b and miR-155 in papillary thyroid cancer. *Oral Oncology., 51*, 77–83.
129. Yu, S., Liu, X., Zhang, Y., Li, J., Chen, S., Zheng, H., Reng, R., Zhang, C., Chen, J., Chen, L., Yu, S., Liu, X., Zhang, Y., Li, J., Chen, S., Zheng, H., Reng, R., Zhang, C., Chen, J., et al. (2016). Circulating microRNA124-3p, microRNA9-3p and microRNA196b-5p may be potential signatures for differential diagnosis of thyroid nodules. *Oncotarget, 7*, 84165–84177.
130. Li, M., Song, Q., Li, H., Lou, Y., & Wang, L. (2015). Circulating miR-25-3p and miR-451a may be potential biomarkers for the diagnosis of papillary thyroid carcinoma R. B. Ray, ed. *PLOS One, 10*, e0132403.
131. Samsonov, R., Burdakov, V., Shtam, T., Radzhabova, Z., Vasilyev, D., Tsyrlina, E., Titov, S., Ivanov, M., Berstein, L., Filatov, M., Kolesnikov, N., Gil-Henn, H., & Malek, A. (2016). Plasma exosomal miR-21 and miR-181a differentiates follicular from papillary thyroid cancer. *Tumor Biology, 37*, 12011–12021.
132. Fuziwara, C. S., & Kimura, E. T. (2014). MicroRNA deregulation in anaplastic thyroid cancer Biology. *International Journal of Endocrinology, 2014*, 743450.
133. Saiselet, M., Pita, J. M., Augenlicht, A., Dom, G., Tarabichi, M., Fimereli, D., Dumont, J. E., Detours, V., Maenhaut, C., Saiselet, M., Pita, J. M., Augenlicht, A., Dom, G., Tarabichi, M., Fimereli, D., Dumont, J. E., Detours, V., & Maenhaut, C. (2015). miRNA expression and function in thyroid carcinomas: A comparative and critical analysis and a model for other cancers. *Oncotarget, 7*, 52475–52492.
134. Boufraqech, M., Klubo-Gwiezdzinska, J., & Kebebew, E. (2016). MicroRNAs in the thyroid. *Best Practice and Research: Clinical Endocrinology and Metabolism., 30*, 603–619.
135. Braun, J., Hoang-Vu, C., Dralle, H., & Hutelmaier, S. (2010). Downregulation of microRNAs directs the EMT and invasive potential of anaplastic thyroid carcinomas. *Oncogene, 29*, 4237–4244.
136. Visone, R., Pallante, P., Vecchione, A., Cirombella, R., Ferracin, M., Ferraro, A., Volinia, S., Coluzzi, S., Leone, V., Borbone, E., Liu, C.-G., Petrocca, F., Troncone, G., Calin, G. A., Scarpa, A., Colato, C., Tallini, G., Santoro, M., Croce, C. M., et al. (2007). Specific microRNAs are downregulated in human thyroid anaplastic carcinomas. *Oncogene, 26*, 7590–7595.
137. Gu, H., Liu, Z., & Zhou, L. (2017). Roles of miR-17-92 cluster in cardiovascular development and common diseases. *BioMed Research International., 2017*, 1–6.
138. Iriki, T., Ohnishi, K., Fujiwara, Y., Horlad, H., Saito, Y., Pan, C., Ikeda, K., Mori, T., Suzuki, M., Ichiyasu, H., Kohrogi, H., Takeya, M., & Komohara, Y. (2017). The cell-cell interaction between tumor-associated macrophages and small cell lung cancer cells is involved in tumor progression via STAT3 activation. *Lung Cancer, 106*, 22–32.
139. Qian, B.-Z., & Pollard, J. W. (2010). Macrophage diversity enhances tumor progression and metastasis. *Cell, 141*, 39–51.
140. Vaňhara, P., & Souček, K. (2013). Mutual cytokine crosstalk between colon cancer cells and microenvironment initiates development of distant metastases. *JAK-STAT., 2*, e23810.
141. Wiseman, B. S., & Werb, Z. (2002). Stromal effects on mammary gland development and breast cancer. *Science, 296*, 1046–1049.
142. Azenshtein, E., Luboshits, G., Shina, S., Neumark, E., Shahbazian, D., Weil, M., Wigler, N., Keydar, I., & Ben-Baruch, A. (2002). The CC chemokine RANTES in breast carcinoma progression: Regulation of expression and potential mechanisms of promalignant activity. *Cancer Research., 62*, 1093–1102.
143. Gianoukakis, A. G., Khadavi, N., & Smith, T. J. (2008). Cytokines, graves' disease, and thyroid associated ophthalmopathy. *Thyroid: Official journal of the American Thyroid Association., 18*, 953–958.

144. Lv, D., Zhang, Y., Kim, H.-J., Zhang, L., & Ma, X. (2013). CCL5 as a potential immunotherapeutic target in triple-negative breast cancer. *Cellular and Molecular Immunology., 10*, 303–310.
145. Aldinucci, D., & Colombatti, A. (2014). The inflammatory chemokine CCL5 and cancer progression. *Mediators of Inflammation, 2014*, 292376.
146. Wolpe, S. D., & Cerami, A. (1989). Macrophage inflammatory proteins 1 and 2: Members of a novel superfamily of cytokines. *FASEB Journal: Official Publication of the Federation of American Societies for Experimental Biology., 3*, 2565–2573.
147. Driscoll, K. E. (1994). Macrophage inflammatory proteins: Biology and role in pulmonary inflammation. *Experimental Lung Research., 20*, 473–490.
148. Xu, J., Futakuchi, M., Iigo, M., Fukamachi, K., Alexander, D. B., Shimizu, H., Sakai, Y., Tamano, S., Furukawa, F., Uchino, T., Tokunaga, H., Nishimura, T., Hirose, A., Kanno, J., & Tsuda, H. (2010). Involvement of macrophage inflammatory protein 1a (MIP1a) in promotion of rat lung and mammary carcinogenic activity of nanoscale titanium dioxide particles administered by intra-pulmonary spraying. *Carcinogenesis, 31*, 927–935.
149. Mantovani, A., Allavena, P., Sica, A., & Balkwill, F. (2008). Cancer-related inflammation. *Nature, 454*, 436–444.
150. Feghali, C. A., & Wright, T. M. (1997). Cytokines in acute and chronic inflammation. *Frontiers in Bioscience: A Journal and Virtual Library., 2*, d12–d26.
151. Hou, Z., Falcone, D. J., Subbaramaiah, K., & Dannenberg, A. J. (2011). Macrophages induce COX-2 expression in breast cancer cells: Role of IL-1β autoamplification. *Carcinogenesis, 32*, 695–702.
152. Kobawala, T. P., Patel, G. H., Gajjar, D. R., Patel, K. N., Thakor, P. B., Parekh, U. B., Patel, K. M., Shukla, S. N., & Shah, P. M. (2011). Clinical utility of serum interleukin-8 and interferon-alpha in thyroid diseases. *Journal of Thyroid Research, 2011*, 270149.
153. David, J., Dominguez, C., Hamilton, D., & Palena, C. (2016). The IL-8/IL-8R Axis: A double agent in tumor immune resistance. *Vaccine, 4*, 22.
154. Ren, J., He, W., Zheng, L., & Duan, H. (2016). From structures to functions: Insights into exosomes as promising drug delivery vehicles. *Biomaterials Science, 4*, 910–921.
155. Tomasetti, M., Lee, W., Santarelli, L., & Neuzil, J. (2017). Exosome-derived microRNAs in cancer metabolism: Possible implications in cancer diagnostics and therapy. *Experimental & Molecular Medicine., 49*, e285.
156. Zhang, J., Zhang, H., Liu, J., Tu, X., Zang, Y., Zhu, J., Chen, J., Dong, L., & Zhang, J. (2012). miR-30 inhibits TGF-β1-induced epithelial-to-mesenchymal transition in hepatocyte by targeting Snail1. *Biochemical and Biophysical Research Communications., 417*, 1100–1105.
157. Kong, W., Yang, H., He, L., Zhao, J.-J., Coppola, D., Dalton, W. S., & Cheng, J. Q. (2008). MicroRNA-155 is regulated by the transforming growth factor β/Smad pathway and contributes to epithelial cell plasticity by targeting RhoA. *Molecular and Cellular Biology., 28*, 6773–6784.
158. Shi, J., & Jian. (2016). Considering Exosomal miR-21 as a biomarker for cancer. *Journal of Clinical Medicine, 5*, 42.
159. Lopes-Ramos, C. M., Habr-Gama, A., De, B., Quevedo, S., Felício, N. M., Cio, M., Bettoni, F., Koyama, F. C., Asprino, P. F., Galante, P. A., Gama-Rodrigues, J., Camargo, A. A., Oliva Perez, R., & Parmigiani, R. B. (2012). Overexpression of miR-21-5p as a predictive marker for complete tumor regression to neoadjuvant chemoradiotherapy in rectal cancer patients. *BMC Medical Genomics, 7*.
160. Yan, L., Cao, R., Liu, Y., Wang, L., Pan, B., Lv, X., Jiao, H., Zhuang, Q., Sun, X., & Xiao, R. (2016). MiR-21-5p links epithelial-mesenchymal transition phenotype with stem-like cell signatures via AKT signaling in keloid keratinocytes. *Scientific Reports, 6*, 28281.
161. Liu, X., Wang, C., Chen, Z., Jin, Y., Wang, Y., Kolokythas, A., Dai, Y., & Zhou, X. (2011). MicroRNA-138 suppresses epithelial-mesenchymal transition in squamous cell carcinoma cell lines. *The Biochemical Journal., 440*, 23–31.
162. Mitomo, S., Maesawa, C., Ogasawara, S., Iwaya, T., Shibazaki, M., Yashima-Abo, A., Kotani, K., Oikawa, H., Sakurai, E., Izutsu, N., Kato, K., Komatsu, H., Ikeda, K., Wakabayashi, G., & Masuda, T. (2008). Downregulation of miR-138 is associated with overexpression of human telomerase reverse transcriptase protein in human anaplastic thyroid carcinoma cell lines. *Cancer Science., 99*, 280–286.
163. Gao, J., & Liu, Q.-G. (2011). The role of miR-26 in tumors and normal tissues (review). *Oncology Letters., 2*, 1019–1023.
164. Bu, Q., You, F., Pan, G., Yuan, Q., Cui, T., Hao, L., & Zhang, J. (2017). MiR-125b inhibits anaplastic thyroid cancer cell migration and invasion by targeting PIK3CD. *Biomedicine & Pharmacotherapy., 88*, 443–448.
165. Ge, S., Wang, D., Kong, Q., Gao, W., & Sun, J. (2017). *Function of MiR-152 as a tumor suppressor in human breast cancer by targeting PIK3CA*. Oncology Research Featuring Preclinical and Clinical Cancer Therapeutics.
166. Liu, X., Li, J., Qin, F., & Dai, S. (2016). miR-152 as a tumor suppressor microRNA: Target recognition and regulation in cancer. *Oncology Letters., 11*, 3911–3939.
167. Sheng, W., Chen, Y., Gong, Y., Dong, T., Zhang, B., & Gao, W. (2016). miR-148a inhibits self-renewal of thyroid cancer stem cells via repressing INO80 expression. *Oncology Reports., 36*, 3387–3396.
168. Colamaio, M., Borbone, E., Russo, L., Bianco, M., Federico, A., Califano, D., Chiappetta, G., Pallante, P., Troncone, G., Battista, S., & Fusco, A. (2011).

miR-191 Down-regulation plays a role in thyroid follicular tumors through CDK6 targeting. *The Journal of Clinical Endocrinology & Metabolism.*, *96*, E1915–E1924.

169. Bednarczyk, R. B. (2016). *Crosstalk between macrophage secretory factors and breast cancer*. New York Medical College.

170. Hébrant, A., Floor, S., Saiselet, M., Antoniou, A., Desbuleux, A., Snyers, B., La, C., de Saint, A. N., Leteurtre, E., Andry, G., & Maenhaut, C. (2014). miRNA expression in anaplastic thyroid carcinomas R. M. Luque, ed. *PLoS One, 9*, e103871.

Disruption of Cell-Cell Communication in Anaplastic Thyroid Cancer as an Immunotherapeutic Opportunity

Sanjukta Chakraborty, Michelle Carnazza, Tara Jarboe, Nicole DeSouza, Xiu-Min Li, Augustine Moscatello, Jan Geliebter, and Raj K. Tiwari

1 Tumor Microenvironment

Carcinogenesis is a multistep process supported by a host of factors that involve not only the aberrant physiology of the malignant cells, but a plethora of changes occurring in the tissue surrounding the tumor during this malignant transformation. Tumor is a heterogeneous mass of resident and infiltrating host cells and various secreted factors that make up the tumor supportive niche, known as the tumor microenvironment (TME). The TME refers to the cellular environment surrounding the tumor that incorporates tumor vasculature and lymphatics, stromal cells such as pericytes and fibroblasts, immune cells, extracellular matrices, the signaling mediators, and secretory factors. The TME plays an extremely crucial role in determining the course of tumor progression and therapeutic response. During later stages of tumorigenesis, the cancer cells reshape the TME in a way that bolsters the tumor development while suppressing antitumor activities, such as immune cell-mediated cytotoxicity. In order to promote indefinite growth, enhanced survival, proliferation, and long-term maintenance, cancer cells rewire their cellular metabolism and secretome composition. This reprogramming is responsible for progressive pathological alterations in nonmalignant components of the TME. These transformed nonmalignant components and the tumor cells collectively decide the therapeutic outcome in the patients. The constant dialogue between the tumor cells and the nonmalignant components of the TME is at the heart of several hallmarks of cancer [1, 2]. In order to develop an effective therapeutic regimen, a holistic understanding of the TME is crucial.

S. Chakraborty
Department of Pathology, Microbiology, and Immunology, New York Medical College, Valhalla, NY, USA

Weill Cornell Medicine, New York, NY, USA

M. Carnazza · T. Jarboe · N. DeSouza · X.-M. Li · J. Geliebter · R. K. Tiwari (✉)
Department of Pathology, Microbiology, and Immunology, New York Medical College, Valhalla, NY, USA
e-mail: Raj_Tiwari@nymc.edu

A. Moscatello
Department of Otolaryngology, Westchester Medical Center, Valhalla, NY, USA

D. Banerjee, R. K. Tiwari (eds.), *Tumor Microenvironment: Cellular, Metabolic and Immunologic Interactions*, Advances in Experimental Medicine and Biology 1350,
https://doi.org/10.1007/978-3-030-83282-7_2

2 Cellular Constituents

The TME is extremely heterogeneous and dynamic in nature. The cellular constituents of the TME can be divided into two broad categories – immune cells and nonimmune cells.

2.1 Immune Cells

The hypothesis of "immune surveillance" was formulated by Frank Macfarlane Burnet and Lewis Thomas in the 1950s [3–6]. The hypothesis suggested that the cells of the immune system should detect and kill the tumor cells. This concept was further developed and the new theory of immunoediting was coined in 2004 by Dr. Old and Dr. Screiber [7]. They suggested that immunoediting is a process that consists of three steps: elimination, equilibrium, and escape [7]. As the field of tumor immunology progressed over time, we have identified specific components of the tumor microenvironment that dictate each of these three steps, and this knowledge has helped us understand the dynamic nature of the immune landscape in different tumors. The immune cell infiltrates and secreted cytokines and chemokines collectively make up the tumor immune microenvironment (TIME). The cellular infiltrates might be composed of all major types of immune cells, such as CD4, CD8, and $\gamma\delta$ T lymphocytes, regulatory T lymphocytes (T_{regs}), regulatory B lymphocytes (B_{regs}), tumor-associated macrophages (TAMs), natural killer (NK) cells, dendritic cells (DC), and mast cells [8]. The proportion of the cellular infiltrates vary greatly not only between but also within cancer types. A recent study that integrated gene expression and clinical outcome data of over 18,000 human tumors noted a stark difference in relative leukocyte composition between different tumors [9]. These immune cells are considered as adjuvant therapeutic targets in cancer and to devise novel strategies to circumvent resistance.

2.1.1 Macrophages

Tumors initiated by extrinsic factors often start out as an uncontrolled inflammatory reaction brought about by the innate cells of the immune system. One of the most prominent innate immune cells is the macrophage. Macrophages are usually found in both the center of the tumor and at the invasive margins and/or tumor stroma. Macrophages can be polarized into inflammatory M1 (classical Th1-activated) or immunosuppressive M2 (Th2-activated) phenotypes. These cells are usually responsible for defending the body against pathogens and aiding in wound healing and tissue repair. Comprehensive lineage tracing has shown that macrophages originate from at least three different embryonic precursors (from erythro-myeloid progenitor (EMP) in the yolk sac and fetal liver and from macrophage/dendritic cell progenitor cells (MDPs) in the bone marrow) and differentiate into tissue resident macrophages [10–12]. These tissue resident macrophages are usually maintained by self-renewal. Recruitment of these immune cells in the TME is largely dictated by the genetic lesions and transcription factors expressed by the tumor cells. Some of the key transcription factors such as STAT3, HIFα, and NFκB are activated by oncogene activation and chronic inflammation which are two of the key events during cancer initiation. Recruitment of macrophages further enriches the mutagenic environment via secretion of pro-inflammatory cytokines like interleukin 6 (IL-6), tumor necrosis factor alpha (TNFα), and interferon gamma (IFNγ). Macrophages are also responsible for secretion of oncogenic growth factors, such as epidermal growth factor (EGFR) and WNTs. The tumor-associated macrophages (TAMs) diversify into a unique population, in terms of cell surface protein expression and transcription factors. The specific population of macrophages are involved in enhanced angiogenesis [13], metastasis [14], invasion [15], tumor cell extravasation [16], and immunosuppression [17]. Each of these functions is carried out by a subpopulation of macrophages with a different transcriptome and cell surface markers.

2.1.2 Dendritic Cells (DCs)

Dendritic cells (DCs) bridge the gap between the innate and adaptive immune system. DCs sequentially develop from common myeloid progenitors

(CMPs) and macrophage DC progenitors (MDPs). These cells are responsible for eliciting pathogen-specific T cell response. DCs stimulate adaptive immune response by sampling the tumor antigens, processing them, and presenting them in the context of MHC class II at the secondary lymphoid organs. During the process, the activated DCs secrete pro-inflammatory cytokines and upregulate the co-stimulatory molecules on their surface that help in activating the T cells in turn. DCs can be subdivided into three main categories, namely, the conventional DCs (cDCs), the plasmacytoid DCs (pDCs), and the monocyte-derived DCs (moDCs). The differentiation of DCs into specific subsets is dictated by specific transcription factors. The differentiation of conventional DCs is driven by Id2 [18], whereas differentiation of pDCs is favored by E2-2 [19]. Under normal physiological conditions, cDCs further differentiate into $CD103^+$, $CD11b^+$, and $CD8^+$ subsets in the lymphoid and non-lymphoid organs. The tumor microenvironment modulates this differentiation, and in this unique condition, pre-DCs differentiate into two rare populations of DCs: $CD11b^+$ DCs (cDC1) and $CD103^+$ DCs (cDC2). cDC1s are specialized in presenting antigens in the context of MHC I molecules to CD8 T cells, while cDC2s specialize in presenting antigens on MHC II molecules to CD4 T cells. The antigen cross-presentation capability of the DCs in the tumor microenvironment is heavily impaired, resulting in poor response to immunotherapeutic strategies that rely on T cell activation via DCs. Some of the factors responsible for this impaired activity of DCs are hypoxia, high concentration of lactate [20–22], low pH [23, 24], and accumulation of adenosine [25].

2.1.3 Natural Killer (NK) Cells

Natural killer cells are a group of cytotoxic innate lymphoid cells (ILCs) that are extremely crucial components of cancer immune surveillance and can eliminate cancer cells very efficiently via secretion of cytotoxic granules or immunomodulatory cytokines upon stimulation. However, the complex cellular architecture of the TME of thyroid tumors interferes with the accessibility of the tumor cells resulting in poor homing and infiltration and low killing efficiency. In vitro analyses confirm susceptibility of TC cells to NK-mediated lysis [26], which suggests their potential as an immunotherapeutic option for the patients where intratumoral NK infiltration has been reported. In contrast to T lymphocytes, which are known as the main players of tumor-specific immune response, NK cells intrinsically express a wide variety of germline encoded activating and inhibiting membrane receptors, hence do not require antigen specificity. An extremely common strategy adopted by tumor cells to evade immune surveillance is downregulation of MHC expression. Interestingly, this phenomenon is responsible for impaired T cell activity which is dependent on TCR/MHC interaction. However, this same phenomenon triggers the activating receptors on NK cells because of "missing self-recognition" on the tumor cells. Thus, NK cell activity complements the antitumor activity of the T cells. Some of the central activating and co-activating NK cell receptors include the NKp46, NKp30, and NKp44, CD16, NKG2D, NKG2C, natural cytotoxicity receptors (NCRs), DNAX accessory molecule-1 (DNAM-1), and 2B4 [27, 28]. A recent study has identified a less functional $CD56^{hi}CD16^{hi/lo}$ NK population which is associated with thyroid malignancy. Interestingly, these NK cells were associated with exhaustion markers programmed cell death protein 1 (PD-1) and T cell immunoglobulin and mucin domain-containing-3 (TIM-3), and blockade of these receptors could reinvigorate the NK cells [29]. Previous studies have shown that these NK cells are associated with unique receptors such as CD62L, CXCR3, CCR7, and CXCR4 that facilitate their homing to inflamed tissues. Some of the common features adopted by the tumor cells to evade NK cells include downregulation of NK cell activating receptor (NKAR) ligands, downregulation of death receptors, increased secretion of immunosuppressive cytokines, hypoxia-dependent autophagy activation, and hypoxia-dependent extracellular adenosine synthesis. In order to fully leverage the antitumor activity of the NK cells, supporting strategies, such as IL-15 agonist, BiKEs, and TRiKEs targeting activating receptors of the NK cells, immune checkpoint inhibitor antagonists, should be introduced in a combinatorial setting.

2.1.4 T Lymphocytes

Tumor-infiltrating T lymphocytes (TILs) are influential in dictating the response of the immune system against the tumor. Most mature T cells circulate in a resting, naïve state. Upon the recognition of cognate antigen, the cells become activated, undergo clonal proliferation, and finally differentiate into effector T cells. Naïve CD8+ T cells differentiate into cytotoxic T cells, while differentiation of CD4+ T cells is largely dictated both spatially and temporally by microenvironmental cues. They can differentiate into an array of different types of helper (i.e., T helper cell type 1 [Th1], Th2, Th17) or regulatory T cells (T_{reg}) depending on the cues. Immunologically, tumors can be classified into two broad categories. T cell-inflamed tumors are characterized by presence of immune activation and extensive T cell infiltration and are amenable to immunomodulatory therapies. Non-T cell-inflamed tumors are devoid of inflammation and T cell infiltration and are refractory to such therapeutic approaches. The former is known as an immunologically "hot" tumor and the latter "cold." The goal of a successful immunotherapy is to turn immunologically cold tumors into hot tumors. Homing of T cells to the tumor site is dictated by various factors. The tissue-specific homing signals for T cells are composed of a specific combination of receptors (e.g., E-selectin and P-selectin ligands and chemokine receptors CXCR3). Stimulation of T cells induces the activation of integrins, primarily LFA-1 and VLA-4 (very late antigen 4), which bind to receptors ICAM-1 and VCAM-1 expressed on inflamed tissues [30]. Inside the tissues, these cells are often organized into cellular aggregates, which are commonly referred to as tertiary lymphoid structures (TLS) or ectopic lymphoid structure (ELS). Within these structures, there is usually a follicular zone with $CD20^+$ B cells, which is surrounded by a mix of $CD3^+$ T cells and lysosome-associated membrane glycoprotein$^+$ ($LAMP1^+$) DCs. This cellular architecture facilitates cross presentation to local tumor antigens by DCs and activation of effector T cells. This also helps with the generation of antibody producing plasma cells. Presence of such cellular architecture inside a solid tumor is often indicative of a favorable prognosis.

2.2 Nonimmune Cells

2.2.1 Neuroendocrine Cells

Neuroendocrine (NE) cells display both nerve and endocrine cell characteristics. They are capable of receiving and interpreting signals from the nervous system and respond to these stimuli through the production and release of hormones directly into the bloodstream.

NE cells frequently inhabit sites of tumor formation. Although these NE cells are nonimmune cells, they have a critical impact on the expression and function of immune system components and contain a highly concentrated cytosolic load of neurosecretory granules that synthesize neuropeptides and receptors [31].

Important immune modulations via NE cells occur through neurotransmitter release. For example, the regulation of migration and cytotoxicity of natural killer (NK) cells occurs through neurotransmitter intervention [8]. Norepinephrine has been attributed to the modulation of T cell activity, through the blocking of tumor necrosis factor alpha (TNFα) synthesis, which inevitably leads to the inhibition of antitumor cytotoxic T lymphocytes (CTLs) [8]. Substance P, a neuropeptide that plays a role in neuromodulation, can also be released by NE cells. This neuropeptide has been shown to induce leukocyte cytokine production. Additionally, substance P has been identified to prevent β1-integrin-mediated T lymphocyte adhesion. This activity leads to an increase in T lymphocyte migration to the tumor site [8]. An important effector function of NE cells regarding the immune modulation of the TME is their role in chemotaxis. The upregulation of tumor-associated macrophages (TAMs) in the TME is attributed to their recruitment by NE cells through chemotactic mechanisms – specifically via secretion of CXCL10 and CXCL11 [32].

The primary markers of NE cells include neuron-specific enolase (NSE), chromogranin A (CgA), and interleukin-2 (IL-2), as well as endothelial growth factor (EGF), which is identified more specifically as a targeting marker. NE cells can lead to the formation of specific tumor types in various physiological realms. For example, in colorectal cancer, differentiation (distribution or dispersion of NE cells within a tumor environment) of NE cells is one of the primary drivers of poor prognosis. This poor prognosis has been speculated to be attributed to an increased amount of tumor-associated macrophages within colorectal adenocarcinomas that express increased NE cell differentiation [33]. Although an NE cell-derived tumor is rare in the thyroid, under specific physiological conditions, this specific form of tumor can still be established. This tumor development is more likely to occur in the event of elevated calcitonin levels, although calcitonin-negative tumors have also been identified. Medullary thyroid carcinoma (MCT) is typically described as the form that persists when discussing NE derivation [34].

TNF-α is an example of a cytokine that can lead to induction of NE cell differentiation within small cell lung cancer (SCLC) cell lines. This increase in NE cell differentiation via TNF-α exposure occurs through the induction of NE cell gene expression, as well as the induction of NE cell-related proteins [35]. Pulmonary NE cells release a specific secretory factor known as gastrin-releasing peptide (GRP). GRP is responsible for the chemoattraction of macrophages and lymphocytes to any site of lung tissue injury, and can serve as a competent biomarker for NE cell differentiation within the TME [35].

Forkhead box A1 (FOXA1) is a transcription factor that is responsible for differentiation of prostate epithelial cells. It has been shown that the absence or loss of FOXA1 can lead to an increase in NE cell differentiation, which occurs through the downstream activation of MAPK, a promoting factor of NE cell differentiation in prostate cancer cells. Therefore, the inhibition of NE cell differentiation can be regulated by the expression of FOXA1. When FOXA1 is present, it binds to an IL-8 promoter leading to an inhibition of its expression, which inevitably leads to a downstream inhibition of mitogen-activated protein kinase (MAPK) activation, decreased enolase 2 (ENO2) expression, and the inhibition of NE cell differentiation [36]. Other signal transduction pathways associated with NE cell differentiation include JAK/STAT3 and PI3K/AKT [36].

2.2.2 Adipose Cells

Adipose cells, or adipocytes, are the primary component of adipose tissue, and are specifically derived from mesenchymal stem cells through a process called adipogenesis. Inflammatory responses generate an influx of immune cells to targeted areas. There is a defined correlation between an increase in adipose tissue and the generation of inflammatory responses. This phenomenon is explained through the correlation between elevated adipose tissue levels and an increased risk in the initial and further development of cancer [37]. Adipocytes have been noted to secrete local and systemic factors that can promote the development of tumors. There is an active interaction that exists between tumor cells and adipose tissue. This can serve as a priming factor in adipocyte alteration, which can lead to the increase in their secretion of adipokines, such as vascular endothelial growth factor (VEGF) and leptin [38].

Adipose tissue can differ in relative density, which categorizes this tissue as either metabolically active (brown adipose) or metabolically inactive (white adipose). Brown adipose tissue (BAT) contains an extensive amount of mitochondria, which supports its critical role in thermogenesis and lipid oxidation. Another distinct characteristic of BAT is the elevated expression of uncoupling protein 1 (UCP1). White adipose tissue (WAT) is associated with the regulation of lipid metabolism, and serves as an energy reservoir. It also can play an endocrine role, as it secretes hormones and chemokines that support inflammation, thus rendering WAT as the primary focus when discussing the TME [38].

Hyperadiposity has been shown to render altered behavior when compared to traditional adipose tissue function, since areas of inflamed adipose tissue greatly resemble tissue injury. Recognition of an injury site is what causes the induction of an inflammatory response, and thus the infiltration of immune-related cells to the area. With this being said, adipose cells are non-immune cells, but they play a critical role in the modulation of immune cell infiltration, activity, and response to inflamed tissue, thus rendering a large impact on the establishment and development of the TME [37]. Adipose inflammation can remodel and impact the TME due to the physiologically established chronic inflammatory response. This is possible because the TME phenotypically resembles the immune environment that is established after tissue injury or wound formation. The infiltration of immune cells and the generation and proliferation of pro-inflammatory mediators occur through adipose tissue induction. As adipocytes increase in number, the adipose tissue will eventually exhibit growth that greatly surpasses their available blood supply. This leads to instances of oxygen deprivation, or hypoxia, which in turn greatly contributes to adipocyte stress, and potentially death. Adipocyte stress and death, in turn, leads to an increase in the production of monocyte chemoattractant protein-1 (MCP-1), which then leads to the upregulation of macrophage proliferation. Macrophage influx leads to the envelopment of adipocytes, forming crown-like structures (CLSs), which are known to serve as an important biomarker of inflammation. Formation of these structures eventually leads to the release of free fatty acids (FFAs) from the internalized adipocyte and can result in the activation of toll-like receptor (TLR) 4. TLR4 activation leads to the initiation of the signal transduction pathway involved in the upregulation of nuclear factor kappa B (NFκB), thus increasing expression levels of NFκB-related genes. These genes include those that encode for the pro-inflammatory cytokines TNF-α and IL-1β, further contributing to the inflammatory environment [37].

2.2.3 Endothelial Cells

Endothelial cells (ECs) are a morphologically and functionally heterogeneous population of cells that form a continuous and uniform monolayer of the inner lining of blood and lymphatic vessels. Under normal physiological conditions, ECs serve critical functions in vascular stabilization, homeostasis, angiogenesis, and immune cell trafficking [39–42]. In a normal, healthy state, ECs are typically non-proliferating, or quiescent. However, upon activation by environmental stressors, activated ECs promote a pro-thrombotic and pro-immunogenic phenotype, with the ability to return to quiescence following removal of the stressor [39]. In the context of cancer, ECs form the inner lining of the blood vessels that make up part of a growing tumor. These tumor endothelial cells (TECs), while not cancer themselves, are essential to cancer progression, becoming dysregulated morphologically and phenotypically, similar to the tumor [40]. TECs are irregular in shape and size, with ruffled margins and long cytoplasmic projections, and their metabolic and genetic phenotype markedly altered. Notably, they are highly proliferative and upregulate proangiogenic, ECM remodeling, and stemness genes, causing enhanced immunomodulatory cytokines and altered cell surface receptors [41]. Some of the TEC-specific markers identified are CD276, CXCR7/ACKR3, VEGF, and EGF when compared to normal ECs [41]. As a consequence of hypoxia, cancer cells express these angiogenic factors and proangiogenic chemokines and receptors to initiate neo-angiogenesis (aka "angiogenic switch") [39]. This angiogenesis is guided by EC proliferation via VEGF, and therefore, the newly formed blood vessels can supply oxygen and nutrients to the tumor, supporting tumor progression and metastasis. In addition to hypoxia, chronic growth factor stimulation also causes endothelial dysfunction, which results in EC turnover 20–2000 times the rate of normal tissues [40]. VEGF-A alone is sufficient to induce most of the morphological changes (tortuosity, excessive branching, and leakiness) observed in the tumor vasculature, as VEGF signaling induced by hypoxia loosens EC tight junctions, leading to tumor cell intravasation during invasion and metastasis [40, 42]. TECs are not only promoting tumor angiogenesis but serve as key mediators of immune regulation in the TME, playing functional roles in immune cell transmigration and affecting T cell priming, activation, and proliferation by acting as antigen-presenting cells. TECs also form a barrier to immune-stimulatory cells promoting "endothelial anergy," the loss of protective anticancer immunity [39]. Therefore, it is evident TECs influence the response to anti-angiogenic and immune checkpoint inhibitor therapies that attempt to re-regulate the TME. Endothelial cells' functions of lining of vasculature, diameter extending, and abnormal growth of the blood vessels promote angiogenesis, extravasation, hypoxia, proliferation, and resistance of tumor cells to therapy. Furthermore, the function in ECM remodeling and alteration of the immune response promotes lymphangiogenesis and cancer progression [39].

2.2.4 Mesenchymal Cells

Mesenchymal stem cells (MSCs) are non-hematopoietic multipotent stem cells existing in a variety of tissues with high differentiation potential and self-renewal abilities [43–45]. Three minimal criteria that define human MSCs are as follows: (1) expression of CD105, CD90, and CD73 and lack of expression of CD45, CD34, CD14 or CD11b, CD79 or CD19, and HLA-DR surface molecules; (2) they must adhere to plastic in culture and differentiate into osteocytes, chondrocytes, and adipocytes; and (3) possess unique immunophenotypic, tissue repair, and immunoregulatory capacities [43]. In addition to their normal residence in areas such as the bone marrow, fat, and dental pulp, MSCs are found in circulation and accumulate in areas of tissue damage [44–45]. Here, they are considered important regulators of tissue homeostasis and integrity. This strong tropism for wounds and damaged tissue to promote regenerative activities also promotes homing to the tumor they are recruited by [44]. Depending on cancer type, the effect of MSCs on tumor progression could be proliferative or inhibitory, depending on the balance between anti- and pro-inflammatory phenotype, respectively. Evidence suggests that the anti-inflammatory MSCs support tumor growth and metastasis via stimulation of proliferation, migration, and invasion while also supporting tumor vasculature by promotion of angiogenesis, and immunosuppression. MSCs have demonstrated interactions with tumor cells, especially via signaling from those that are hypoxic and necrotic, facilitating cancer progression via direct contact and secretion of cytokines, chemokines, growth factors, and soluble factors and mediators, such as TGFB, OPN, CCL5, SDF1a, and lactate [45]. These pro-tumorigenic activities of MSCs are enhanced in response to tumor perturbation, therefore explaining tumor regrowth and resistance to therapy. While it is widely accepted that MSCs tend to be more pro-tumorigenic than anti-tumorigenic, MSCs have antitumor effects including suppression of proliferation and angiogenesis. Anticancer immunity is induced by promotion of a massive inflammatory cell infiltration. This is also achieved via the secretion of cytokine and chemokines by MSCs [43]. However, an explanation for this could be a polarization of MSCs, similar to macrophages, in response to secreted factors by the tumor driving tumor-promoting or tumor suppressive functions of MSCs [45]. In summation, MSCs form the fibrovascular network that maintains the TME via secretion of cytokines and differentiation of fibroblasts and vascular pericytes.

2.2.5 Fibroblasts

Fibroblasts are the most common type of cell found in connective tissue, in which their classical function is to produce extracellular matrix components responsible for maintaining the tissue structural integrity, and subsequently tissue homeostasis and function, via the synthesis of collagen proteins [46–48]. These include fibrillar collagens, proteoglycans, fibronectin, glycosaminoglycans, and other glycoproteins and fibrils. Fibroblasts are non-epithelial, nonimmune cells with a likely mesenchymal origin. In normal tissues, they are commonly present in the interstitial space and exhibit a spindle-shaped morphology. Moreover, in normal tissues, they are usually indolent, with insignificant metabolic and transcriptomic activity, and considered to be in a quiescent state. In this context, they are identified by α-smooth muscle actin (αSMA; also known as ACTA2) expression, a cytoskeletal protein associated with smooth muscle cells [46]. Their ability to become activated is demonstrated in the process of wound healing and tissue fibrosis. They are important for the deposition of extracellular matrix and scar tissue is formed via fibroblast over proliferation [47]. Furthermore, they generate cytokines and chemokines that recruit immune cells, and exert physical forces to modify tissue architecture [46]. Classic wound healing recruits inflammation, immune cells, and fibroblasts to promote angiogenesis and deposition of ECM. Once the tissue is repaired, the activated fibroblasts undergo apoptosis. However, under chronic wound healing, or tissue fibrosis, fibroblasts exhibit continuous activation controlled partly epigenetically by enhancing anti-apoptotic pathways and promoting proliferation [46]. Normal fibroblasts are considered antitumor due to the "neighbor suppression phenomenon" in which upon contact, will inhibit the growth of adjacent abnormal or transformed cells [48]. However, fibroblasts can also act as tumor promoters. Within a dominant part of the tumor stroma, studies have suggested a role of fibroblasts in cancer initiation, progression, and metastasis. Tumors are considered "wounds that do not heal" and initiate the chronic wound healing response mentioned previously, initiating signaling cascades altering cancer cell proliferation, invasion, metastasis, EMT, tumor-promoting inflammation, and angiogenesis [46]. This also is considered to require epigenetic modifications. These fibroblasts are called cancer-associated fibroblasts (CAFs), which can be identified by expression of PDGFRα/β, αSMA, fibroblast-associated protein (FAP), and fibroblast-specific protein 1 (FSP1) [48]. Their recruitment to the tumor is largely due to growth factors secreted by cancer cells and infiltrating immune cells, including TGFB, PDGF, and FGF2 [48]. There, CAFs hijack the physiological functions of normal fibroblast in the TME, as these irreversibly activated fibroblasts are more migratory due to their constant exposure to different stimuli. They exhibit functions including secretion of cytokines, chemokines, growth factors, matricellular proteins, and production of ECM to change the physical, biomechanical, and biochemical properties of the microenvironment. CAFs are emerging as central players in immune regulation that shapes the TME to be more immunosuppressive and growth-promoting. The mechanism by which this occurs is the orchestration of immune cell recruitment, such as myeloid cells and regulatory T cells, driving an immunosuppressive function of these immune cells, including TAMs, MDSCs, T cells, and DCs, and directly inhibiting cell-mediated killing of cytotoxic lymphocytes, including NK cells and T cells [49]. An immunosuppressive environment is also a direct result of the ECM remodeling and fibrosis. All in all, the secretion of cytokines, ECM proteases, and other factors results in the tumor drug resistance, proliferation, metastasis, and promotion of angiogenesis, ECM remodeling, immunosuppression, and cancer progression through the targeting of tumor cells, endothelial cells, T lymphocytes, and other cells of the TME [49].

3 Dynamic Nature of the Tumor Microenvironment

Cancer progression coincides with a dynamically evolving TME. It has been demonstrated that the acellular components, immune cells, and nonimmune cells are together perpetuating the different stages of cancer progression via interaction with the growing tumor. Regarding tumors as complex tissues in which cancer cells have recruited and manipulated normal cells to conspire in their neoplastic agenda, it is evident these interactions between the genetically altered malignant cells and these supporting co-conspirators are critical in cancer pathogenesis [1]. Therefore, it can be said that this milieu evolves functionally and acts synergistically in cancer progression as the intrinsic factors of the cancer cells and the TME together determine the tumor trajectory [50]. The TME is not only the tumor and supporting cells, but the environmental changes that accompany this interaction, including oxygen tension, nutrient composition, pH/redox potential, and interstitial pressure [1, 51]. The cancer cells can adapt to these nutritional changes and restrictions via modulation of their metabolism [52]. This crosstalk can alter the growth and therapeutic resistance of the tumor cells, such as by induction of the Warburg phenotype of cancer cells [52]. Typically, oxygen nutrients, pH, and drugs are mostly concentrated at the outer zones, while their concentration decreases as they diffuse inside the tumor mass, where waste and CO_2 are highly concentrated [53]. This leads to TME acidification and subsequently metabolic reprogramming, tumor malignancy, and immunosuppression, resulting in cancer progression [52].

Together with the CAFs, MSCs, immune infiltrate, epithelium, environmental pressures, vascular and nervous networks, and ECM and proteases, the dynamical balance can be tipped toward a tumor-promoting or tumor-suppressing TME [1]. The TME should be considered a multispecies ecosystem in which the cytokines, chemokines, growth factors, and proteases are intricately secreted to provide a positive feedback loop to the growing tumor [54]. For example, PDGF, TGFB, and IL1B, to name a few, are affecting the ECM, CAFs, endothelial cells, pericytes, and immune cells surrounding the tumor [54]. In turn, proliferation is induced by providing an environment rich in growth factors, interventions are resisted, and tumors can remain dormant over long periods [54]. This coincides with the view that carcinogenesis is both an ecological and evolutionary process whereby the accumulation of advantageous mutations selects for a permissive TME for the tumor cells to grow [50]. The genetic and epigenetic alterations of the surrounding cells can act on cell intrinsic and extrinsic factors of the tumor. The tumor cells are dependent on the aid of these cells and therefore can create an ecosystem where they can thrive [57] as the epigenetic dysregulation of these cells reshapes the TME from an antitumor environment to an immunosuppressive environment [55]. The plasticity is exhibited through cell polarization, driven by distinct transcriptional programs enabling cells with the functions that are essential during tissue regeneration or for tumor development [56]. This leads to a microenvironment induced by CAFs, TAMs, growth factors, cytokines, etc. that can manipulate the growing tumor via inflammation, senescence, or injury [51]. The TME is accompanied by a dynamic inflammatory process that supplies these molecules and factors that stimulate tumor growth and progression. This is evident in persistent infections causing chronic inflammation, which leads to recruitment of the immune cells secreting pro-inflammatory factors in the tissue microenvironment that causes DNA damage in the proliferating cells. These can permanently alter the genetic makeup of the proliferating cells by ways of point mutations, deletion, or rearrangements, triggering tumor promotion. Inflammation drives tumor initiation, growth, progression, and metastasis as the entirely altered immune environment plays a significant role in cancer progression [56]. Immunoediting is the dynamic process by which immune cells modulate tumor progression, creating a selective pressure leading to immune-resistant tumor cells [57]. This, in turn, leads to the inhibition of eradication of the tumor [57]. Editing the TME, therefore, provides great potential for sensitizing cancer immunotherapy to augment the antitumor response [55].

This extensive crosstalk is also pertinent to the metastatic dissemination of the primary tumor. The supportive stroma of the primary tumor fuels the progression to an invasive carcinoma. Ultimately, this results in the capability for activation of invasion and metastasis of the cancer cells. Metastasis, responsible for 90% of cancer-related deaths, requires angiogenesis and the escape of epithelial cancer cells from the primary tumor site. Following metastatic dissemination, when micrometastases reach a permissive niche, stromal cells are recruited to the seeded metastasis. Then, macrometastases signal metastatic growth, and establish a supportive stroma. The local invasion, the first step of metastatic dissemination, can be achieved through the process of epithelial-mesenchymal transition (EMT). A number of genetic and epigenetic changes that occur inside a cancer cell make it conducive to EMT induction by heterotypic tumor microenvironment signals [59–62]. During tumorigenesis, tumor stromal mediators may amplify a number of oncogenic pathways, which promote EMT. This is associated with a malignant transformation increasing the motility and invasiveness of the tumor cells. Mesenchymal cells also possess a lot of ECM proteins that are more resistant to apoptosis and senescence, making them more aggressive and difficult to control, in comparison to epithelial cells. Collectively, the transcription factors and cytoskeletal proteins function to transition cells from a less aggressive polarized phenotype to a more motile one. These inter- and intracellular changes take place based on the extracellular signals the cell receives, and hence, EMT is not a direct lineage switch but rather encompasses a spectrum of changes that are not always seen all together. The completion of EMT is denoted by the degradation of the basement membrane, which creates the passage for the mesenchymal cells to migrate away from the primary site.

These invasive-metastatic tumor cells have the capability to break loose, enter the bloodstream or lymphatics, and form tumors at distant secondary systemic sites where they go through the reverse, mesenchymal-epithelial transition (MET). It is this property to metastasize that majorly influences the prognosis of the disease, and the TME components play this vital role in the establishment of a favorable environment that allows for tumor growth and survival [58]. Metastasis promotes drug resistance and therefore, disease recurrence [51].

The transition of cells from one state to another during such processes as EMT, cell migration, MET, and metastasis is strongly influenced and regulated by inflammation, cytokines, and growth factors [56]. The cells of the TME are involved in reciprocal activation, inhibition, and differentiation that influence plasticity and consequently tipping the scale to promotion of tumor development [56]. It is evident the TME can be critical to several of the established hallmarks of cancer [53].

4 Specificity of the Thyroid Tumor Microenvironment

4.1 Immune Landscape in Anaplastic Thyroid Cancer

The genetic lesion BRAFV600E and transcription factor STAT3, which is frequently linked to aberrant oncogenic signaling, have been shown to drive expression of IL-6, IL-10, and VEGF, cytokines that encourage a tolerogenic monocyte-derived DC phenotype in vitro [63], a phenomenon that could potentially modulate their antigen presentation efficiency and dampen antitumor T cell response in vivo. This process is facilitated by BRAFV600E-mediated upregulation of WNT/β-catenin which induces ATF3, a transcriptional suppressor of the chemokine CCL4. A diminished amount of this cytokine is associated with polarization of dendritic cells (DCs) toward a tolerogenic phenotype which is incapable of optimal antigen presentation. Also, two reports have suggested immunosuppressive cytokine secretion by tumor cells harboring the KRASG12D mutation. These studies have shown that cells with these mutations secrete granulocyte-macrophage colony-stimulating factor (GM-CSF), which in turn recruits myeloid-derived suppressor cells (MDSCs) and leads to poor prognosis in mouse models of pancreatic adenocarcinoma [64]. In this study, this mutation was associated with recruitment of Gr1+CD11b+ double-positive cells which represent a heterogeneous population composed of MDSCs, monocytes, and immature myeloid cells in mice. At the molecular level, KRAS induces expression and secretion of the suppressive cytokines IL10 and TGFβ-1 by cancer cells in a MEK/ERK/AP-1 dependent way which promote Treg induction [65]. A recent study by Julianna et al. has shown that tumor-specific loss of P53 can reorchestrate the immune microenvironment toward an immune suppressive type where CD8+T cell activity is diminished [66]. Interestingly, these are some of the high-ranking somatic mutations identified in ATCs by multiple studies. Activation of oncogenic pathways drives production of cytokines triggering recruitment of innate immune cells, namely, macrophages. These macrophages in turn contribute to cancer progression by producing pro-inflammatory mediators such as IL-6, tumor necrosis factor (TNF), and interferon-γ (IFNγ) and growth factors including epidermal growth factor (EGF) and WNTs which create a highly mutagenic microenvironment. These cytokines upregulate transcription factors promoting tumorigenesis. This complex cytokine milieu controls the immune surveillance in TC via recruitment of immune cells conducive to tumor progression. Conception of this pro-tumorigenic niche precludes the tumor cells from immune surveillance via recruitment of tolerogenic immune cells that secrete primarily immune suppressive cytokines dampening T cell response leading to immune escape.

4.2 Immune Surveillance in Thyroid Cancer

During the process of tumorigenesis, from the early stages of transformation to the emergence of clinically detectable full-blown neoplasia, the tumor cells are aided by avoidance or subversion of detection by the immune system, known as immune surveillance. Cells of both innate and adaptive immune systems are engaged in the process of immune surveillance in thyroid cancer. Tumor-associated macrophages (TAMs) are one of the most crucial cell types possessing divergent roles in tumor progression, which has been reported in thyroid carcinogenesis [67]. In PTCs, TAMs correlated with lymph node metastasis, larger tumor size, and poor survival [68–70]. In PDTC, TAM density correlated with capsular invasion, extrathyroidal extension, and poor survival [70]. TAMs represent more than 50% of immune cells in ATCs, forming a "microglia-like" interconnected cellular supportive network in close contact with cancer cells [71]. These TAMs secrete inflammatory cytokines such as IL-23 and IL-17 that trigger tumor-elicited inflammation that in turn promote tumor growth. TAMs also provide essential support required for tumor metastasis.

DCs are responsible for sampling tumor antigens and presenting them to T cells in the draining lymph nodes. Unfortunately, tumor-associated DCs are usually immature with impaired antigen presentation skill. Presence of CD1a+ DCs is reported in PTC, which supports the hypothesis of immature DC and inadequate antigen presentation in TC [72].

As discussed in the previous section, MDSCs are attracted to tumor site by multiple factors and impart a strong local as well as global immune suppressive environment. An increase in peripheral blood MDSC level was observed in ATC patients compared to healthy controls which correlated with the serum IL-10 level, pointing toward a correlation between MDSCs and systemic immunosuppression [73]. Other immune cells involved in immune surveillance, like natural killer (NK) cells, are also sparse in ATC compared to DTC and FTC.

Optimally primed CD8+ T cells execute antitumor activity via perforin- and granzyme-mediated lysis of tumor cells. Hence, tumor-infiltrating T lymphocytes (TILs) are instrumental for mounting a potent antitumor immune response. In a study conducted with a wide cohort of DTC patients, including PTC and FTC, immunohistochemical analysis revealed that the combined enrichment of CD8+ cells and Cox-2 overexpression correlated with the highest risk of disease relapse. In most of the tumor samples analyzed (68%), CD8+ cells were granzyme B negative, suggesting an anergic state [74]. TILs are often associated with better prognosis as observed in melanoma [75], ovarian cancer [76], lung cancer [77], bladder cancer [78], and colorectal cancer [79]. Interestingly, a low intratumoral CD8+/Foxp3+ ratio was reported in human BRAFV600E PTC, which was also associated with an increased expression of the immunosuppressive molecules arginase-1, indoleamine 2,3-dioxygenase 1 (IDO1), and programmed death-ligand 1 (PD-L1) [80]. A recent study reported data on the PD-L1 expression in 407 primary TCs with a median 13.7 years of follow-up, studying the associations between PD-L1 expression and clinicopathologic features, such as TERT promoter, disease progression, and BRAF status. Tumoral PD-L1 expression was observed in 6.1% of PTCs, 7.6% of follicular thyroid cancer (FTCs), and 22.2% of ATCs. Another study noted that the proportions of PD-L1-positive follicular cells in ATCs were more than 80% [81]. These observations confirm the lack of effective immune surveillance in ATC that might promote immune escape and progression of the cancer via upregulation of the checkpoint molecule PD-L1. This molecule interacts with PD-1 on T cells and is responsible for induction of T cell exhaustion. Immune checkpoint molecules physiologically prevent excessive immune responses and the development of autoimmunity [82]. These molecules are largely responsible for immune evasion observed in aggressive immunogenic cancer.

4.3 Evolution of the Metastatic Phenotype

Anaplastic thyroid cancer and advanced differentiated thyroid cancers are aggressive and metastatic in nature. At the time of diagnosis, most of the patients with anaplastic thyroid cancer present with either lymph node metastasis or distant metastasis. Such metastasis of tumor cells requires the escape of epithelial cancer cells from the primary tumor site, which relates to the plasticity of the cellular phenotypes in thyroid cancer. The local invasion, the first step of metastatic dissemination, exploits this plasticity when the thyroid cancer cells gain a mesenchymal phenotype. This can be achieved through a process called epithelial-mesenchymal transition (EMT). EMT is a complex biological process by which polarized epithelial cells, with their basal surface interacting with the basement membrane, acquire mesenchymal cell-like properties resulting in various cellular phenotypic changes – such as increased migratory and invasive properties – necessary for cell metastasis.

Epithelial cells have an apicobasal polarity and are closely adjoined to each other forming layers. Distributed throughout the epithelial cells are membrane structures such as tight junctions, desmosomes, adherens, and gap junctions and adhesion molecules, including cadherins and integrins, that provide stationary stability. The actin cytoskeleton offers polarity to the epithelial cells, and the basal lamina forms the basal surface that interacts with the basement membrane. The cell surface adhesion proteins are present on the lateral cell-cell junctions which prevent detachment. Alternatively, this polarization, cell-cell adhesion, and basement membrane attachment are absent in the mesenchymal cells, making them more motile with the ability to penetrate the ECM compartment. Mesenchymal cells possess a lot of ECM proteins, such as fibronectin and vimentin, and are more resistant to apoptosis and senescence. This makes them more aggressive and difficult to control, in comparison to epithelial cells. During the process of EMT, epithelial cells undergo complex changes in cellular architecture as well as behavior. A loss of epithelial characteristics like apicobasal polarity and cell-cell contact surface proteins leads to cytoskeleton remodeling. At the same time, the cells gain this mesenchymal phenotype, manifesting greater migratory and invasive properties. These inter- and intracellular changes take place based on the extracellular signals the cell receives [59–62]. Hence, EMT is not a direct lineage switch but rather encompasses a spectrum of changes that are not always seen all together.

One of the most prominent hallmarks of EMT is the loss of E-cadherin protein. E-cadherin is a calcium-dependent transmembrane glycoprotein important for cell-cell adhesion. E-cadherin is also considered a tumor suppressor since its transcriptional loss was noticed in several carcinomas and re-expression of the protein in some cancers transformed them to their less aggressive forms. Adherens junction proteins such as zona occludens-1 (ZO-1), occludin, and claudin are also essential in maintaining the epithelial integrity required for cell-cell adhesion. Initiation of EMT leads to destabilization of these junction proteins. E-cadherin is cleaved from the membrane surface and ultimately degraded. β-catenin, no longer in association with E-cadherin, localizes to the nucleus and acts as a transcription factor [83, 84]. Downregulation of genes encoding the other adherens junction and tight junction proteins along with loss of desmosomes during

EMT results in detachment of the cells from the basement membrane. They are now free to invade the ECM and migrate to distant sites. E-cadherin and β-catenin disruption during EMT causes reorganization of actin filaments to form membrane projections that facilitate cell mobility. Another hallmark associated with EMT is cadherin switch, whereby the decrease in E-cadherin is counter-adjusted by an increase in N-cadherin (mesenchymal neural cadherin) expression. Simultaneous to the loss of epithelial factors is the gain of mesenchymal characteristics such as scattering and elongation of cells, as well as the acquisition of mesenchymal markers like vimentin, FSP-1, fibronectin, and smooth muscle actin. A number of transcription factors regulate each other and also regulate E-cadherin. Snail, Slug, Twist, NFκB, SIP1, FOXC2, E47/E2A, and ZEB (zinc-finger E-box-binding protein) are some of the transcription factors that regulate the expression of epithelial and/or mesenchymal genes on initiation of EMT [59, 83–85]. Snail is a DNA binding factor that recognizes and binds to the E-box motif of the E-cadherin promoter. Slug, a closely related gene to Snail, also targets the same E-box motif. Similarly, Zeb and Twist transcription factors, when overexpressed, repress E-cadherin. Hence, these transcription factors negatively regulate E-cadherin-mediated cell-cell adhesion, promoting cellular migration and invasion [86–90]. However, downregulation or suppression of E-cadherin and other adhesion proteins is not solely sufficient for EMT to occur. A proper balance between the loss of epithelial factors and procurement of mesenchymal features is necessary for the initiation and maintenance of EMT state in a cell [59, 91]. Thus, EMT is initiated by various essential transcription factors such as Snail, Slug, Twist, and cell surface proteins like cadherins and catenin; rearrangement of the cellular cytoskeleton proteins such as vimentin and cadherin; as well as ECM degrading enzymes, all of which are all involved in increasing cell migration and invasiveness. The completion of EMT is denoted by the degradation of the basement membrane, which creates the passage for the mesenchymal cells to migrate away from the primary site. Collectively, the transcription factors and cytoskeletal proteins function to transition cells from a less aggressive polarized phenotype to a more motile one. These factors also act as a biomarker to represent the occurrence of EMT in cells. However, there might be concomitant expression of epithelial and mesenchymal markers in the cell undergoing EMT. The lineage switch between epithelial and mesenchymal phenotype may not be sudden or immediate but is rather a continuous process where intermediary cells expressing both phenotypes in differing ratios may be present, indicating that transition is taking place [92, 93]. In summation, the cellular changes associated with EMT are loss of cytokeratin expression, E-cadherin protein, and epithelial cell polarity, with acquisition of a fibroblast – like shape, motility, invasiveness, mesenchymal gene expression, N-cadherin, protease secretion, vimentin expression, fibronectin, PDGF receptor, and αVβ6 integrin expression. This coincides with the progression from cell-cell adhesion with low motility, or static, characteristics of the epithelial cells to the highly motile mesenchymal cells with high matrix production and cell-matrix interactions. These malignant transformations disrupt and weaken cell-cell adhesion and instead promote cell membrane movement via cell-ECM adhesion molecules such as integrins, laminin receptors, and CD44, and motility via RhoGTPase regulation.

The signal transduction pathway for EMT goes hand in hand with its regulation. All the oncogenic signaling and regulation pathways converge at repression of E-cadherin. A number of growth factors such as EGF, FGF, HGF, and IGF2 can induce EMT by binding to their respective RTKs (receptor tyrosine kinases). The downstream signaling is mediated by numerous different effectors. The SRC family of effector molecules rearranges the cellular architecture by phosphorylating cytoskeletal and focal adhesion proteins. WNT/β-catenin signaling, commonly activated in cancer, leads to translocation of β-catenin to the nucleus, activates Snail-Slug, and represses the transcription of E-cadherin. Some other pathways such as Notch signaling and integrin linked kinase signaling downregulate the epithelial genes and induce EMT [83, 90, 94]. Oxidative damage, Oxidative damage which leads to production of reactive oxygen species also induces transcription of Snail and EMT [95]. RAS is a very important downstream effector of receptor tyrosine kinases. Signaling from RAS involves the PI3K-AKT as well as the RAF-MEK-ERK pathway to activate NFκB, Snail, and Slug, and consequently induces EMT [96]. TGFβ, a potent inducer of EMT, mediates the process through the PI3K-AKT pathway. Bakin et al. used a murine mammalian cell line to demonstrate the molecular and cellular changes under the effect of TGFβ [97]. PI3K-AKT pathway activation leads to regression of E-cadherin, ZO-1, and other tight junction cell-adhesion proteins as well as morphological changes, whereby cuboidal cells gain spindle-like elongated morphology [94]. Tumor necrosis factor alpha (TNFα) is a very important mediator of cancer-related inflammation and is also an inducer of EMT by contributing to cellular transformation. It has angiogenic and tumor-promoting effects. It is produced abundantly by the tumor stromal cells such as fibroblasts, macrophages, astrocytes, and tumor cells as well. Multiple studies on TNFα suggest that this cytokine activates the AKT signaling pathway leading to NFκB stimulation. This in turn upregulates and stabilizes Snail, ultimately inducing EMT, further encouraging the migration and invasion of tumor cells [90, 98, 99]. Thus, in a cell going through EMT, a number of signaling pathways cross their path with the transcription factors under the influence of inter- and intracellular mediators. This offers more complexity in an already intricate cellular transition process.

Development of metastasis is a multistep process, and EMT is the starting step. The cells that undergo the process of EMT are usually located at the invasive front of the tumor and eventually undergo invasion and metastasis. Regarding the stages that occur for this process, the primary tumor undergoes localized invasion. Invasion involves translocation across ECM barriers and cell migration via lysis of matrix proteins with proteases. Matrix metalloproteinases (MMPs) are calcium-dependent proteases controlled by an increase in transcriptional expression. This localized invasion is followed by intravasation and release into circulation. Hence, angiogenesis is required for metastasis. Following circulation survival and transport, tumor cells arrest in microvessels of capillary beds at various distant organs. Here, extravasation can occur where they penetrate and colonize the secondary site. A micrometastasis is formed and colonization occurs, forming a macrometastasis. An interesting aspect about EMT is its reversibility, as cells frequently undergo a reverse process called mesenchymal-epithelial transition (MET). So, these invasive-metastatic tumor cells have the capability to break loose, enter the bloodstream or lymphatics, and form tumors at distant secondary systemic sites where it goes through the reverse MET. Hence, the secondary tumors histologically resemble the primary tumor they arose from. It is this property to metastasize that majorly influences the prognosis of the disease. This is important to consider when it comes to the theories of organ selectivity. The two major theories are mechanistic via blood flow/lymphatics and "seed and soil" via metastatic tropisms. This argues that there is a need for appropriate growth factors or an ECM environment with compatible adhesion sites and selective chemotaxis attracting tumor cells. This is why different carcinomas metastasize to different secondary locations. Furthermore, different carcinomas have varied tendencies toward malignancy. However, ATC is known to be very malignant and rapidly gives rise to secondary metastasis making it a difficult target for treatment. Hence, it becomes necessary to explore all possible avenues that can direct us to the mechanisms involved in rendering high degree of malignancy and poor prognosis to some cancers.

During tumorigenesis, tumor stromal mediators such as HGF, EGF, PDGF, TGFβ, and TNFα may amplify a number of oncogenic pathways, which promote EMT. This is associated with a malignant transformation increasing the motility and invasiveness of the tumor cells. In tumor cells, the aberrant signaling causes the Ras pathways to be constitutively active. A number of epithelial cancers have shown activated AKT signaling, which affects the epithelial morphology by downregulating the cell adhesion proteins and inducing EMT [100]. An in vitro study done by Baquero et al. indicated that the BRAFV600E mutation mediates an upregulation of transcriptional repressor Snail by activation of the MEK-ERK pathway, thus inducing EMT in aggressive thyroid cancer [101]. TGFβ has dual roles in tumorigenesis. On one hand, it induces senescence and apoptosis, and on the other hand, it suppresses epithelial cell proliferation and induces EMT-mediated metastasis of tumor cells.

The exploration of EMT for thyroid cancer advancement started about a decade ago. Very few studies have been done correlating EMT with differentiated thyroid cancer and even fewer in ATC. Hardy and colleagues [102] found the presence of the transcription factors Snail and Slug in a significant percent of tumors from well-differentiated thyroid carcinoma patients. Moreover, increased expression of vimentin in PTC was associated with enhanced invasion and lymph node metastasis [103]. A study by the Wiseman team demonstrated higher downregulation of E-cadherin and beta-catenin expression in anaplastic thyroid carcinomas compared to differentiated carcinomas [104]. To fortify this result, an in vitro study was performed in anaplastic thyroid cancer cell lines and showed upregulation in Twist, a repressor of E-cadherin [105]. Another in vitro study demonstrated the role of N-cadherin in the promotion of growth and invasiveness of PTC via activation of MAPK/ERK, PI3K/AKT, and p16/Rb signaling pathways [106]. It is believed that triggering EMT in thyroid tumor cells depends on an assortment of external signals [107, 108]. These signals are present in the tumor microenvironment in the form of various secretory mediators such as cytokines, chemokines, or secretory molecules – exosomes. The inflammatory microenvironment plays an important role in thyroid cancer occurrence and advancement. Patients with preexisting chronic inflammatory conditions tend to get advanced thyroid cancer denoting some link between inflammatory microenvironment and increased migratory capacity of the thyroid cancer cells. Hence, there is increasing interest to decipher the patterns of secretory factors (the secretome) of inflammatory cells in the thyroid tumor microenvironment [109, 110]. In order to understand the initiation and progression of thyroid cancer, it is important to assess the role of major secretory players which induce EMT. Moreover, the regulators of EMT do not just initiate the tumor progression, but rather influence the increase in cell survival and resistance to apoptosis/senescence making the current therapies inadequate to treat aggressive invasive thyroid cancer. Hence, innovative therapy strategies are needed to be explored that will target EMT regulators to curb the advanced thyroid cancer, especially anaplastic thyroid cancer.

4.4 Interacting Molecules

4.4.1 ATC Has a Complex Cytokine Milieu

The association between an inflammatory microenvironment and DTC has been implicated in multiple studies [111, 112]. The immune microenvironment in TC is extremely complex in nature with a combination of pro- and anti-inflammatory cytokines and immune cell infiltrates [113]. Our study revealed an immunosuppressive microenvironment in ATC with high expression of IL10 and IDO1. IL10 is an extremely potent immunosuppressive cytokine secreted by TAMs and tumor cells themselves in both PTC and ATC [114]. This cytokine has pleiotropic effects in both immunoregulation and inflammation. It dampens the expression of Th1 cytokines, MHC class II antigen presentation, and co-stimulatory molecules on macrophages. IDO1 is an enzyme that catalyzes the first and rate-limiting step in tryptophan catabolism to N-formylkynurenine. Expression of this enzyme in DCs, monocytes, and macrophages regulates T cell activity by controlling pericellular catabolism of tryptophan and limiting its availability to T cells. This is a prominent immunosuppressive cytokine responsible for dampening antitumor T cell response. High expression of IDO1 in our clinical samples corroborates with previous reports of upregulated IDO1 during thyroid carcinogenesis [115]. In this study, the authors observed five- to tenfold higher expression of IDO1 and more Treg polarization in ATC compared to PTC. The study also confirmed that expression of IDO1 in the tumor cells was IFNγ inducible. This depicts another possible mechanism of induction of immune tolerance in ATC.

4.4.2 Immune Targets on the Tumor and Its Tripartite Cell-Cell Communication

The complex immune contexture of ATC tumor microenvironment involves dynamic interaction between the tumor cells and the components of the adaptive immune system, such as various subsets of T cells and antigen-presenting cells. This interaction is facilitated by several cell surface receptors and their cognate ligands expressed on the T cells, antigen-presenting cells, and the tumor cells. These molecules are under stringent spatial and temporal regulation and help in the formation of immunological synapse between these different cellular subtypes. In the next section, we would focus on these unique molecules, which are responsible for shaping the local and systemic antitumor immune response.

4.4.3 T Cell Co-signaling Molecules

T cell activation, differentiation, and effector function are intricate processes, controlled by molecular interactions and biochemical signaling pathways triggered by interaction between co-stimulatory receptors and their cognate ligands (Fig. 1). These molecules belong to two major families, the TNF receptor superfamily (TNFRSF) and immunoglobulin superfamily (IgSF). CTLA4 and PD-1 belong to IgSF. These receptors and ligands usually interact within families, as evidenced by interaction of CTLA4 and CD28 or CD80/86 or PD-1 with PD-L1. However, co-signaling molecule from TNFRSF, herpesvirus entry mediator (HVEM) interacts with members of both families, and each interaction uniquely shapes T cell activation status.

Currently, it is evident that the expression of many co-stimulatory and co-inhibitory molecules on the T cell surface is induced following activation and their expression pattern changes in an overlapping manner as T cells continue to proliferate and differentiate. This underscores the importance of understanding their regulation and unique signal transduction mechanisms.

4.4.4 Immune Checkpoint Molecules in Cancer

Immune checkpoint molecules physiologically prevent excessive immune responses and the development of autoimmunity. Optimal T cell responses require three signals, which are transduced via formation of a functional immune synapse between naïve T cells and an antigen-presenting cell through surface receptors and ligands (Fig. 1). The first activation signal comes through ligation of MHCI/II and T cell receptor (TCR). APCs process foreign antigens into small peptides which are presented to the T cell in an MHC-bound form. This interaction is followed by ligation of co-stimulatory molecule CD28 on T cells and their cognate ligands CD80/86 on APCs. This interaction provides the second signal for optimal stimulation of the T cells. Only signal 1 in the absence of signal 2 leads to T cell anergy, when T cells lose their functionality for a prolonged period and cannot be restimulated. These two signals are also not enough for optimal T cell activity. The third signal comes via the cytokines secreted by APCs that help in T cell differentiation and proliferation. IL-6, IL-12, and TGF-β are some of the cytokines produced by APCs that help in T cell differentiation. This is the third signal for optimal T cell activation. Interestingly, in order to put a brake on T cell activity, there are certain activation induced checkpoint molecules in place controlling T cell activity. Unfortunately, prolonged expression of these immune checkpoint molecules is often observed on the T cells, especially in the case of cancer. This leads to a generalized dampening of antitumor T cell response and promotes immune escape. Cytotoxic T lymphocyte antigen 4 (CTLA4) was the first such molecule that was characterized for its immune checkpoint activity in cancer. CTLA4 is an activation induced immune checkpoint molecule that competes with CD28 for binding to CD80/86 [116]. Unfortunately, CTLA4 binds

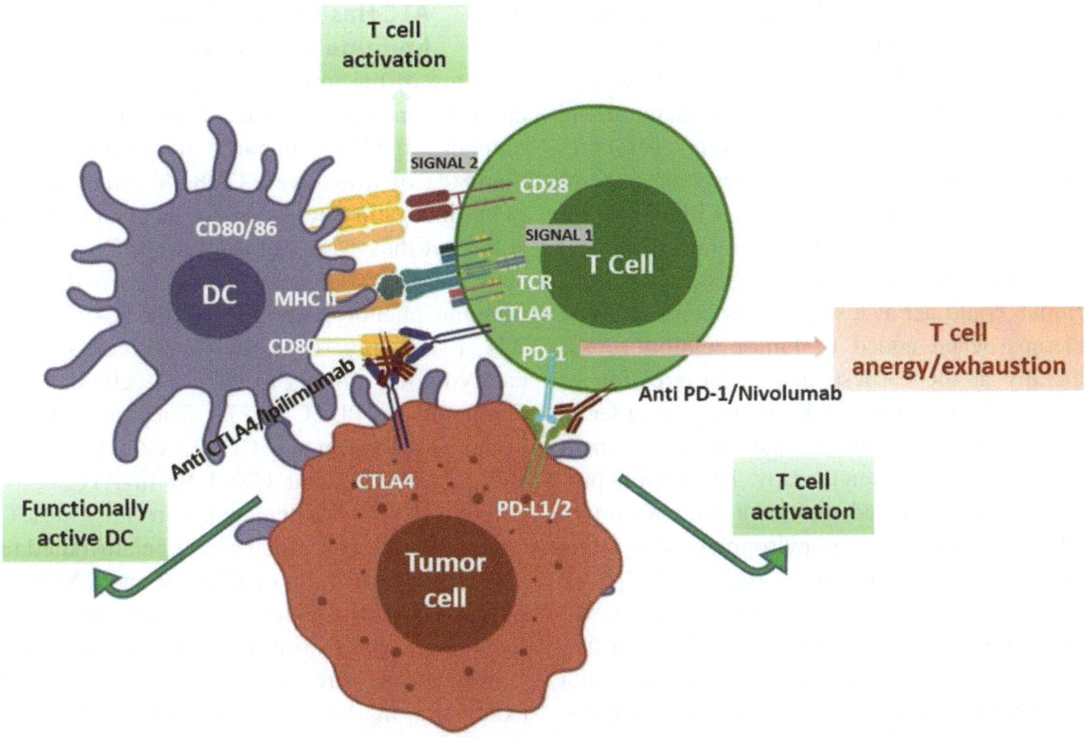

Fig. 1 Immune synapse between T cells, APC, and tumor cells

CD80/86 with much higher avidity than CD28. This leads to absence of signal 2 during T cell activation eventually leading to T cell anergy. Interestingly, ligation of CTLA4 on CD4+ T cells with DCs has been shown to trigger induction of IDO1 in DCs which in turn dampens CD8+ T cell responses [117]. Subsequently, another immune checkpoint molecule PD-1 was discovered on T cells which interacted with PD-L1 on APCs. PD-1/PD-L1 interaction was initially implicated in case of viral infection-mediated chronic exhaustion of T cells [118]. Subsequent investigations revealed that the distribution and functionality of these two molecules extend far beyond viral infection and autoimmune conditions. Targeting these molecules in cancer has revolutionized the field of tumor immunotherapy. The therapeutic antibody ipilimumab, targeting CTLA-4, was the first checkpoint inhibitor to be approved by US FDA in 2011 for clinical use in metastatic melanoma [119, 120]. It is undergoing clinical trials for the treatment of non-small cell lung carcinoma (NSCLC), small cell lung cancer (SCLC), bladder cancer, and metastatic hormone-refractory prostate cancer. Unfortunately, patients on ipilimumab therapy soon developed severe immune-related adverse effects (IrAE) including but not limited to diarrhea, colitis, enterocolitis, large and small intestinal perforations, rash, hypothyroidism, and hypopituitarism. Most of the IrAEs were dermatological, followed by gastrointestinal and then endocrine [121]. This promptly called for the development of a second immune checkpoint inhibitor targeting PD-1/PD-L1 interaction. The rationale behind this was that these two molecules activate two unique downstream pathways in order to execute their effect which suggested a possible difference in their toxicity profile also. Two drugs, pembrolizumab and nivolumab targeting PD-1, were approved by US FDA for unresectable melanoma in December 2014. So far, nivolumab has been approved for NSCLC, renal cell carcinoma, Hodgkin's lymphoma, head and neck cancer, urothelial carcinoma, and small cell lung cancer

[122]. This drug has not been approved for metastatic advanced thyroid cancers, like PDTC and ATC. This could be due to the failure of successful clinical trials with these patients due to rapid progression and mortality. However, several preclinical studies noted moderate response to pembrolizumab in combination with a BRAFV600E inhibitor in animal models of immune competent ATC [123]. A recent report suggested pembrolizumab could act as a safe and effective salvage therapy when added to kinase inhibitor (KI) therapy at the earliest sign of progression or sooner in the course of KI therapy in order to attain maximum clinical and survival benefit from this combination therapy. The authors proposed that prolonged treatment with KI might alter the immune microenvironment into a less permissive type during progression [124]. Currently, pembrolizumab is undergoing phase 2 clinical trials for ATC patients (NCT02688608). Nivolumab-associated toxicities are also not uncommon, and they also include dermatologic toxicity, gastrointestinal toxicity, and endocrine toxicity. Unfortunately, late onset of neurological toxicities is also being reported with nivolumab treatment [125, 126]. IrAEs take at least weeks to months to appear and usually present as a rash initially, but they often persist even after discontinuation of treatment. This points toward a systemic reprogramming of the immune system during these checkpoint inhibitions that is not reversed after treatment termination and might have a debilitating consequence.

CTLA4 and PD-1 are not the only molecules involved in regulation of T cell activity. There are a plethora of such immunomodulatory molecules which act in their unique way to modulate T cell responses. Most of these molecules are under strict spatiotemporal regulation which suggests that they could be tapped in a combinatorial treatment regimen, depending on the patient's response. This warrants a thorough characterization of these molecules in the context of T cell activation and inhibition and identification of novel targets which might be able to circumvent the problem of IrAE experienced with ipilimumab and nivolumab.

4.4.5 ATC Has T Cell-Inflamed Immune Microenvironment

Profiling of the immune infiltrate in our clinical ATC samples revealed a significantly higher number of TILs compared to normal, more than 80% of which were CD8+ T cells. Studies in our laboratory noted the presence of CD4+ T cells, but they were not intratumoral. A recent study suggests the existence of two distinct immune phenotypes in TC – PDTC-like and ATC-like. In this study, they observed a significantly higher number of CD8+ T cells in ATC, compared to PDTC [127]. They also noted higher expression of CCL2, CCL3, CCL4, CCL5, CXCL9, and CXCL10 in ATC compared to PDTC. We detected more TILs in ATC compared to PTC, which might be attributed to preferential secretion of CXCL9 and CXCL10 by the ATC cells, which act as chemoattractant for T cells. Interestingly, their study detected simultaneous upregulation of several T cell exhaustion markers such as TIM3, LAG3, and TIGIT and co-stimulatory molecules, like GITR, 4-1BB, and OX40 at a high extent ATC, and to a lesser extent in PTC, but not at all in PDTC. Our observation corroborated this study, and we believe the immune microenvironment of ATC should be categorized as T cell-inflamed or "hot" as opposed to the traditional belief of being "cold" (Fig. 2). This observation opens the immense possibility of immune checkpoint blockade therapy for these patients. One of our primary objectives was to explore this new avenue to find a novel therapeutic approach.

4.4.6 Immune Modulatory Molecules in ATC: An Unexplored Realm

The last decade of immune checkpoint inhibitor therapy has revolutionized the field of tumor immunotherapy. Ipilimumab, an anti-CTLA-4 antibody, was the first immune checkpoint inhibitor (ICI) to be FDA-approved in 2011 for metastatic melanoma. Subsequently, five other immune checkpoint-targeted therapies have been approved, all directed against PD-1 or PD-L1, for the treatment of melanoma, non-small cell lung

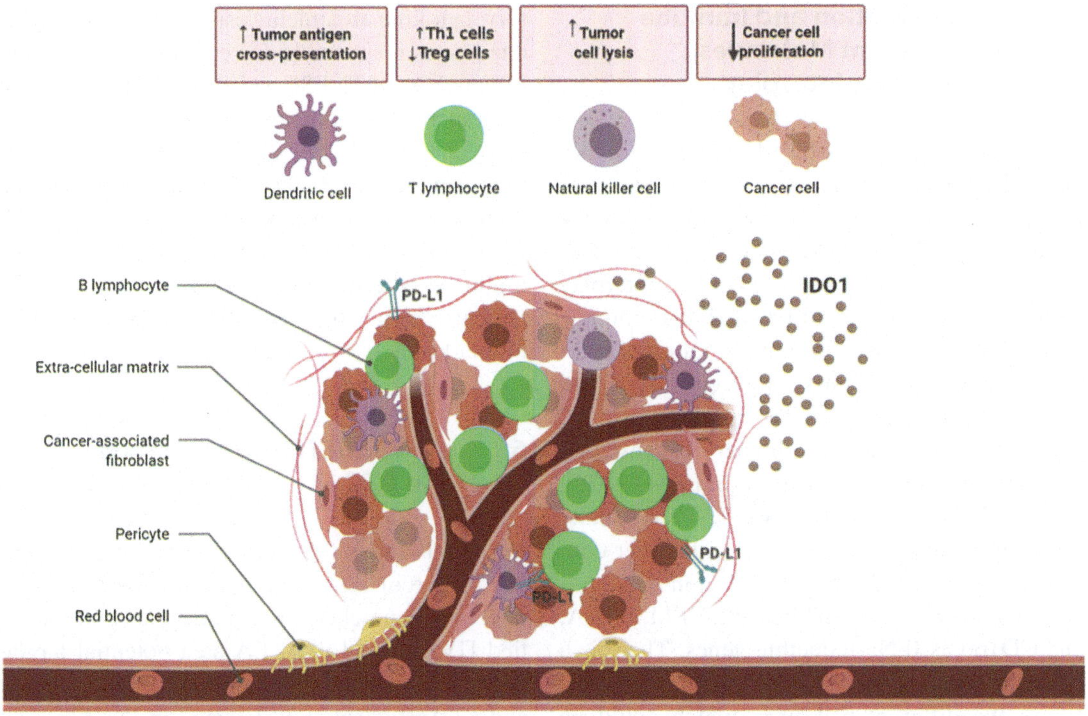

Fig. 2 Characteristic features of immunologically hot tumor microenvironment (made with BioRender)

cancer (NSCLC), renal cell carcinoma (RCC) and several other tumor types, in monotherapy and combinatorial regimen. Several clinical trials investigating PD-1/PD-L1 inhibitors as monotherapy or in combination in ATC are presently underway (NCT02688608, NCT03181100, NCT03211117, NCT03246958). One of the major hallmarks of immunotherapy is the durability of the responses that can be translated into survival benefit for the patient. ICI prolonged survival in patients; however, the response was not universal.

A substantial variation in responsiveness toward ICI is observed among patients with same malignancy and among different malignancies. The degree of responsiveness often correlates with tumor mutational burden (TMB), though it alone is not sufficient to predict clinical response. High TMB with additional elevated levels of tumor neoantigen expression plays a crucial role in antitumor immunity. However, there are several tumor-intrinsic and tumor-extrinsic factors that shape the final response. Extrinsic factors include quality of T cell infiltrates, composition of cytokines, and percentage of immune suppressor cells such as MDSCs. All these eventually shape the immune response in a highly individualized manner. High percentage of TAMs and immune suppressive cytokines are well-established features of the immune landscape in ATC. Some preliminary studies have shown promising results with PD-1 blockade, but they are not yet approved for ATC.

5 Consequences of Three-Way Communication

The outcome of this three-way communication described above is dependent on not only the strength and affinity of the receptor-ligand interaction but also the cytokine milieu as we will see in the following sections.

5.1 Inflammation and Immune Checkpoint Molecules: A Complex Interplay

Until recently, the crosstalk between cytokines and immune checkpoint proteins was underappreciated. Recent reports focusing on a complex regulation of PD-L1 by IL-6 and IL-8 reinvigorated the perception of a complex interplay between the cytokine milieu and the immune checkpoint molecules. The concentration of cytokines varies significantly between serum and tumor tissues. A study by Young et al. on CRC reported almost four times higher concentration of intratumoral IL-8 than its serum level [128]. Serum concentration of IL-8 and TNFα is usually higher in inflammatory cancers, and higher concentration of IL-8 has been reported in ATC.

Our study has also established HVEM, BTLA, and CD160 as IFNγ-inducible genes. There is a heterogeneous level of sensitivity observed across the different cell lines which could be attributed to the inherently heterogeneous nature of the tumor cells. This was an interesting observation, and it points toward the possibility of upregulation of these molecules in the presence of IFNγ secreted by activated T cells and other immune cells in the T cell-inflamed TME. Previous study in our lab has shown that the thyroid cancer cells secrete several pro-inflammatory cells that have pleotropic functions and can support tumor growth and upregulate proliferation. IL-8 and TNFα are two most prominent pro-inflammatory cytokines secreted by TC cells and the tumor-infiltrating M1 macrophages commonly observed in ATC. We observed a complex regulation of HVEM in ATC cell lines by IL-8 and TNFα. In our study, IL-8 and TNFα upregulated HVEM expression at transcript level which can be attributed to multiple binding sites for STAT3 and RELA/NFκB p65 in the promoter of HVEM. Interestingly, we observed solubilization of HVEM post-IL-8 and TNFα treatment. HVEM ELISA confirmed presence of soluble HVEM in the conditioned media from ATC cell lines. Interestingly, we observed increased expression of a metalloprotease ADAM17 in the ATC cell lines when subjected to the inflammatory cytokine treatment, especially TNFα. This enzyme is responsible for ectodomain shedding of members of TNFSF and TNFRSF [129]. There is an increasing appreciation of ADAM17 in carcinogenesis and is being implicated in different malignancies such as lung adenocarcinoma, breast cancer, colon cancer, and so on [130–133]. Our preliminary observation suggests that we might be able to detect soluble HVEM in ATC patients' sera which could potentially act as a biomarker.

6 HVEM/CD160/BTLA Axis in ATC

In our laboratory, we performed a thorough profiling of four ATC cell lines for expression of novel immune checkpoint molecules and identified HVEM/CD160/BTLA as a potential target. Constitutively high expression of HVEM, BTLA, and CD160 genes was detected in the ATC cell lines. HVEM acts as a bidirectional switch which can transduce either co-stimulatory or inhibitory signal into the T cells depending on the receptor/ligand it is interacting with. HVEM itself is a ligand for the TNF superfamily members LIGHT. Binding of T cell-expressed LIGHT to HVEM expressed by APCs results in enhanced T cell proliferation and cytokine production. On the contrary, when HVEM engages BTLA – a member of the immunoglobulin superfamily – or CD160 on T cells, it triggers inhibitory signals resulting in decreased T cell proliferation and cytokine production [134].

Tumor cell expression of HVEM has recently been reported in ovarian serous adenocarcinoma tissues. In this study, expression of HVEM was evaluated in 40 ovarian serous adenocarcinoma tissue samples by IHC. 72.5% of the cases were positive for expression of HVEM. Tumors at stage III and IV had significantly higher cytoplasmic expression of HVEM, and the expression also positively correlated with lymph node metastasis [135]. In our study, HVEM expression was identified in both the cytoplasm and plasma membrane of follicular cancer cells in ATC tissues, but there was no expression in normal thyroid follicular cells. High HVEM expression was also observed in the PTC tissues in our study which were aggressive variants with previous history of thyroiditis and with capsular invasion and extrathyroidal extensions. Takashi et al. looked at HVEM expression in 234 colorectal cancers (CRCs) by IHC. 49.6% of the cases had intermediate expression of HVEM and 19.2% of the cases had strong HVEM expression. They also found that HVEM positivity correlated with disease stage, and they concluded that HVEM could act as an independent prognostic factor for CRC [136]. The authors observed a graded expression pattern of HVEM, where normal colonic epithelium had a minimal expression followed by 24% adenomas positive for HVEM and more than 50% of CRC samples had high HVEM expression [136]. Expression of these proteins in the aggressive forms of TC indicates that HVEM/BTLA pathway might be actively involved in development and progression of aggressive variants of PTCs into ATC. This pathway is capable of successful induction of immune evasion in the tumor cells, which is one of the novel hallmarks of cancer.

6.1 Novel Targets of Therapeutic Intervention

The Cancer Research Institute (https://app.emergingmed.com/cri/trials/#partnerhome) Clinical Trials for adult cancer treatment of thyroid cancer indicated 15 ongoing clinical trials in Phase 1 and 2 utilizing immunotherapy, chemotherapy, monoclonal antibodies, and cell therapy. Some molecular targets include CD279, CTLA4, PD1, PDCD1, and BRAF, to name a few (Table 1).

7 HVLA/BTEM Axis as Potential Therapeutic Target

Overexpressed in ATC, common drug targets are serine-threonine kinases and tyrosine kinases such as BRAFV600E, VEGFR, EGFR, PDGFR, and RET. The presence of multiple genetic lesions in ATC including BRAFV600E, the third most common after TERT and P53, makes ATC patients suitable candidates for BRAFV600E-directed targeted therapy with small molecule inhibitors. BRAFV600E-positive PTCs display the constitutively activated RAF/ERK pathway which leads to repression of downstream pathways responsible for regulation of many thyroid-specific genes, leading to cellular dedifferentiation, tumor progression, and acquisition of more aggressive phenotypes eventually leading to ATC. The BRAFV600E mutation is closely associated with aggressive clinical and pathologic features of thyroid cancer such as aggressive and highly proliferative cancers, lymphatic metastases, extrathyroidal capsular invasion, advanced clinical stage, recurrence, and morbidity. Vemurafenib is a widely used anticancer drug that targets constitutively active BRAFV600E. Unfortunately, reports of acquired resistance are extremely common. As a ligand-independent activator of MAPK, BRAFV600E is thought to induce "oncogene addiction" in thyroid cancer and melanoma. In previous sections, we have discussed the small molecule inhibitors currently in use and in clinical trials for ATC. However, eventual development of resistance is inevitable. Resistance against small molecule inhibitors can manifest itself in three different forms: innate, acquired, and adaptive. Innate and acquired resistance are often associated with novel mutations and expansion of mutated clonal population in response to the drug, respectively. Adaptive resistance is very interesting in that they rewire the signaling mechanism to bypass the effect of the specific inhibitor. Adaptive resistance is often associated with reactivation of the same molecular pathway or activation of compensatory pathways which transform the tumor into a more resistant phenotype and alter its microenvironment at the same time. One such mechanism responsible for acquired resistance against BRAFV600E inhibitors in ATC is activation of the HGF/MET axis [137]. Interestingly, this study noted a higher expression of HGF with increased copy number of MET in murine model of ATC, suggesting the activation of an autocrine loop supporting tumor

Table 1 Ongoing clinical trials with immunotherapeutic agents in thyroid cancer

Title	Phase	Modalities	Interventions	Molecular Targets	Location
Pembrolizumab in Anaplastic/Undifferentiated Thyroid Cancer	2	Immunotherapy, Monoclonal Antibody	pembrolizumab	CD279, PD1, PDCD1	USA - TX - Dallas
Pembrolizumab in Treating Patients With Rare Tumors That Cannot Be Removed by Surgery or Are Metastatic	2	Immunotherapy, Monoclonal Antibody…	pembrolizumab	CD279, PD1, PDCD1	USA - TX - Houston
Study of Pembrolizumab (MK-3475) in Participants With Advanced Solid Tumors (MK-3475-158/KEYNOTE-158)	2	Immunotherapy, Monoclonal Antibody	pembrolizumab	CD279, PD1, PDCD1	View Locations
Nivolumab and Ipilimumab in Treating Patients With Rare Tumors	2	Immunotherapy, Monoclonal Antibody	ipilimumab, nivolumab	CD279, CTLA4, PD1, PDCD1	View Locations
Pembrolizumab With Chemotherapy for Poorly Chemo-responsive Thyroid and Salivary Gland Tumors	2	Chemotherapy, Immunotherapy,…	pembrolizumab, docetaxel	CD279, PD1, PDCD1, Tubulin	USA - IL - Chicago
Pembrolizumab in With Liver-Directed or Peptide Receptor Radionuclide Therapy in Neuroendocrine Tumors With…	2	Immunotherapy, Monoclonal Antibody…	pembrolizumab	CD279, PD1, PDCD1	USA - CA - San Francisco
Atezolizumab With Chemotherapy in Treating Patients With Anaplastic or Poorly Differentiated Thyroid Cancer	2	Chemotherapy, Immunotherapy,…	nab-paclitaxel, bevacizumab,…	B7H1, BRAF, CD274, MAP2K1, MEK1, ME…	USA - TX - Houston
Testing the Combination of Cabozantinib, Nivolumab, and Ipilimumab (CaboNivoIpi) for Advanced Differentiated…	2	Immunotherapy, Monoclonal Antibody…	cabozantinib, cabozantinib s-malat…	CD279, CTLA4, MET, PD1, PDCD1, VEGF,…	View Locations
PDR001 Combination Therapy for Radioiodine-Refractory Thyroid Cancer	2	Immunotherapy, Monoclonal Antibody…	trametinib, spartalizumab,…	BRAF, MAP2K1, MEK, MEK1, PD1	View Locations
Enapotamab Vedotin (HuMax-AXL-ADC) Safety Study in Patients With Solid Tumors	1/2	Immunotherapy	HuMax-AXL-ADC	AXL	View Locations
BMS-986156, Ipilimumab, and Nivolumab With or Without Stereotactic Body Radiation Therapy in Treating Patients…	1/2	Immunotherapy, Monoclonal Antibody…	BMS-986156, ipilimumab, nivolumab	CD279, CTLA4, GITR, PD1, PDCD1	USA - TX - Houston
Avelumab With Radiotherapy in Patients With Leptomeningeal Disease	1	Immunotherapy, Monoclonal Antibody…	avelumab	PD1	USA - FL - Tampa
First-in-Human Study of XMT-1536 in Cancers Likely to Express NaPi2b	1	Immunotherapy, Monoclonal Antibody	XMT-1536	NaPi2b	View Locations
Pembrolizumab With Intratumoral Injection of Clostridium Novyi-NT	1	Antimicrobial Therapy, Immunomodulatory…	doxycycline monohydrate,…	30S ribosomal subunits, CD279, PD1, PDCD1	USA - TX - Houston
Study of AIC100 in Relapsed/Refractory Thyroid Cancer	1	CAR T Cells, Cell Therapy,…	autologous CAR T cells directed against ICA…	[Not available]	USA - NY - New York

growth. Increasing reports of acquired and intrinsic resistance against the small molecule inhibitors emphasize the need for development of alternative therapeutic approaches for ATC patients. A good indicator of development of adaptive resistance is reactivation of the MAPK pathway via activation of CRAF. Remarkably, most of the studies on resistance mechanism against PLX4032 focus on reactivation of MAPK pathways during development of resistance, but there is a paucity of studies characterizing immunological implications of this treatment and their contribution to development of therapeutic resistance from the perspective of tumor cells (Fig. 3).

Owing to the extremely refractory nature of ATC, we began examining the feasibility of a combinatorial therapeutic approach with MEK inhibitor and antagonistic antibodies in ATC. We saw that vemurafenib treatment modulates expression of multiple immunomodulatory molecules including HVEM, BTLA, and CD160 in thyroid cancer cell lines at transcript level. However, transient treatment with vemurafenib does not change the expression of these proteins in the cells. This points toward induction of an immunosuppressive molecular signature in ATC during treatment with PLX4032. This type of immunosuppressive environment usually correlates with worse clinical outcomes. This phenomenon supports the rationale for monitoring the immune profile of the patients alongside clinical course and clinical responses to treatments and tailors the therapeutic regimen based on the patient-specific molecular and immune signature.

We observed a significantly higher expression of active CRAF in PLX4032 resistant phenotype compared to the sensitive phenotype in our study. Immunological consequences of this adaptive resistance are not well characterized and completely unknown in ATC. We believed a better understanding of the adaptive resistant phenotype would help us identify better actionable targets in these patients that could be targeted in a combinatorial therapeutic approach. Two BRAFV600E inhibitor (PLX4032) resistant cell lines were generated in the lab over 7 months of slowly escalated drug treatment. BRAFV600Ei –

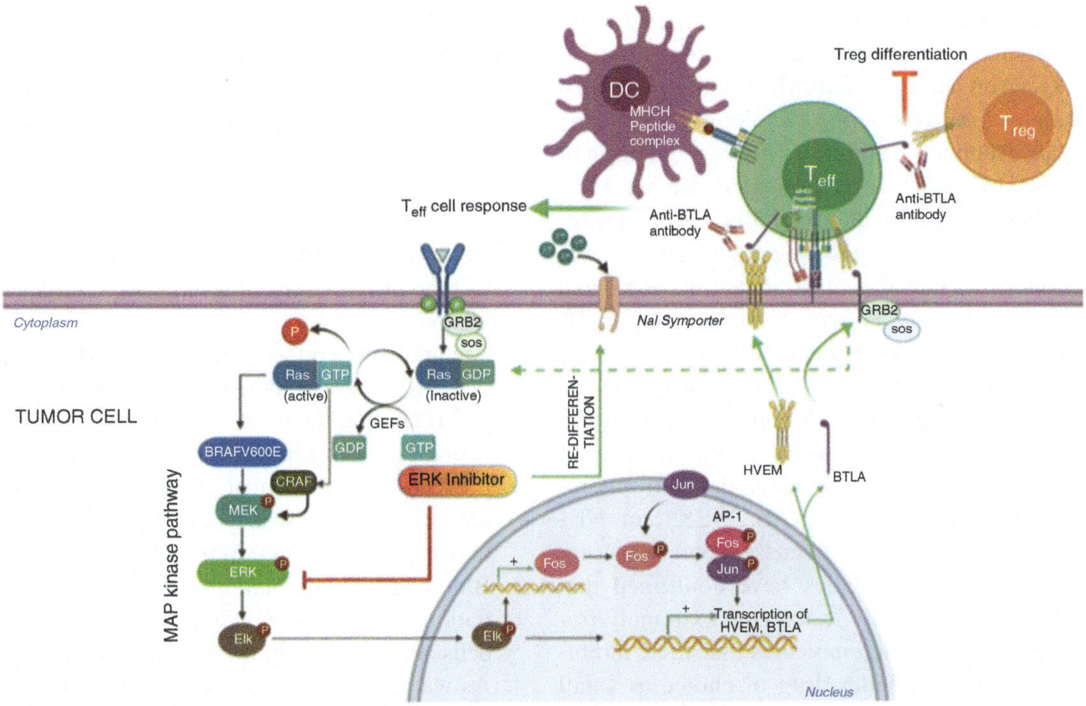

Fig. 3 Rationale for targeting the HVEM/BTLA axis with small molecule inhibitors of the MAPK pathway in anaplastic thyroid cancer

PLX4032 – resistant ATC cell lines in our study had a completely different expression profile of the immunomodulatory compared to the sensitive phenotype. We saw that acquired resistance to PLX4032 or vemurafenib is associated with increased expression of HVEM, BTLA, CD160, TIM3, and LGALS9B in BRAFV600E-positive ATC cell lines at transcript level. Expression of HVEM was more than 100-fold higher in the resistant cell lines compared to the sensitive cell lines. BTLA had more than tenfold upregulation in the resistant cell lines compared to normal. PD-L1, TIM3, and LGALS9B expressions were highly upregulated in the resistant phenotype. Resistance-associated increase in surface expression of HVEM suggests an increased immunomodulatory potential of the PLX4032 resistant ATC cells in the tumor microenvironment which might support immune evasion. This suggests activation of cellular processes during development of resistance that finally culminates into upregulation of these immunomodulatory molecules. These observations underscore the importance of a multipronged approach while considering a new treatment modality for a patient who started out as a BRAFV600Ei-sensitive phenotype but eventually developed resistance. It is of utmost importance to profile the tumor intermittently as the patient is on one specific small molecule inhibitor for a prolonged period. The development of adaptive resistance might alter the tumor phenotype in a way that the tumor becomes more amenable to another type of therapeutic intervention.

Combination therapy, including BRAFV600E inhibitor PLX4032 and MEK inhibitor trametinib, has modest impact on expression of HVEM in the PLX4032-sensitive tumor cells, as the expression was mildly dampened but was persistent in the resistant cells. However, once the cells acquire resistance against BRAFV600Ei, this combination therapy is not sufficient to control the expression of HVEM, and the patient might develop a unique and unforeseen immune interaction at the tumor site. Most of the compensatory pathways activated during development of BRAFV600Ei resistance eventually leads to upregulation of ERK. Activation of HGF/MET pathway or activation of STAT3 during development of resistance eventually culminates into upregulation of ERK [137–140]. This indicates that an ERK inhibitor might be more suitable for hyperproliferative cancers where the patients are prone to develop resistance against standard BRAF and MEK inhibitors. A recent study using ERK inhibitor LY3214996 in a panel of cell lines, including melanoma, colorectal cancer, pancreatic cancer, and NSCLC, demonstrated preferential in vitro sensitivity toward the inhibitor in the cell lines harboring ERK pathway alterations (BRAF, KRAS, NRAS, MEK1, or NF1 mutations) [141]. As discussed before, recent multicenter NGS studies have confirmed that most of these genetic lesions are extremely frequent in ATC, which indicates that ERK inhibitors might be a better drug of choice as small molecule inhibitors. A careful examination needs to be done to assess the potential off target effect of ERK inhibitors in ATC. Expression of HVEM and BTLA in ATC patients, and their further upregulation in the resistant phenotype, suggests that these patients might benefit from a combination of antagonistic antibodies targeting HVEM/BTLA signaling axis and ERK inhibitors depending on their tumor profile. Overall, we have concluded that transient treatment with vemurafenib or PLX4032 upregulates expression of certain immunomodulatory genes and a significantly higher constitutive surface expression of HVEM persists in PLX4032 resistant cells upon combination therapy with BRAFV600Ei and MEKi. Our studies have concluded that HVEM fundamentally supports tumorigenesis and its interaction with the cognate ligand LIGHT triggers activation of tumor associated MAPK signaling in ATC.

The expression profile of the components of the HVEM/BTLA/CD160 axis in ATC strongly suggests an alternate therapeutic avenue that could be explored in these patients. The ideal outcome of this therapeutic approach should be increased activation of effector T cells accompanied with diminished tumor cell proliferation and redifferentiation. A combination of ERK inhibitor and antagonistic antibodies targeting the HVEM/BTLA axis seems to be a rational combination based on the following observations:

1. Anaplastic thyroid cancer cells have high constitutive expression of HVEM, BTLA, and CD160 on their surface which can be targeted by antibodies.
2. Antagonistic antibody targeting BTLA can disrupt the cis interaction between HVEM and BTLA on the tumor cells and trans interaction between tumor cells and T cells, thus preventing activation of NFκB in the tumor cells in the first case and dampening of antitumor immune response in the latter.
3. Blocking BTLA would also prevent differentiation of effector T cells into regulatory T cells and in turn help immune activation.
4. As we observed in our study, anaplastic thyroid cancer cells can develop resistance against BRAFV600E inhibitor, and the resistant cells have much higher expression of HVEM, BTLA, CD160, TIM3, and galectin9 genes and significantly higher surface expression of HVEM protein.
5. A combination of BRAFV600E inhibitor vemurafenib (PLX4032) and MEK inhibitor (trametinib) does not modulate the expression of HVEM in the resistant tumor cells 205.
6. Introduction of an ERK inhibitor with anti-B 6. Introduction of an ERK inhibitor with anti-BTLA antibody might help induce redifferentiation in the dedifferentiated follicular cells which would be accompanied with increased expression of NIS and re-sensitize the patient toward radioiodine ablation therapy.
7. Also, inhibition of ERK would downregulate the transcription of crucial transcription factors responsible for upregulation of HVEM and BTLA in the tumor cells, such as cJun, STAT3, c-fos, ATF2, and c-Myc. Our study has identified the HVEM/BTLA axis as a potential immunotherapeutic target in anaplastic thyroid cancer.

8 Importance of TME Interacting Components Targets

Development of adaptive resistance to targeted therapies is inevitable, and a combination therapy targeting the immune microenvironment can forestall therapeutic resistance in ATC and provide a promising outcome. The dynamic nature of the TME including the immune cells, nonimmune cells, and acellular components can be valuable combination therapy targets in ATC. It has been demonstrated that the cells in the TME serve as double-edged swords in which they could be tumor-suppressing or tumor-promoting depending on the context. Studies have examined the positive and negative feedback loops affecting signal transduction and gene expression of cancer cells and the cells in the tumor stroma. Recent insights on this plasticity in cancer progression and relapse have demonstrated the need for new and combinatorial therapies. The goal of these would be to inhibit specific cell markers, interfere with stemness and EMT signaling, and affect the components of the TME. It is evident that the polarization of the cells in the TME is functionally and structurally different but also expresses different genes and cell surface markers. Therefore, these different phenotypes specifically can potentially provide the generation of novel biomarkers that provide an insight into the interaction with cancer cells and therefore guide the stage of cancer development and subsequently the treatment. Tipping the scale to an immunogenic TME will come with immunotherapy, antiangiogenic therapy, and stroma normalizing. The immunoactivation can be achieved via decreasing the tortuosity and permeability while increasing the blood perfusion of the vasculature. The decrease in immune checkpoint expression along with increase in immune activation of DCs and antigen presentation can further promote an immunogenic tumor suppressive TME. The recruitment of immune cells such as the increase of CD8+ T cells and the decrease of Tregs and MDSCs while polarizing immune cells and nonimmune cells alike to their tumor suppressive phenotype should also be considered. This can potentially be achieved by blocking of the tumor-promoting polarized cells via their specific cell surface markers with mAbs.

This will not only promote a normoxic environment but one in which the tumor cytokines and chemokines are immune-activating rather than immune-suppressing. Many are pleiotropic in nature and may alter their specific effects based on tumor type and other factors. But, for example, this can include secretion of IFNY and IL-2 while tipping the scale away from secretion of IL-6, CCL2, IL-10, CCL5, and CXCL12.

9 Further Studies in ATC: Cytokines, miRNAs, Exosomes, etc.

Reciprocal communication exists between the cancer and stromal cells in the tumor microenvironment as witnessed in a number of cancers [142, 143]. This crosstalk is facilitated by a number of secretory factors which comprise of soluble mediators – cytokines/chemokines, growth factors, as well as exosomes (nanovesicles packed with miRNA cargo). The secretory profile we obtained from the thyroid cancer cells and the macrophages clearly suggests the presence of pro-inflammatory chemokines and cytokines in the tumor microenvironment. All of these cytokines have major implications for regulating the signaling cascade in cancer cells to promote tumorigenesis. Other means of cellular crosstalk are reactive oxygen species and exosomes. Oxidative stress generates reactive oxygen species, which cause recruitment of infiltrating immune cells as well as damage the cellular DNA. The latter results in initiation of repair mechanisms that lead to further accumulation of genetic mutations and activation of oncogenic pathways, promoting tumorigenesis. Our work elucidated that anaplastic thyroid cancer cells generate ROS which aids in tumor progression and recruitment of macrophages. This effect of ROS along with the secreted chemotactic cytokines by ATC indicates an additive effect in recruiting the macrophages at the tumor site.

Additionally, we characterized the miRNA content of the exosomes secreted by the thyroid cancer cells. Researchers are now concentrating on the miRNA functionality for diagnosis and treatment modalities. However, most of the studies performed are focused on the circulating miRNA. Exosomes can be isolated from bodily fluids in a noninvasive way and hence can become a very important diagnostic marker based on their content. The exosomal cargo predominantly consists of miRNAs, which are highly conserved noncoding RNA that regulate the posttranscriptional or translation protein expression. The cells in tumor microenvironment secrete exosomes that are shuttled from primary to secondary recipient cells. They carry within them these functional miRNAs, which are transcribed and translated to biologically relevant proteins that regulate cellular processes. This implies that cellular crosstalk is mediated by soluble mediators and exosomes, ultimately promoting tumorigenesis. Previous studies have revealed the profile and functionality (to some extent) of the deregulated miRNAs in ATC tissues [144, 145]. The three major families of miRNAs downregulated in ATC are miR-200 family, miR-30 family, and let-7 family. In our comparative analysis between the various thyroid cancer secreted exosomal miRNAs, we did not observe any variation in expression profile of miR-200 family, or let-7 family. Common miRNAs upregulated in ATC tissues consist of miR-146, miR-221/222, and cluster miR-17-92 [144–146]. These miRNAs were not observed to be upregulated in anaplastic thyroid cancer secreted exosomes compared to other thyroid cancers. Thus, we can say that the profile of miRNAs obtained from ATC secreted exosomes can be different from that obtained from the tissue. The pro-tumorigenic functions of the exosome-derived miRNAs, through the regulation of genes in the recipient cells, have recently started to gain research interest. The role of exosomes as a drug delivery system and for diagnostic purposes has further added to their clinical relevance. However, only a handful of studies have examined the miRNA profile of circulating tumor-derived exosomes in FTC or PTC [147]. Exosomal miRNA cargo is understudied in anaplastic thyroid cancer.

In our study, we have come across a group of miRNA present in the exosomes secreted by anaplastic thyroid cancer cells that have tumor suppressive effects. The fact that these miRNAs are downregulated suggests a profile of a huge set of genes that are regulated by these miRNAs, contributing to the metastatic phenotype in ATC. The studies here are a clear indication that phenotype is regulated by epigenetic phenomenon of which miRNAs constitute a major cargo. We have defined the ATC phenotype based on miRNAs – miR-125b, miR-138, miR-148a, miR-152, miR-191, and miR-26b – that play a functional role in suppressing the ATC phenotype. Their downregulation paves the way for procurement of metastatic ATC phenotype, and as such can be considered as "tumor suppressors." Their biological function and specificity to ATC however remain to be determined. The other mode to establish whether PTC to ATC phenotype is linked is to examine the presence and gradual disappearance of these markers in the serum of patients. The steady disappearance of these miRNAs from the serum designates them as a transition biomarker for early detection of ATC phenotype, and should be pursued further.

The molecular therapies that target genetic mutations and aberrant signaling pathways are paving ways toward a cure of the disease. Current therapies target the bulk of well-differentiated thyroid cancer but fail to address the aggressive resilient cancer cells. This leads to high recurrence and relapse of thyroid cancer. Targeted therapies are being used for DTC, but undifferentiated ATC still remains unresponsive to the newer available drugs. Microarray analysis and genomic screening has helped us in understanding the complex molecular profile associated with ATC. Thus, determining the effect of various tumor microenvironmental factors will help in defining the spectrum of molecular mechanisms fundamental to the signaling in metastatic thyroid cancer. We have established that there exists a reciprocal relationship between the immune infiltrates and the cancer cells in the thyroid TME that aids in cancer progression as the thyroid TME secretome characterizes and polarizes the tumor infiltrates. Additionally, the distinct exosomal miRNA profile of anaplastic thyroid cancer can be used as an important diagnostic and prognostic marker. The chemokine and cytokine profile of ATC is also characteristic as the tumor infiltrates, and cancer cells regulate the secretory factors. Monitoring the serum levels of these pro-inflammatory soluble mediators can aid in assessing prognosis of the disease.

Therapies can also be devised against the secretory mediators of thyroid TME that promote cancer progression. Anti-cytokine therapies as well as silencing miRNAs can be used to dampen their pro-tumorigenic effect. Drugs targeting pro-inflammatory cytokines such as TNFα, IL-6, and IL-1 and their receptors are being tested for inflammatory diseases such as rheumatoid arthritis, Crohn's disease, and certain cancers such as multiple myeloma and renal cell cancer with promising results [148]. Moreover, overexpression of the distinct tumor suppressor miRNAs is proposed to revert the metastatic properties of the ATC cells. Though this approach is in its initial stages, cellular model studies of transfecting these miRNAs in cancer cells result in the transition of the cells to more differentiated phenotype, making them more receptive to standard therapies [149–154]. The secretory mediators of thyroid cancer modulate the thyroid cancer phenotype by inducing EMT leading to increased migration and invasion of cancer cells. Molecular markers that define the process of EMT can help in the identification of early markers of thyroid cancer cell differentiation as well as allowing for the possible development of targeted therapy designed at inhibiting EMT and subsequent suppression of thyroid cancer metastasis and dissemination. Thus, targeting the metastatic thyroid carcinoma microenvironment could offer potential additional therapeutic benefits and should be explored further in preclinical/translational models of human metastatic thyroid cancer.

References

1. Hanahan, D., & Weinberg, R. A. (2000). The hallmarks of cancer. *Cell, 100*(1), 57–70. https://doi.org/10.1016/S0092-8674(00)81683-9
2. Hanahan, D., & Weinberg, R. A. (2011). Hallmarks of cancer: The next generation. *Cell, 144*, 646–674. https://doi.org/10.1016/j.cell.2011.02.013
3. Thomas, L. (1959). Discussion. In H. S. Lawrence (Ed.), *Cellular and humoral aspects of the hypersensitive states.* (pp. 529–532). Hoeber-Harper.
4. Burnet, F. M. (1971). Immunological surveillance in neoplasia. *Immunological Reviews, 7*(1), 3–25. https://doi.org/10.1111/j.1600-065X.1971.tb00461.x
5. Möller, G., & Möller, E. (1976). The concept of immunological surveillance against neoplasia. *Immunological Reviews, 28*(1), 3–17. https://doi.org/10.1111/j.1600-065X.1976.tb00189.x
6. Sirmbomfr, S. (1959). *Immunological factors in the process of carcinogenesis* (pp. 1959–1963). SIS.
7. Dunn, G. P., Old, L. J., & Schreiber, R. D. (2004). The immunobiology review of cancer immunosurveillance and immunoediting. *Immunity, 21*, 137–148.
8. Wang, M., Zhao, J., Zhang, L., Wei, F., Lian, Y., Wu, Y., Gong, Z., Zhang, S., Zhour, J., Cao, K., Li, X., Xiong, W., Li, G., Zeng, Z., & Guo, C. (2017). Role of tumor microenvironment in tumorigenesis. *Journal of Cancer, 8*(5), 761–773.
9. Gentles, A. J., Newman, A. M., Liu, C. L., et al. (2015). The prognostic landscape of genes and infiltrating immune cells across human cancers. *Nature Medicine, 21*(8), 938–945. https://doi.org/10.1038/nm.3909
10. Lavin, Y., Mortha, A., Rahman, A., & Merad, M. (2015). Regulation of macrophage development and function in peripheral tissues. *Nature Reviews. Immunology, 15*(12), 731–744. https://doi.org/10.1038/nri3920
11. Perdiguero, E. G., & Geissmann, F. (2016). The development and maintenance of resident macrophages. *Nature Immunology, 17*(1), 2–8. https://doi.org/10.1038/ni.3341
12. Hoeffel, G., & Ginhoux, F. (2015). Ontogeny of tissue-resident macrophages. *Frontiers in Immunology, 6*(Sep), 1. https://doi.org/10.3389/fimmu.2015.00486
13. Lin, E. Y., & Pollard, J. W. (2007). Tumor-associated macrophages press the angiogenic switch in breast cancer. *Cancer Research, 67*(11), 5064–5066. https://doi.org/10.1158/0008-5472.CAN-07-0912
14. Mazzieri, R., Pucci, F., Moi, D., et al. (2011). Targeting the ANG2/TIE2 axis inhibits tumor growth and metastasis by impairing angiogenesis and disabling rebounds of proangiogenic myeloid cells. *Cancer Cell, 19*(4), 512–526. https://doi.org/10.1016/j.ccr.2011.02.005
15. Lin, Y., Xu, J., & Lan, H. (2019). Tumor-associated macrophages in tumor metastasis: Biological roles and clinical therapeutic applications. *Journal of Hematology & Oncology, 12*(1). https://doi.org/10.1186/s13045-019-0760-3
16. Strilic, B., & Offermanns, S. (2017). Intravascular survival and extravasation of tumor cells. *Cancer*

Cell, 32(3), 282–293. https://doi.org/10.1016/j.ccell.2017.07.001
17. DeNardo, D. G., & Ruffell, B. (2019). Macrophages as regulators of tumour immunity and immunotherapy. *Nature Reviews. Immunology, 19*(6), 369–382. https://doi.org/10.1038/s41577-019-0127-6
18. Chopin, M., Allan, R. S., & Belz, G. T. (2012). Transcriptional regulation of dendritic cell diversity. *Frontiers in Immunology, 3*(FEB). https://doi.org/10.3389/fimmu.2012.00026
19. Cisse, B., Caton, M. L., Lehner, M., et al. (2008). Transcription factor E2-2 is an essential and specific regulator of plasmacytoid dendritic cell development. *Cell, 135*(1), 37–48. https://doi.org/10.1016/j.cell.2008.09.016
20. Santos, N., Nunes-Pereira, A., Baltazar, F., & Granja, S. (2019). Lactate as a regulator of cancer inflammation and immunity. *Immunometabolism, 1*(e190015), 1–18. https://doi.org/10.20900/immunometab20190015
21. Mishra, D., & Banerjee, D. (2019). Lactate dehydrogenases as metabolic links between tumor and stroma in the tumor microenvironment. *Cancers (Basel), 11*(6), 750. https://doi.org/10.3390/cancers11060750
22. de la Cruz-López, K. G., Castro-Muñoz, L. J., Reyes-Hernández, D. O., García-Carrancá, A., & Manzo, M. J. (2019). Lactate in the regulation of tumor microenvironment and therapeutic approaches. *Frontiers in Oncology, 9*, 1143. https://doi.org/10.3389/fonc.2019.01143
23. Singer, K., Cheng, W. C., Kreutz, M., Ho, P. C., & Siska, P. J. (2018). Immunometabolism in cancer at a glance. *Disease Models & Mechanisms, 11*(8), dmm034272. https://doi.org/10.1242/dmm.034272
24. Lacroix, R., Rozeman, E. A., Kreutz, M., Renner, K., & Blank, C. U. (2018). Targeting tumor-associated acidity in cancer immunotherapy. *Cancer Immunology, Immunotherapy, 67*(9), 1331–1348. https://doi.org/10.1007/s00262-018-2195-z
25. Vigano, S., Alatzoglou, D., Irving, M., et al. (2019). Targeting adenosine in cancer immunotherapy to enhance T-cell function. *Frontiers in Immunology, 10*(June), 925. https://doi.org/10.3389/fimmu.2019.00925
26. Wennerberg, E., Pfefferle, A., Ekblad, L., et al. (2014). Human anaplastic thyroid carcinoma cells are sensitive to NK cell-mediated lysis via ULBP2/5/6 and chemoattract NK cells. *Clinical Cancer Research, 20*(22), 5733–5744. https://doi.org/10.1158/1078-0432.CCR-14-0291
27. Vivier, E., Raulet, D. H., Moretta, A., et al. (2011). Innate or adaptive immunity? The example of natural killer cells. *Science (80-), 331*(6013), 44–49. https://doi.org/10.1126/science.1198687
28. Moretta, L., & Moretta, A. (2004). Unravelling natural killer cell function: Triggering and inhibitory human NK receptors. *The EMBO Journal, 23*(2), 255–259. https://doi.org/10.1038/sj.emboj.7600019
29. Yin, M., Di, G., & Bian, M. (2018). Dysfunction of natural killer cells mediated by PD-1 and Tim-3 pathway in anaplastic thyroid cancer. *International Immunopharmacology, 64*(June), 333–339. https://doi.org/10.1016/j.intimp.2018.09.016
30. Masopust, D., & Schenkel, J. M. (2013). The integration of T cell migration, differentiation and function. *Nature Reviews. Immunology, 13*(5), 309–320. https://doi.org/10.1038/nri3442
31. Liu, Y., He, J., Xu, J., Li, J., Jiao, Y., Bei, D., Hu, Y., Chen, H., Xiao, Q., & Ding, K. (2017). Neuroendocrine differentiation is predictive of poor survival in patients with stage II colorectal cancer. *Oncology Letters, 13*(4), 2230–2236. https://doi.org/10.3892/ol.2017.5681
32. Zeng, Y., Lai, W., Wu, H., Liu, L., Xu, H., Wang, J., & Chu, Z. (2016). Neuroendocrine-like cells-derived CXCL10 and CXCL11 induce the infiltration of tumor-associated macrophage leading to the poor prognosis of colorectal cancer. *Oncotarget, 7*(19), 27394–27407.
33. Cai, H., Wang, H., Cao, N., Huang, B., Kong, F., Lu, L., Huang, Y., & Wang, W. (2020). Calcitonin-negative neuroendocrine tumor of the thyroid with metastasis to liver-rare presentation of an unusual tumor: A case report and review of literature. *World Journal of Clinical Cases, 8*(1), 179–187.
34. Chorny, J., Orrego, J., & Cameselle-Teijeiro, J. (2018). Primary high-grade calcitonin-negative neuroendocrine carcinoma of the thyroid: A very rare cancer. *Endocrinology, Diabetes & Metabolism., 1*, 1–4.
35. Haley, K., Patidar, K., Zhang, F., Emanuel, R., & Sunday, M. (1998). Tumor necrosis factor induces neuroendocrine differentiation in small cell lung cancer cell lines. *The American Journal of Physiology, 275*(2), L311–L321.
36. Kim, J., Jin, H., Zhao, J., Yang, Y., Li, Y., Yang, X., Dong, X., & Yu, J. (2017). FOXA1 inhibits prostate cancer neuroendocrine differentiation. *Oncogene, 36*, 4072–4080.
37. Iyengar, N., Gucalp, A., Dannenberg, A., & Hudis, C. (2016). Obesity and cancer mechanisms: tumor microenvironment and inflammation. *Journal of Clinical Oncology, 34*(35), 4270–4276.
38. Guaita-Esteruelas, S., Guma, J., Masana, L., & Borras, J. (2017). The peritumoral adipose tissue microenvironment and cancer. The roles of fatty acid binding protein 4 and fatty acid binding protein 5. *Molecular and Cellular Endocrinology, 462*, 107–118.
39. Nagl, L., Horvath, L., Pircher, A., & Wolf, D. (2020). Tumor endothelial cells (TECs) as potential immune directors of the tumor microenvironment – New findings and future perspectives. *Frontiers in Cell and Development Biology, 8*, 766. https://doi.org/10.3389/fcell.2020.00766
40. Salazar, N., & Zabel, B. A. (2019). Support of tumor endothelial cells by chemokine receptors. *Frontiers*

in Immunology, 10, 147. https://doi.org/10.3389/fimmu.2019.00147
41. Dudley, A. C. (2012). Tumor endothelial cells. *Cold Spring Harbor Perspectives in Medicine, 2*(3), a006536. https://doi.org/10.1101/cshperspect.a006536
42. Hida, K., Maishi, N., Annan, D. A., & Hida, Y. (2018). Contribution of tumor endothelial cells in cancer progression. *International Journal of Molecular Sciences, 19*(5), 1272. https://doi.org/10.3390/ijms19051272
43. Lin, W., Huang, L., Li, Y., Fang, B., Li, G., Chen, L., & Xu, L. (2019). Mesenchymal stem cells and cancer: Clinical challenges and opportunities. *BioMed Research International, 2820853*. https://doi.org/10.1155/2019/2820853
44. Ridge, S. M., Sullivan, F. J., & Glynn, S. A. (2017). Mesenchymal stem cells: Key players in cancer progression. *Molecular Cancer, 16*(1), 31. https://doi.org/10.1186/s12943-017-0597-8
45. Timaner, M., Tsai, K. K., & Shaked, Y. (2020). The multifaceted role of mesenchymal stem cells in cancer. *Seminars in Cancer Biology, 60*, 225–237. https://doi.org/10.1016/j.semcancer.2019.06.003
46. Kalluri, R. (2016). The biology and function of fibroblasts in cancer. *Nature Reviews. Cancer, 16*, 582–598. https://doi.org/10.1038/nrc.2016.73
47. Ichim, T. E., O'Heeron, P., & Kesari, S. (2018). Fibroblasts as a practical alternative to mesenchymal stem cells. *Journal of Translational Medicine, 16*, 212. https://doi.org/10.1186/s12967-018-1536-1
48. Alkasalias, T., Moyano-Galceran, L., Arsenian-Henriksson, M., & Lehti, K. (2018). Fibroblasts in the tumor microenvironment: Shield or spear? *International Journal of Molecular Sciences, 19*, 1532. https://doi.org/10.3390/ijms19051532
49. Monteran, L., & Erez, N. (2019). The dark side of fibroblasts: Cancer-associated fibroblasts as mediators of immunosuppression in the tumor microenvironment. *Frontiers in Immunology, 10*, 1835. https://doi.org/10.3389/fimmu.2019.01835
50. LeBleu, V. (2015). Imaging the tumor microenvironment. *Cancer Journal, 21*, 174–178. https://doi.org/10.1097/PPO.0000000000000118
51. Jiang, X., & Tomlinson, I. (2020). Why is cancer not more common? A changing microenvironment may help explain why, and suggests strategies for anticancer therapy. *Open Biology, 10*, 190297. https://doi.org/10.1098/rsob.190297
52. Fanelli, G. N., Naccarato, A. G., & Scatena, C. (2020). Recent advances in cancer plasticity: Cellular mechanisms, surveillance strategies, and therapeutic optimization. *Frontiers in Oncology, 10*, 569. https://doi.org/10.3389/fonc.2020.00569
53. Avagliano, A., Fiume, G., Pelagalli, A., Sanita, G., Ruocco, M. R., Montagnani, S., & Arcucci, A. (2020). Metabolic plasticity of melanoma cells and their crosstalk with tumor microenvironment. *Frontiers in Oncology, 10*, 722. https://doi.org/10.3389/fonc.2020.00722
54. Burgos-Panadero, R., Lucantoni, F., Gamero-Sandemetrio, E., de la Cruz-Merino, L., Alvaro, T., & Noguera, R. (2019). The tumour microenvironment as an integrated framework to understand cancer biology. *Cancer Letters, 461*, 112–122. https://doi.org/10.1016/j.canlet.2019.07.010
55. Bolouri, H. (2015). Network dynamics in the tumor microenvironment. *Seminars in Cancer Biology, 30*, 52–59. https://doi.org/10.1016/j.semcancer.2014.02.007
56. Pan, X., & Zheng, L. (2020). Epigenetics in modulating immune functions of stromal and immune cells in the tumor microenvironment. *Cellular and molecular immunology, 17*, 940–953. https://doi.org/10.1038/s41423-020-0505-9
57. Greten, F., & Grivennikov, S. (2019). Inflammation and cancer: Triggers, mechanisms, and consequences. *Immunity, 51*, 27–41. https://doi.org/10.1016/j.immuni.2019.06.025
58. Perez-Romer, K., Rodriguez, R. M., Amedei, A., Barcelo-Coblijn, G., & Lopez, D. H. (2020). Immune landscape in tumor microenvironment: Implications for biomarker development and immunotherapy. *International Journal of Molecular Sciences, 21*, 5521. https://doi.org/10.3390/ijms21155521
59. Kang, Y., & Massague, J. (2004). Epithelial – mesenchymal transitions: Twist in development and metastasis. *Cell, 118*, 277–279. https://doi.org/10.1016/j.cell.2004.07.011
60. Thiery, J. P., & Lim, C. T. (2013). Tumor dissemination: An EMT affair. *Cancer Cell, 23*, 272–273. https://doi.org/10.1016/j.ccr.2013.03.004
61. Kalluri, R., & Weinberg, R. A. (2009). The basics of epithelial-mesenchymal transition. *The Journal of Clinical Investigation, 119*, 1420–1428. https://doi.org/10.1172/JCI39104
62. Thiery, J. P., & Sleeman, J. (2006). Complex networks orchestrate epithelial-mesenchymal transitions. *Nature Reviews Molecular Cell Biology, 7*, 131–142. https://doi.org/10.1038/nrm1835
63. Sumimoto, H., Imabayashi, F., Iwata, T., & Kawakami, Y. (2006). The BRAF-MAPK signaling pathway is essential for cancer-immune evasion in human melanoma cells. *Journal of Experimental Medicine, 203*, 1651–1656. https://doi.org/10.1084/jem.20051848
64. Pylayeva-Gupta, Y., Lee, K. E., Hajdu, C. H., Miller, G., & Bar-Sagi, D. (2012). Oncogenic Kras-induced GM-CSF production promotes the development of pancreatic neoplasia. *Cancer Cell, 21*, 836–847. https://doi.org/10.1016/j.ccr.2012.04.024
65. Zdanov, S., Mandapathil, M., Eid, R. A., Adamson-Fadeyi, S., Wilson, W., Quian, J., Carnie, A., Tarasova, N., Mkrtichyan, M., Berzofsky, J. A., Whiteside, T. L., & Khleif, S. N. (2016). *Cancer Immunology Research, 4*, 354–365. https://doi.org/10.1158/2326-6066.CIR-15-0241
66. Blagih, J., Buck, M. D., & Vousden, K. H. (2020). P53, cancer and the immune response. *Journal of*

Cell Science, 133, 1–13. https://doi.org/10.1242/jcs.237453
67. Park, S., Zhu, J., Altan-Bonnet, G., & Cheng, S.-Y. (2019). Monocyte recruitment and activated inflammation are associated with thyroid carcinogenesis in a mouse model. *American Journal of Cancer Research, 9*(7) www.ajcr.us/
68. Fang, W., Ye, L., Shen, L., Cai, J., Huang, F., Wei, Q., Fei, X., Chen, X., Guan, H., Wang, W., Li, X., & Ning, G. (2014). Tumor-associated macrophages promote the metastatic potential of thyroid cancer by releasing CXCL8. *Carcinogenesis, 35*, 1780–1787. https://doi.org/10.1093/carcin/bgu060
69. Kim, S., Cho, S. W., Min, H. S., Kim, K. M., Yeom, G. J., Kim, E. Y., Lee, K. E., Yun, Y. G., Park, D. J., & Park, Y. J. (2013). The expression of tumor-associated macrophages in papillary thyroid carcinoma. *Endocrinology and Metabolism, 28*, 192–198. https://doi.org/10.3803/EnM.2013.28.3.192
70. Ryder, M., Ghossein, R. A., Ricarte-Filho, J. C., Knauf, J. A., & Fagin, J. A. (2008). Increased density of tumor-associated macrophages is associated with decreased survival in advanced thyroid cancer. *Endocrine-Related Cancer, 15*, 1069–1074. https://doi.org/10.1677/ERC-08-0036
71. Caillou, B., Talbot, M., Weyemi, U., Pioche-Durieu, C., Ghuzlan, A. A., Bidart, J. M., Chouaib, S., Schlumberger, M., & Dupuy, C. (2011). Tumor-associated macrophages (TAMs) form an interconnected cellular supportive network in anaplastic thyroid carcinoma. *PLoS One, 6*, 22567. https://doi.org/10.1371/journal.pone.0022567
72. Tsuge, K., Takeda, H., Kawada, S., Maeda, K., & Yamakawa, M. (2005). Characterization of dendritic cells in differentiated thyroid cancer. *The Journal of Pathology, 205*, 565–576. https://doi.org/10.1002/path.1731
73. Suzuki, S., Shibata, M., Gonda, K., Kanke, Y., Ashizawa, M., Ujiie, D., Suzushino, S., Nakano, K., Fukushima, T., Sakurai, K., Tomita, R., Kumamoto, K., & Takenoshita, S. (2013). Immunosuppression involving increased myeloid-derived suppressor cell levels, systemic inflammation and hypoalbuminemia are present in patients with anaplastic thyroid cancer. *Molecular and Clinical Oncology, 1*, 959–964. https://doi.org/10.3892/mco.2013.170
74. Cunha, L. L., Marcello, M. A., Nonogaki, S., Morari, E. C., Soares, F. A., Vassallo, J., & Ward, L. S. (2015). CD8+ tumour-infiltrating lymphocytes and COX2 expression may predict relapse in differentiated thyroid cancer. *Clinical Endocrinology, 83*(2), 246–253. https://doi.org/10.1111/cen.12586
75. Antohe, M., Nedelcu, R. I., Nichita, L., et al. (2019). Tumor infiltrating lymphocytes: The regulator of melanoma evolution (Review). *Oncology Letters, 17*(5), 4155–4161. https://doi.org/10.3892/ol.2019.9940
76. Sato, E., Olson, S. H., Ahn, J., Bundy, B., Nishikawa, H., Qian, F., Jungbluth, A. A., Frosina, D., Gnjatic, S., Ambrosone, C., Kepner, J., Odunsi, T., Ritter, G., Lele, S., Chen, Y., Ohtani, H., Old, L. J., & Odunsi, K. (2005). Intraepithelial CD8+ tumor-infiltrating lymphocytes and a high CD8+/regulatory T cell ratio are associated with favorable prognosis in ovarian cancer. *Proceedings of the National Academy of Sciences of the United States of America, 102*, 185038–118543. https://doi.org/10.1073/pnas.0509182102
77. Ye, S., Li, X., Zhao, K., & Feng, T. (2017). High expression of CD8 predicts favorable prognosis in patients with lung adenocarcinoma. *Medicine, 96*, e6472. https://doi.org/10.1097/MD.0000000000006472
78. Joseph, M., & Enting, D. (2019). Immune responses in bladder cancer – Role of immune cell populations, prognostic factors and therapeutic implications. *Frontiers in Oncology, 9*, 1–15. https://doi.org/10.3389/fonc.2019.01270
79. Glaire, M. A., Domingo, E., Sveen, A., Bruun, J., Nesbakken, A., Nicholson, G., Novelli, M., Lawson, K., Oukrif, D., Kildal, W., Danielsen, H. E., Kerr, R., Kerr, D., Tomlinson, I., Lothe, R. A., & Church, D. N. (2019). Tumour- infiltrating CD8+ lymphocytes and colorectal cancer recurrence by tumour and nodal stage. *British Journal of Cancer, 121*, 471–482. https://doi.org/10.1038/s41416-019-0540-4
80. Angell, T. E., Lechner, M. G., Jang, J. K., LoPresti, J. S., & Epstein, A. L. (2014). MHC class I loss is a frequent mechanism of immune escape in papillary thyroid cancer that is reversed by interferon and selumetinib treatment in Vitro. *Clinical Cancer Research, 20*(23), 6034–6044. https://doi.org/10.1158/10780432
81. Ahn, S., Kim, T. H., Kim, S., Ki, C., Jang, H. W., Kim, J. S., Kim, J. H., Choe, J., Shin, J., Hahn, S., Oh, Y., & Chung, J. H. (2017). Comprehensive screening for PD-L1 expression in thyroid cancer. *Endocrine-Related Cancer, 24*, 97–106. https://doi.org/10.1530/ERC-16-0421
82. Ribas, A., & Wolchok, J. D. (2018). Cancer immunotherapy using checkpoint blockade. *Science, 359*, 1350–1355. https://doi.org/10.1126/science.aar4060
83. Lamouille, S., Xu, J., & Derynck, R. (2014). Molecular mechanisms of epithelial-mesenchymal transition. *Nature Reviews. Molecular Cell Biology, 15*, 178–196. https://doi.org/10.1038/nrm3758
84. Micalizzi, D., Farabaugh, S. M., & Ford, H. L. (2010). Epithelial-mesenchymal transition in cancer: Parallels between normal development and tumor progression. *Journal of Mammary Gland Biology and Neoplasia, 15*, 117–134. https://doi.org/10.1007/s10911-010-9178-9
85. Vleminckx, K., Vakaet, L. J., Mareel, M., Fiers, W., & Van Roy, F. (1991). Genetic manipulation of E-cadherin expression by epithelial tumor cells reveals an invasion suppressor role. *Cell, 66*, 107–119.
86. Villarejo, A., Cortes-Cabrera, A., Molina-Ortiz, P., Portillo, F., & Cano, A. (2013). Differential role of Snail1 and Snail2 Zinc fingers in E-cadherin repres-

sion and epithelial to mesenchymal transition. *The Journal of Biological Chemistry, 289*, 930–941. https://doi.org/10.1074/jbc.M113.528026

87. Molina-Ortiz, P., Vilarejo, A., MacPherson, M., Santos, V., Montes, A., Souchelnytskyi, S., Portillo, F., & Cano, A. (2012). Characterization of the SNAG and SLUG domains of Snail2 in the repression of E-cadherin and EMT induction: Modulation by Serine 4 phosphorylation. *PLoS One, 7*, e36132. https://doi.org/10.1371/journal.pone.0036132
88. Kumar, K., Raza, S. S., Knab, L. M., Chow, C. R., Kwok, B., Bentrem, D. J., Popovic, R., Ebine, K., Licht, J. D., & Minshi, H. G. (2015). GLI2-dependent c-MYC upregulation mediates resistance of pancreatic cancer cells to the BET bromodomain inhibitor JQ1. *Scientific Reports, 5*, 9489. https://doi.org/10.1038/srep09489
89. Phillips, S., Prat, A., Sedic, M., Proia, T., Wronski, A., Mazumdar, S., Skibinski, A., Shirley, S. H., Perou, C. M., Gill, G., Gupta, P. B., & Kupperwasser, C. (2014). Cell-state transitions regulated by SLUG are critical for tissue regeneration and tumor initiation. *Stem Cell Reports, 2*, 633–647. https://doi.org/10.1016/j.stemcr.2014.03.008
90. Wu, Y., & Zhou, B. P. (2010). TNF-α/NF-κB/Snail pathway in cancer cell migration and invasion. *British Journal of Cancer, 102*, 639–644. https://doi.org/10.1038/sj.bjc.6605530
91. Yang, J., Mani, S. A., Donaher, J., Ramaswamy, S., Itzykson, R., Come, C., Savagner, P., Gitelman, I., Richardson, A., & Weinberg, R. A. (2004). Twist, a master regulator of morphogenesis plays an essential role in tumor metastasis. *Cell, 117*, 927–939. https://doi.org/10.1016/j.cell.2004.06.006
92. Ye, X., & Weinberg, R. A. (2015). Epithelial-mesenchymal plasticity: A central regulator of cancer progression. *Trends in Cell Biology, 25*, 675–686. https://doi.org/10.1016/j.tcb.2015.07.012
93. Tsai, J. H., & Yang, J. (2013). Epithelial – Mesenchymal plasticity in carcinoma metastasis. *Genes and Development, 27*, 2192–2206. https://doi.org/10.1101/gad.225334.113
94. Larue, L., & Bellacosa, A. (2005). Epithelial-mesenchymal transition in development and cancer: Role of phosphatidylinositol 3′kinase/AKT pathways. *Oncogene, 24*, 7443–7454.
95. Radisky, D. C. (2005). Epithelial-mesenchymal transition. *Journal of Cell Science, 118*, 4325–4326. https://doi.org/10.1242/jcs.02552
96. Edme, N., Downward, J., Thiery, J. P., & Boyer, B. (2002). Ras induces NBT-II epithelial cell scattering through the coordinate activities of Rac and MAPK pathways. *Journal of Cell Science, 115*, 2591–2601.
97. Bakin, A., Tomlinson, A., Bhowmick, N. A., Moses, H. L., & Arteaga, C. L. (2000). Phosphatidylinositol 3-kinase function is required for transforming growth factor β- mediated epithelial to mesenchymal transition and cell migration. *Journal of Biological Chemistry, 275*, 36803–36810. https://doi.org/10.1074/jbc.M005912200
98. Wu, Y., Deng, J., Rychahou, P., Qiu, S., Evers, B. M., & Zhou, B. P. (2009). Stabilization of snail by NF-κB is required for inflammation-induced cell migration and invasion. *Cancer Cell, 15*, 416–428. https://doi.org/10.1016/j.ccr.2009.03.016
99. Julien, S., Puig, I., Caretti, E., Bonaventure, J., Nelles, L., van Roy, F., Dargemont, C., Garcia de Herreros, A., Bellacosa, A., & Larue, L. (2007). Activation of NF-κB by Akt upregulates snail expression and induces epithelium mesenchyme transition. *Oncogene, 26*, 7445–7456. https://doi.org/10.1038/sj.onc.1210546
100. Grille, S. J., Bellacosa, A., Upson, J., Klein-Szanto, A., van Roy, F., Lee-Kwon, W., Donowitz, M., Tsichlis, P. N., & Larue, L. (2003). The protein Kinase Akt induces epithelial mesenchymal transition and promotes enhances motility and invasiveness of squamous cell carcinoma lines. *Cancer Research, 63*, 2172–2178.
101. Banquero, P., Sanchez-Hernandez, I., Jimenez-Mora, E., Orgaz, J., Jimenez, B., & Chiloeches, A. (2013). V600EBRAF promotes invasiveness of thyroid cancer cells by decreasing E-cadherin expression through a Snail-dependent mechanism. *Cancer Letters, 335*, 232–241. https://doi.org/10.1016/j.canlet.2013.02.033
102. Hardy, R. G., Vicente-Dueñas, C., González-Herrero, I., Anderson, C., Flores, T., Hughes, S., Tselepis, C., Ross, J. A., & Sánchez-García, I. (2007). Snail family transcription factors are implicated in thyroid carcinogenesis. *The American Journal of Pathology, 171*, 1037–1046.
103. Vasko, V., Espinosa, A. V., Scouten, W., He, H., Auer, H., Liyanarachchi, S., Larin, A., Savchenko, V., Francis, G. L., de la Chapelle, A., Saji, M., & Ringel, M. D. (2007). Gene expression and functional evidence of epithelial-to-mesenchymal transition in papillary thyroid carcinoma invasion. *Proceedings of the National Academy of Sciences of the United States of America, 104*, 2803–2808.
104. Wiseman, S. M., Masoudi, H., Niblock, P., Turbin, D., Rajput, A., Hay, J., Filipenko, D., Huntsman, D., & Gilks, B. (2006). Derangement of the E-cadherin/catenin complex is involved in transformation of differentiated to anaplastic thyroid carcinoma. *The American Journal of Surgery, 191*, 581–587.
105. Salerno, P., Garcia-Rostan, G., Piccinin, S., Bencivenga, T. C., Di Maro, G., Doglioni, C., Basolo, F., Maestro, R., Fusco, A., Santoro, M., & Salvatore, G. (2011). TWIST1 plays a pleiotropic role in determining the anaplastic thyroid cancer phenotype. *The Journal of Clinical Endocrinology & Metabolism, 96*, E772–E781.
106. Da, C., Wu, K., Yue, C., Bai, P., Wang, R., Wang, G., Zhao, M., Lv, Y., Hou, P., Da, C., Wu, K., Yue, C., Bai, P., Wang, R., Wang, G., Zhao, M., Lv, Y., Hou, P., Da, C., et al. (2017). N-cadherin promotes thyroid tumorigenesis through modulating major signaling pathways. *Oncotarget, 8*, 8131–8142.

107. Sabbah, M., Emami, S., Redeuilh, G., Julien, S., Prévost, G., Zimber, A., Ouelaa, R., Bracke, M., De Wever, O., & Gespach, C. (2008). Molecular signature and therapeutic perspective of the epithelial-to-mesenchymal transitions in epithelial cancers. *Drug Resistance Updates, 11*, 123–151.
108. Moustakas, A., & Heldin, C.-H. (2007). Signaling networks guiding epithelial-mesenchymal transitions during embryogenesis and cancer progression. *Cancer Science, 98*, 1512–1520.
109. Mathias, R. A., Wang, B., Ji, H., Kapp, E. A., Moritz, R. L., Zhu, H.-J., & Simpson, R. J. (2009). Secretome-based proteomic profiling of Ras-transformed MDCK cells reveals extracellular modulators of epithelial-mesenchymal transition. *Journal of Proteome Research, 8*, 2827–2837.
110. Palena, C., Hamilton, D. H., & Fernando, R. I. (2012). Influence of IL-8 on the epithelial-mesenchymal transition and the tumor microenvironment. *Future Oncology (London, England), 8*, 713–722.
111. Cunha, L. L., Marcello, M. A., & Ward, L. S. (2014). The role of the inflammatory microenvironment in thyroid carcinogenesis. *Endocrine-Related Cancer, 21*, R85–R103.
112. Graceffa, G., Patrone, R., Vieni, S., Campanella, S., Calamia, S., Laise, I., Conzo, G., Latteri, M., & Cipolla, C. (2019). Association between Hashimoto's thyroiditis and papillary thyroid carcinoma: A retrospective analysis of 305 patients. *BMC Endocrine Disorders, 19*, 4–9. https://doi.org/10.1186/s12902-019-0351-x
113. Varricchi, G., Loffredo, S., Marone, G., Modestino, L., Fallahi, P., Ferrari, S. M., De Paulis, A., Antonelli, A., & Galdiero, M. R. (2019). The immune landscape of thyroid cancer in the context of immune checkpoint inhibition. *International Journal of Molecular Sciences, 20*. https://doi.org/10.3390/ijms20163934
114. Todaro, M., Zerilli, M., Ricci-Vitiani, L., Bini, M., Alea, M. P., Florena, A. M., Miceli, L., Condorelli, G., Bonventre, S., Di Gesù, G., De Maria, R., & Stassi, G. (2006). Autocrine production of interleukin-4 and interleukin-10 is required for survival and growth of thyroid cancer cells. *Cancer Research, 66*, 1491–1499. https://doi.org/10.1158/0008-5472.CAN-05-2514
115. Moretti, S., Menicali, E., Voce, P., Morelli, S., Cantarelli, S., Sponziello, M., Colella, R., Fallarino, F., Orabona, C., Alunno, A., De Biase, D., Bini, V., Mameli, M. G., Filetti, S., Gerli, R., Macchiarulo, A., Melillo, R. M., Tallini, G., Santoro, M., … Puxeddu, E. (2014). Indoleamine 2,3-Dioxygenase 1 (IDO1) is up-regulated in thyroid carcinoma and drives the development of an immunosuppressant tumor microenvironment. *Journal of Clinical Endocrinology and Metabolism, 99*. https://doi.org/10.1210/jc.2013-3351
116. Linsley, P. S., Brady, W., Urnes, M., Grosmaire, L. S., Damle, N. K., & Ledbetter, J. A. (1991). CTLA4 is a second receptor for the B cell activation antigen B7. *The Journal of Experimental Medicine, 174*, 561–569.
117. Munn, D. H., Sharma, M. D., & Mellor, A. L. (2004). Ligation of B7-1/B7-2 by human CD4+ T cells triggers indoleamine 2,3-dioxygenase activity in dendritic cells. *Journal of Immunology (Baltimore, Md.: 1950), 172*, 4100–4110. https://doi.org/10.4049/JIMMUNOL.172.7.4100
118. Barber, D. L., Wherry, E. J., Masopust, D., Zhu, B., Alison, J. P., Sharpe, A. H., Freeman, G. J., & Ahmed, R. (2005). Restoring function in exhausted CD8 T cells during chronic viral infection. *Nature, 439*, 682–687.
119. Lipson, E. J., & Drake, C. G. (2011). Ipilimumab: An anti-CTLA-4 antibody for metastatic melanoma. *Clinical Cancer Research, 17*, 6958–6962. https://doi.org/10.1158/1078-0432.CCR-11-1595
120. Mansh, M. (2011). Ipilimumab and cancer immunotherapy: A new hope for advanced stage melanoma. *Yale Journal of Biology and Medicine, 84*, 381–389.
121. Tarhini, A. (2013). Immune-mediated adverse events associated with Ipilimumab CTLA-4 blockade therapy: The underlying mechanisms and clinical management. *Scientifica, 2013*, 1–19. https://doi.org/10.1155/2013/857519
122. Drugs.com. (2020). Opdivo FDA approval history. *Drugs.com*. https://www.drugs.com/history/opdivo.html
123. Brauner, E., Gunda, V., Vanden Borre, P., Zurakowski, D., Kim, Y. S., Dennett, K. V., Amin, S., Freeman, G. J., & Parangi, S. (2016). Combining BRAF inhibitor and anti PD-L1 antibody dramatically improves tumor regression and anti tumor immunity in an immunocompetent murine model of anaplastic thyroid cancer. *Oncotarget, 7*. www.impactjournals.com/oncotarget
124. Iyer, P. C., Dadu, R., Gule-Monroe, M., Busaidy, N. L., Ferrarotto, R., Habra, M. A., Zafereo, M., Williams, M. D., Gunn, G. B., Grosu, H., Skinner, H. D., Sturgis, E. M., Gross, N., & Cabanillas, M. E. (2018). Salvage pembrolizumab added to kinase inhibitor therapy for the treatment of anaplastic thyroid carcinoma. *Journal for Immunotherapy of Cancer, 6*, 1–10. https://doi.org/10.1186/s40425-018-0378-y
125. Diamantopoulos, P. T., Gaggadi, M., Kassi, E., Benopoulou, O., Anastasopoulou, A., & Gogas, H. (2017). Late-onset nivolumab-mediated pneumonitis in a patient with melanoma and multiple immune-related adverse events. *Melanoma Research, 27*, 391–395. https://doi.org/10.1097/CMR.0000000000000355
126. Mirabile, A., Brioschi, E., Ducceschi, M., Piva, S., Lazzari, C., Bulotta, A., Viganò, M. G., Petrella, G., Gianni, L., & Gregorc, V. (2019). PD-1 inhibitors-related neurological toxicities in patients with non-small-cell lung cancer: A literature review. *Cancers, 11*(3) MDPI AG. https://doi.org/10.3390/cancers11030296

127. Giannini, R., Moretti, S., Ugolini, C., Macerola, E., Menicali, E., Nucci, N., Morelli, S., Colella, R., Mandarano, M., Sidoni, A., Panfili, M., Basolo, F., & Puxeddu, E. (2019). Immune profiling of thyroid carcinomas suggests the existence of two major phenotypes: An ATC-like and a PDTCLike. *The Journal of Clinical Endocrinology and Metabolism, 104*, 3557–3575. https://doi.org/10.1210/jc.2018-01167
128. Kim, Y. W., Kim, S. K., Kim, C. S., Kim, I. Y., Cho, M. Y., & Kim, N. K. (2014). Association of serum and intratumoral cytokine profiles with tumor stage and neutrophil lymphocyte ratio in colorectal cancer. *Anticancer Research, 34*, 3481–3487.
129. Ward-Kavanagh, L. K., Lin, W. W., Šedý, J. R., & Ware, C. F. (2016). The TNF receptor superfamily in co-stimulating and co-inhibitory responses. *Immunity, 44*(5), 1005–1019. https://doi.org/10.1016/j.immuni.2016.04.019
130. Düsterhöft, S., Lokau, J., & Garbers, C. (2019). The metalloprotease ADAM17 in inflammation and cancer. *Pathology Research and Practice, 215*, 152410. https://doi.org/10.1016/j.prp.2019.04.002
131. Moss, M. L., & Minond, D. (2017). Recent advances in ADAM17 research: A promising target for cancer and inflammation. *Mediators of Inflammation, 2017*. https://doi.org/10.1155/2017/9673537
132. Pavlenko, E., Cabron, A. S., Arnold, P., Dobert, J. P., Rose-John, S., & Zunke, F. (2019). Functional characterization of colon cancer-associated mutations in ADAM17: Modifications in the prodomain interfere with trafficking and maturation. *International Journal of Molecular Sciences, 20*, 1–18. https://doi.org/10.3390/ijms20092198
133. Saad, M. I., Rose-John, S., & Jenkins, B. J. (2019). ADAM17: An emerging therapeutic target for lung cancer. *Cancers, 11*. https://doi.org/10.3390/cancers11091218142
134. del Rio, M. L., Lucas, C. L., Buhler, L., Rayat, G., & Rodriguez-Barbosa, J. I. (2009). HVEM/LIGHT/BTLA/CD160 cosignaling pathways as targets for immune regulation. *Journal of Leukocyte Biology, 87*, 223–235. https://doi.org/10.1189/jlb.0809590
135. Fang, Y., Ye, L., Zhang, T., He, Q. Z., & Zhu, J. L. (2017). High expression of herpesvirus entry mediator (HVEM) in ovarian serous adenocarcinoma tissue. *Journal of B.U.ON., 22*, 80–86. www.jbuon.com
136. Inoue, T., Sho, M., Yasuda, S., Nishiwada, S., Nakamura, S., Ueda, T., Nishigori, N., Kawasaki, K., Obara, S., Nakamoto, T., Koyama, F., Fujii, H., & Nakajima, Y. (2015). HVEM expression contributes to tumor progression and prognosis in human colorectal cancer. *Anticancer Research, 35*, 1361–1368.
137. Knauf, J. A., Luckett, K. A., Chen, K. Y., Voza, F., Socci, N. D., Ghossein, R., & Fagin, J. A. (2018a). Hgf/Met activation mediates resistance to BRAF inhibition in murine anaplastic thyroid cancers. *Journal of Clinical Investigation, 128*, 4086–4097. https://doi.org/10.1172/JCI120966
138. Brighton, H. E., Angus, S. P., Bo, T., Roques, J., Tagliatela, A. C., Darr, D. B., Karagoz, K., Sciaky, N., Gatza, M. L., Sharpless, N. E., Johnson, G. L., & Bear, J. E. (2018). New mechanisms of resistance to MEK inhibitors in melanoma revealed by intravital imaging. *Cancer Research, 78*, 542–557. https://doi.org/10.1158/0008-5472.CAN-17-1653
139. Byeon, H. K., Na, H. J., Yang, Y. J., Kwon, H. J., Chang, J. W., Ban, M. J., Kim, W. S., Shin, D. Y., Lee, E. J., Koh, Y. W., Yoon, J. H., & Choi, E. C. (2016). c-Met-mediated reactivation of PI3K/AKT signaling contributes to insensitivity of BRAF(V600E) mutant thyroid cancer to BRAF inhibition. *Molecular Carcinogenesis, 55*, 1678–1687. https://doi.org/10.1002/mc.22418
140. Titz, B., Lomova, A., Le, A., Hugo, W., Kong, X., Ten Hoeve, J., Friedman, M., Shi, H., Moriceau, G., Song, C., Hong, A., Atefi, M., Li, R., Komisopoulou, E., Ribas, A., Lo, R. S., & Graeber, T. G. (2016). JUN dependency in distinct early and late BRAF inhibition adaptation states of melanoma. *Cell Discovery, 2*. https://doi.org/10.1038/celldisc.2016.28
141. Bhagwat, S. V., McMillen, W. T., Cai, S., Zhao, B., Whitesell, M., Shen, W., Kindler, L., Flack, R. S., Wu, W., Anderson, B., Zhai, Y., Yuan, X. J., Pogue, M., Van Horn, R. D., Rao, X., McCann, D., Dropsey, A. J., Manro, J., Walgren, J., … Peng, S. B. (2020). ERK inhibitor LY3214996 targets ERK pathway-driven cancers: A therapeutic approach toward precision medicine. *Molecular Cancer Therapeutics, 19*, 325–336. https://doi.org/10.1158/1535-7163.MCT-19-0183
142. Vaňhara, P., & Souček, K. (2013). Mutual cytokine crosstalk between colon cancer cells and microenvironment initiates development of distant metastases. *JAK-STAT., 2*, e23810.
143. Wiseman, B. S., & Werb, Z. (2002). Stromal effects on mammary gland development and breast cancer. *Science, 296*, 1046–1049.
144. Hébrant, A., Floor, S., Saiselet, M., Antoniou, A., Desbuleux, A., Snyers, B., La, C., de Saint, A. N., Leteurtre, E., Andry, G., & Maenhaut, C. (2014). miRNA expression in anaplastic thyroid carcinomas. *PLoS One, 9*, e103871.
145. Fuziwara, C. S., & Kimura, E. T. (2014). MicroRNA deregulation in anaplastic thyroid cancer biology. *International Journal of Endocrinology, 2014*, 743450.
146. Visone, R., Pallante, P., Vecchione, A., Cirombella, R., Ferracin, M., Ferraro, A., Volinia, S., Coluzzi, S., Leone, V., Borbone, E., Liu, C.-G., Petrocca, F., Troncone, G., Calin, G. A., Scarpa, A., Colato, C., Tallini, G., Santoro, M., Croce, C. M., et al. (2007). Specific microRNAs are downregulated in human thyroid anaplastic carcinomas. *Oncogene, 26*, 7590–7595.
147. Samsonov, R., Burdakov, V., Shtam, T., Radzhabova, Z., Vasilyev, D., Tsyrlina, E., Titov, S., Ivanov, M., Berstein, L., Filatov, M., Kolesnikov, N., Gil-Henn, H., & Malek, A. (2016). Plasma exosomal miR-21

and miR-181a differentiates follicular from papillary thyroid cancer. *Tumor Biology, 37*, 12011–12021.
148. Tayal, V., & Kalra, B. S. (2008). Cytokines and anti-cytokines as therapeutics – An update. *European Journal of Pharmacology, 579*, 1–12.
149. Mitomo, S., Maesawa, C., Ogasawara, S., Iwaya, T., Shibazaki, M., Yashima-Abo, A., Kotani, K., Oikawa, H., Sakurai, E., Izutsu, N., Kato, K., Komatsu, H., Ikeda, K., Wakabayashi, G., & Masuda, T. (2008). Downregulation of miR-138 is associated with overexpression of human telomerase reverse transcriptase protein in human anaplastic thyroid carcinoma cell lines. *Cancer Science, 99*, 280–286.
150. Boufraqech, M., Klubo-Gwiezdzinska, J., & Kebebew, E. (2016). MicroRNAs in the thyroid. *Best Practice & Research. Clinical Endocrinology & Metabolism, 30*, 603–619.
151. Song, J., & Li, Y. (2017). miR-25-3p reverses epithelial-mesenchymal transition via targeting Sema4C in cisplatin-resistance cervical cancer cells. *Cancer Science, 108*, 23–31.
152. Sheng, W., Chen, Y., Gong, Y., Dong, T., Zhang, B., & Gao, W. (2016). miR-148a inhibits self-renewal of thyroid cancer stem cells via repressing INO80 expression. *Oncology Reports, 36*, 3387–3396.
153. Liu, X., Wang, C., Chen, Z., Jin, Y., Wang, Y., Kolokythas, A., Dai, Y., & Zhou, X. (2011). MicroRNA138 suppresses epithelial-mesenchymal transition in squamous cell carcinoma cell lines. *The Biochemical Journal, 440*, 23–31.
154. Kong, W., Yang, H., He, L., Zhao, J.-J., Coppola, D., Dalton, W. S., & Cheng, J. Q. (2008). MicroRNA155 is regulated by the transforming growth factor/Smad pathway and contributes to epithelial cell plasticity by targeting RhoA. *Molecular and Cellular Biology, 28*, 6773–6784.

Exosomes in the Healthy and Malignant Bone Marrow Microenvironment

Caitlyn A. Moore, Alejandra I. Ferrer, Sara Alonso, Sri Harika Pamarthi, Oleta A. Sandiford, and Pranela Rameshwar

1 The Bone Marrow Microenvironment

The adult hematopoietic system is primarily located in the bone marrow (BM). BM is contained within the central cavity of long and axial bones (e.g., femur, tibia, ribs) and intra-trabecular spaces of spongy bones [1]. In healthy BM, hematopoietic stem cells (HSCs) are the most primitive cells within the hematopoietic hierarchy. Throughout an individual's lifespan, HSCs are the source of blood and immune cells. The differentiation process is regulated by cells of the BM microenvironment, via molecular and environmental cues [2]. In order to sustain this process over the long term, HSC numbers are maintained through asymmetric division, enabling these cells to self-renew [3]. In other reports, it appears that HSCs ensure their survival by a percentage remaining quite dormant unless needed by hematopoietic stress.

Our understanding of the hematopoietic system has improved dramatically over recent decades, challenging the concept of a more traditional hematopoietic hierarchy on the basis of studies that have stem cell fate are governed on a single-cell level or by cell autonomous method [4–7]. Together, such studies suggest that lineage commitment may not be as rigid as previously believed and that there are several ways by which stem cell fate can be regulated. This concept is underscored by contemporary studies that reveal a high degree of interdependency between HSCs and the BM microenvironment (BMM) [8].

As a whole, BMM includes but is not limited to hematopoietic cells (e.g., HSCs, hematopoietic progenitors), cells that comprise the BM stromal compartment (e.g., endothelial cells, osteolineage cells, adipocytes, sympathetic neurons, non-myelinating Schwann cells, mesenchymal stem cells (MSCs), CXCL12-abundant reticular (CAR) cells, macrophages, and megakaryocytes), extracellular matrix, and secreted factors (e.g., secretome). More specifically, HSC fate is orchestrated by discrete regions of the BMM known as "niches" which exhibit distinct cellular and physical compositions [9–11]. This highly complex system supports the number, location,

C. A. Moore · A. I. Ferrer · O. A. Sandiford · P. Rameshwar (✉)
Rutgers New Jersey Medical School, Rutgers University, Newark, NJ, United States

Rutgers School of Graduate Studies at New Jersey Medical School, Rutgers University, Newark, NJ, United States
e-mail: rameshwa@njms.rutgers.edu

S. Alonso
Rutgers School of Graduate Studies at New Jersey Medical School, Rutgers University, Newark, NJ, United States

S. H. Pamarthi
Rutgers New Jersey Medical School, Rutgers University, Newark, NJ, United States

D. Banerjee, R. K. Tiwari (eds.), *Tumor Microenvironment: Cellular, Metabolic and Immunologic Interactions*, Advances in Experimental Medicine and Biology 1350,
https://doi.org/10.1007/978-3-030-83282-7_3

proliferation, self-renewal capacity, and differentiation of HSCs. The relationship between the major BM niches - endosteal and perivascular - and HSC maintenance is briefly explored in the following sections.

1.1 Endosteal Niche

HSCs were first shown to reside close to the bone surface, or endosteal niche, in 1975 [12]. Later reports demonstrated that HSCs are in close contact with the endosteum and that this contact is responsible for the seemingly unlimited proliferative capacity and maturation inhibition of HSCs [13]. Further, scanning electron microscopy and histology of opened rat bone provided morphological evidence of the presence of HSC niches in association with the endosteum [14]. In the subsequent years, these phenotypic studies were bolstered by functional studies, which revealed that the endosteal HSCs have long cycling times with approximately one division every 30–60 days [15, 16]. Together, these results provide irrefutable evidence of the presence of non-proliferative, dormant HSCs as well as multipotent progenitors in the endosteal region of the BM, suggesting that the endosteal niche is the site for long-term maintenance of the quiescent HSCs.

1.2 Perivascular Niche

The BM perivascular niche is considered to be the region surrounding the arterioles and sinuses, the intersection between the systemic circulation and the BM cavity [17]. Due to the large number of perivascular HSCs, the vascular niche is widely considered to be the area of HSC proliferation and self-renewal [18]. HSCs from this niche are generally considered to be "active" or highly proliferative and are predisposed to differentiation since they are conveniently located for subsequent mobilization in the bloodstream [19]. However, this has been challenged by the idea that there may indeed be distinct vascular niches for quiescent and non-quiescent HSCs. Studies have shown that by ablating the arteriolar vascular niche, HSCs localized to sinusoidal niches where the HSCs became proliferative [20, 21].

2 Exosomes

To reiterate, there is an immense amount of heterotypic cell-cell communication within the BMM that regulates cell fate. Communication can be direct (e.g., gap junction, adhesion molecules) or indirect interactions (e.g., secretome). The "secretome" encompasses all soluble (e.g., cytokine, chemokines, growth factors, neuronal peptides, hormones) and insoluble factors (e.g., extracellular vesicles, exosomes) released from cells. Although all modes of communication are vital to proper function, the secretome, and its microvesicles in particular, is emerging as a critical player in hematopoietic regulation [9, 22–24]. Microvesicles are lipid bilayer-delimited particles released from cells that serve as a means of indirect intercellular communication by fusing to and incorporating with nearby cells [25]. Importantly, extracellular vesicles are found in all biological fluids and can also be collected from cells in vitro [25]. In this section, exosomes, a specific subclassification of extracellular vesicles, are discussed.

2.1 Characterization

To reiterate, there are various classes of extracellular vesicles, including microvesicles, apoptotic bodies, and exosomes. Each subcategory is distinguished based on size and membrane-bound markers. Exosomes range in diameter from 30 to 150 nm and express several membrane markers: CD63 (a membrane-bound protein), ALG2 (an interacting protein), TSG101 (tumor susceptibility gene 101), and HSC10 (a proteasome component) [26]. Further, exosomes have more recently been divided into two subpopulations: small exosomes (Exo-S) with diameters from 60 to 80 nm and large exosomes (Exo-L) with diameters from 90 to 120 nm [27].

2.2 Biogenesis

As compared to other subclasses of extracellular vesicles, exosomes originate in the endosome. Early endosomes are formed through inward budding of the plasma membrane and mature into late endosomes and multivesicular bodies (MVBs) [28]. MVBs are endosomes that contain internalized portions of the limiting membrane, forming "intraluminal vesicles" (ILVs) [29]. MVBs are then transported to the plasma membrane where they fuse and release their ILVs into the extracellular space as exosomes [28].

The biogenesis of exosomes is primarily controlled by the endosomal sorting complex required for transport (ESCRT) [30]. The ESCRT family is comprised of four proteins (ESCRT-0, ESCRT-I, ESCRT-II, and ESCRT-III) which act to sort ILVs into endosomes. Briefly, the endosome sorting cycle begins when ESCRT-0 is recruited to the endosome, subsequently recruiting ESCRT-I, ESCRT-II, and ESCRT-III to the endosomal membrane, forming a large complex [31, 32]. AAA ATPase Vps4 complex breaks apart the ESCRT-III subunit causing the rest of the complex to dissociate from the membrane, recycling the ESCRT machinery for subsequent cycles of sorting [33].

The ability of ILVs to form in the absence of ESCRT components has led researchers to investigate alternate ESCRT-independent pathways for vesicle formation [34]. Tetraspanins, a class of transmembrane proteins enriched in exosomes, have also been implicated for their involvement in ESCRT-independent exosome biogenesis [35–37]. Furthermore, small integral membrane proteins of the lysosome/late endosome (SIMPLE) have also been suggested to play a role in exosome formation [38]. Additionally, it is thought that the organization of certain lipids, such as lysobisphosphatidic acid and ceramides, into specialized regions results in changes in membrane curvature, leading to inward bending of the endosomal membrane and the subsequent formation of ILVs [39, 40]. Several studies have shown the involvement of lipids by targeting specific lipid-modifying enzymes, such as neural sphingomyelinase 2 (nSMase2) and phospholipase D2 (PLD2) [39, 41–43]. In total, it is important to note that due to challenges of separating these machineries experimentally, it is possible that ESCRT-dependent and ESCRT-independent pathways may be synergistic rather than discrete. Moreover, specific subpopulations of exosomes could be derived through these processes as well as cell type and microenvironmental conditions.

2.3 Cargo

Exosomes were originally proposed to be cellular waste receptacles [44]. However, contemporary studies have uncovered the important role of exosomes as crucial intercellular couriers that deliver messages through distinct molecular contents. Exosome content has been shown to vary depending on the cell from which they are released, indicating that their cargo is directly related to the cell of origin [45–47]. Exosomes contain a wide variety of proteins, lipids, metabolites, and nucleic acids, including messenger RNA (mRNA), microRNA (miRNA), noncoding RNAs (ncRNA), circular RNA (cRNA), and DNA [48, 49]. The exosomal contents change depending on growth conditions, treatments, and external factors [50]. The selectivity underlying packaging of discrete cargo into exosomes remains unclear. However, a sequence that controls the loading of miRNAs into exosomes through sumoylated heterogeneous nuclear ribonucleoprotein A2B1 (hnRNPA2B1) has been identified [51]. In addition, KRAS has been implicated in loading of miRNA and associated regulatory proteins into exosomes [52, 53]. Regarding exosomal mRNA, these molecules have enriched 3' UTRs which may guide their preferential sorting into exosomes [54]. Also, studies have demonstrated that ubiquitinated proteins are highly enriched within exosomal cargo, suggesting that ubiquitin tagging may serve as a mechanism for sorting of proteins into exosomes [55, 56]. The idea of selective exosomal packing is further supported by the differences in cargo between Exo-S and Exo-L exosome subclassifications. Exo-S contain proteins associated with endosomes and

MVBs, while Exo-L contain proteins associated with the plasma membrane, cell-cell contacts, Golgi network proteins, and the remnants of late endosomes [27].

2.4 Docking and Release

MVBs are transported from the cytoplasm for docking on the plasma membrane through interactions with the cytoskeletal network of actin and microtubules [57, 58]. Upon their arrival, MVBs must fuse with the plasma membrane in order to release exosomes into the extracellular environment. Proteins involved in membrane fusion include soluble N-ethylmaleimide-sensitive factor attachment protein receptors (SNAREs) and Rab GTPases. SNARE proteins are well-known for their role in fusion of vesicles with various target membranes [59]. Studies have shown impairment of MVB fusion with the plasma membrane, and ultimate exosome release, when interfering with the SNARE complex formation [60–63]. Also, the Rab GTPase family of proteins has been well characterized for its regulatory role in exosome secretion [64]. For instance, studies have shown that silencing of Rab27a and Rab27b prevents exosome secretion [65]. In addition, through studies using dominant-negative Rab11 mutant K562 leukemia cells, exosome release was shown to be inhibited [66]. This observation has been more recently supported through Rab11 depletion studies in *Drosophila* [60].

The question of whether all MVBs can fuse with the plasma membrane or whether there is specificity in this process remains unanswered. It has been shown that only MVBs with higher cholesterol content fuse with the membrane and release their exosomes [67]. Furthermore, it has been determined that exosomes secreted from the apical and basolateral side of polarized cells differ in composition, supporting the existence of distinct MVB populations [68–70]. Although interesting, additional studies are required to confidently resolve this issue.

2.5 Uptake and Downstream Effects

Exosomes are rapidly taken up by target cells [71]. Endocytosis is a broad term that applies to a range of pathways through which exosomes can be internalized, including clathrin-mediated endocytosis, caveolin-dependent endocytosis, micropinocytosis, and phagocytosis [72, 73]. Tetraspanins are proteins that are known to be important for mediating exosome endocytosis [74]. For instance, blocking of CD81 or CD9 on target cells using antibodies led to reduced vesicle uptake [75]. Moreover, overexpression of Tspan8 was accompanied by enhanced vesicle uptake [36]. In addition to protein-receptor interactions, exosomes are capable of fusing directly with the plasma membrane of target cells to deliver their cargo since exosomes also exhibit lipid bilayer membranes [76, 77].

Once incorporated into the target cell, exosomes regulate specific downstream pathways through their molecular cargo, giving them the ability to modulate local and distant microenvironments through paracrine and autocrine signaling [78]. The role of exosomes in the healthy BMM is illustrated in Fig. 1. In the context of cancer, however, exosomes play a major role in tumor progression and metastasis. Exosomes have been implicated in the formation of pre-metastatic niche and support of tumor progression through the promotion of angiogenesis, immune system modulation, and parenchymal tissue remodeling [79]. Cancer cells secrete exosomes that can activate receptors or change miRNA or general RNA expression in healthy neighboring cells that alter their biological phenotypes [80]. Additionally, exosomes originating from cancer cells have been shown to alter the immune response by inactivating the proliferation of lymphocytes and natural killer cells while also triggering the immune response to create an inflammatory microenvironment [81]. During metastasis, cancer cells release exosomes that led to the cells undergoing epithelial-to-mesenchymal transition (EMT). These

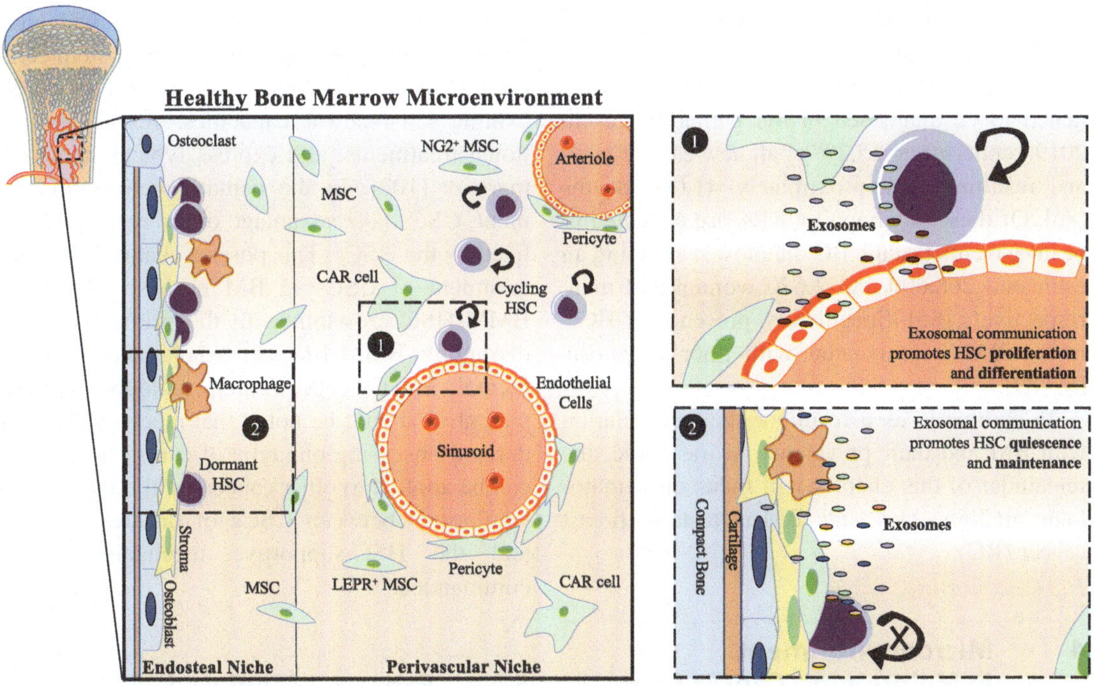

Fig. 1 Exosomes in the healthy bone marrow microenvironment. The healthy bone marrow microenvironment (BMM) is comprised of a heterogeneous population of cells that are distributed across the perivascular and endosteal niches. BMM cells communicate with hematopoietic stem cells (HSCs) in these niches to regulate their stemness and differentiation. (1) HSCs in the perivascular niche are more proliferative than those in the endosteal niche, a phenotype that is regulated through the bidirectional exchange of exosomes between mesenchymal stem cells (MSCs), CXCL12-abundant reticular (CAR) cells, endothelial cells, and HSCs. (2) In the endosteal niche, HSCs exhibit a dormant phenotype in which they are cycling quiescent. This is regulated through the exchange of exosomes between macrophages, MSCs, stroma, osteoblasts, and HSCs

changes led to mobilization and ultimately, metastasis of the EMT cells [82]. In the following sections, bidirectional exosome-mediated communication will be discussed in through the lens of specific BMM cells and malignant cells, hematologic malignancies, and BC.

3 Bone Marrow-Associated Cancers

Worldwide, one in three men and one in five women are expected to be diagnosed with cancer in their lifetime, contributing to over 200 million disability-adjusted life years [83]. The BM is an organ associated with several malignancies due to its abundance of cells and signaling factors. Not surprisingly, cancers of the hematopoietic system, referred to as hematologic malignancies, originate in the BM. Furthermore, cancer cells from other solid tumors elsewhere in the body are reported to metastasize to BM, including cells from breast, gastric, prostate, colon, and lung cancers [84]. In order to narrow the scope of this chapter, we will specifically focus on BC in BM herein.

In addition to the putative role of the BMM in their progression, these malignancies affect substantial populations of Americans each year. Hematologic malignancies ("BM cancers," "blood cancers," or "liquid tumors"), such as leukemias (acute myelogenous leukemia [AML], chronic myelogenous leukemia [CML], acute lymphoblastic leukemia [ALL], chronic lymphoblastic leukemia [CLL]), lymphomas, and myelodysplastic disorders (multiple myeloma [MM]), were the subject of 176,000 new diagnoses and 56,000 American deaths in 2019 alone [85]. Moreover, in BC, over 315,000 cases are estimated to be diagnosed in the United States in 2019, representing 15.2% of all new cancer cases and resulting in approximately 41,000 deaths [86]. Of these, a whopping 81% are expected to be invasive/metastatic BC diagnoses, affecting an estimated 268,600 and 2,670 women and men, respectively [86]. Specifically, presence of BCC in the BM is associated with poor prognosis [87–89].

In summary, as a result of their association with BM and their prevalence in the clinic, the remainder of this chapter will focus on hematologic malignancies and BM-metastatic breast cancer (BC).

4 Microenvironment in Maintaining Cancer Stem Cells

The tumor microenvironment has been described as a "complex adaptive system" due to its unique and dynamic characteristics [9, 90]. Moreover, there is mounting evidence to suggest an intricate relationship between cancer cells and cells native to the BMM. In particular, cancer cells are able to appropriate the established mechanisms used for the BM to support healthy HSCs to promote their own survival. For example, leukemia cells have been shown to hijack the secretome of the BMM to induce leukemogenesis, progression, and therapy resistance [22, 23, 91]. Also, experimental models have established a variety of alterations in the BMM perturb normal hematopoiesis and promote malignant transformation [92–97]. Furthermore, in terms of BM-metastatic BC, disseminated BC cells (BCCs) have also been reported to hijack the BMM. The BMM confers BCCs with a dormant phenotype, characterized by cell cycling quiescence and chemoresistance [98–101]. By displaying this dormant phenotype, BCCs can evade the immune system and persist within the marrow for decades. Upon eventual activation, dormant BCCs can metastasize to tertiary sites and lead to cancer resurgence.

Additionally, dormant BCCs, like leukemia stem cells, exhibit properties of cancer stem cells (CSCs); they act as tumor-initiating cells which exhibit self-renewal capacities, resist conventional treatments, and express typical stem cell markers [102]. In the hematopoietic compartment, CSCs take advantage of the resources utilized by the HSCs. This poses a challenge for the treatment of CSCs in BM because disrupting BMM-HSC crosstalk with the primary aim of disrupting BMM-BCC crosstalk can be detrimental for the HSCs and, undoubtebly, the patient. It should be noted that much of the data derived observing one type of cancer in the BM can be applied to other cancers in the BM due to similarities between CSCs of different origins and the HSC-supportive mechanisms they commandeer.

5 Exosome-Mediated Communication: Hematologic Malignancies

5.1 Endothelial Cells

ECs promote normal HSC maintenance in vitro and in vivo [103–107]. This is thought to occur both indirectly through soluble factors and directly through SLAM receptors [108–110]. More recently, EC-derived exosomes, specifically, have also been shown play an important role in hematologic cancer progression. In terms of angiogenesis, exosomes from K562 CML cells induce angiogenic activity in human umbilical endothelial cells (HUVECs) via transfer of miR-92a and inhibition of oncogenic signaling via the mutated Src kinase BCR-ABL [111–113]. In vitro tube formation and tube length were twice that of control ECs. Importantly, another study found that CML exosomes released under hypoxic conditions promote more robust tube formation due to increased levels of miR-210 which downregulates ERNA3, a known inhibitor of angiogenesis [114]. This is consistent with the current understanding that hypoxia is a driver of angiogenesis. Alternatively, MM cells secrete exosomes enriched with miR-135b [112]. This miRNA targets the FIH-1 gene in ECs, increasing hypoxic tube formation via HIF-FIH pathway in vitro and enhancing neovascularization in vivo [112]. Furthermore, hypoxia upregulates expression of the miR-17-92 family, stimulating angiogenesis in tumor-associated ECs via direct repression of secreted antiangiogenic molecules TSP-1 and CTGF [115].

The importance of exosomal interactions with ECs is not limited to angiogenesis. Recent studies consider EC-derived miR-126 to be a regulator of self-renewal in leukemia SCs in CML [116]. Additionally, exosomes from CLL cells have been shown to be incorporated by ECs and MSCs inducing inflammatory phenotype and transformation into cancer-associated fibroblast cells [117]. Increases were observed in the proliferation and inflammatory cytokine secretion as well as angiogenic capacities of exposed BMM cells [117].

5.2 Mesenchymal Stem Cells (MSCs)

Normal perivascular HSCs are supported by a variety of mesenchymal cells, such as MSCs, CXCL12-abundant reticular (CAR) cells, and pericytes. These cells are located adjacent to sinusoids and are co-localized with HSCs. The niche cells exert significant effects within the BMM, including synthesis of factors to regulate HSC functions, such as the production of stem cell factor (SCF) and CXCL12 [118–121]. Nestin$^+$ MSCs can be further categorized as periarteriolar (NG2$^+$) or perisinusoidal (LEPR$^+$). Activation of HSC cycling was shown mediate the relocation of HSCs from NG2$^+$ periarteriolar niches to LEPR$^+$ perisinusoidal niches, indicating that periarteriolar niches are critical for HSC quiescence while sinusoidal niches support HSC proliferation [20].

In addition to their role in normal hematopoiesis, several studies implicate MSCs and their exosomes in hematologic malignancies. PKH26-labeled AML-derived exosomes have been shown to be taken up readily by BM-derived MSCs [122]. These exosomes carry several RNA transcripts relevant to leukemia pathogenesis, including FLT3, NPM1, CXCR4, MMP9, or IGF-1R, as well as miR-150 which directly targets CXCR4 [122]. MSCs and other stromal cells release CXCL12, the ligand CXCR4 expressed on HSCs and leukemic SCs homing to the BM [123]. Due to increased abundance of miR-150, migration toward CXCL12 decreased as a result of reduced CXCR4 surface expression in target cells, suggesting that leukemia exosomes promote their own growth through modulation of MSCs [122]. This finding is highlighted in studies that compare MSCs before and after exposure to malignant cells. For instance, exosomes released from BM-MSCs, which were exposed to multiple myeloma (MM), contained higher levels of oncogenic proteins, cytokines, and adhesion molecules relative to exosomes from unexposed BM-MSC [124]. When taken up by MM cells, MM-exposed BM-MSC exosomes promote MM growth, while MM-naïve BM-MSC exosomes inhibited cell growth [124]. In addition, another study showed BM stromal cells promoting MM cell migration through exosomal transfer of chemotactic proteins [125].

MSCs are well-known for their ability to modulate the immune response, a characteristic that is leveraged by malignant cells to promote their own survival. Chronic lymphoid leukemia (CLL)-derived exosomes transfer miRNAs and proteins into MSCs that induce an inflammatory phenotype and transform MSCs into cancer-associated fibroblasts [117]. MSC-derived exosomes have also been shown to inhibit proliferation of activated lymphocytes [126]. Moreover, like MSC plasma membranes, MSC exosomes express galectin-1 [127, 128]. Galectin-1 has been shown to induce apoptosis of activated T cells and promote the generation of regulatory T cells (Tregs) [129, 130]. Similarly, PD-L1, a negative costimulatory molecule for PD-1, is expressed on MSC exosomes, promoting proliferation and function of Tregs [131, 132]. In addition, exosomes from MSCs express TGF-β which is a notable inducer of Tregs [133, 134]. Altogether, these studies demonstrate that MSC exosomes promote immune tolerance and cancer progression through their cargo and surface proteins.

5.3 Macrophages

The role of macrophages in maintenance of normal and malignant hematopoietic cells continues to be investigated. Previous studies demonstrated that macrophages inhibit osteoblast function and elicit a robust HSPC mobilization [135]. In addition, macrophages treated with CML-derived exosomes exhibited reduced levels of nitric oxide and reactive oxygen species and increased levels of TNF-α and IL-10, suggesting that these exosomes may alter the local BMM to become leukemia-reinforcing [136].

5.4 Osteoblasts

Osteoblasts within the BM endosteal niche can also support hematopoiesis [137–139]. Interestingly, the number of HSCs is increased in areas where new trabecular bone is formed, and, as such, its surface is enriched with osteoblasts [140]. Although these studies were performed in the context of normal hematopoiesis, the information can be extrapolated to understand how osteoblasts contribute to BM niche-mediated support of dysregulated hematopoiesis and hematological malignancy. Hematological malignancy can influence BMM, including cancer-derived exosomes as mediators. For instance, MM can survive in within bone lesions, consequent to imbalanced osteoblast-osteoclast ratio. This imbalance has been shown to be caused by MM cell-derived exosomes, resulting in increased IL-6 production in MSCs. The IL-6 then suppressed osteoblastic differentiation, resulting in increased osteoclasts [141]. This observation has been corroborated by other studies that demonstrated dysregulation of osteoblast differentiation and function with enhanced osteoclast through exosomal transfer of Dickkopf WNT signaling pathway inhibitor-1 (DKK-1) [142]. Also, AML-derived exosomes downregulated normal osteogenesis-related genes and upregulate genes associated with AML survival and growth [23].

6 Exosome-Mediated Communication: Bone Marrow-Metastatic Breast Cancer

6.1 Endothelial Cells

The primary BC microenvironment is highly vascularized and facilitates BC metastasis to secondary organs, such as BM. Nonmetastatic BCCs induce vascular permeability through secretion of miR-105 which targets the tight junction protein ZO-1, facilitating metastasis to secondary organs, such as BM [143]. Conversely, inhibition of miR-105 in highly metastatic BCCs mitigates vascular permeability and metastasis [143]. As such, miR-105 levels in the circulation and tumor during clinical premetastatic stages correlate to ZO-1 expression, serving as a potential diagnostic biomarker for metastatic progression in early-stage BC. Furthermore, similar to the primary tumor, upon metastasis to BM, vascularity of BM increases [144]. Exosomes from BCCs activate VEGF signaling in endothelial cells promoting angiogenesis within the tumor niche. Inhibition of exosome release by direct targeting of HSP90 potentiated the function of bevacizumab, a VEGF inhibitor [145]. However, it has been shown that MSC exosomes can suppress proliferation and migration of ECs through the downregulation of VEGF expression in BCCs [146].

6.2 Mesenchymal Stem Cells

The role of MSC-derived exosomes in metastasis, invasion, and premetastatic niche formation has been studied. The low invasive/metastatic MCF7 BCCs exhibit enhanced migratory capacity following treatment with MSC exosomes. Furthermore, exosome treatment led to significant increases in β-catenin mRNA and protein levels and expression of WNT target genes, suggesting that MSC exosomes promote BCC migration [147]. Furthermore, CAR cells, a subtype of MSCs, are located on the abluminal region of the vasculature and are characterized primarily by high expression of CXCL12. As discussed previously, the CXCL12-CXCR4 signaling axis is critical for homing of normal and malignant SCs to the bone marrow [123]. Additionally, CXCL12-CXCR4 signaling is critical for recruitment of BCCs into the BM [148, 149].

Similar to hematologic malignancies, MSCs are implicated in regulating immune phenotype, differentiation, cycling quiescence, and chemoresistance of BCCs. Increased miR-23b and decreased myristoylated alanine-rich protein C-kinase substrate (MARCKS) in BM-MSC exosomes have been shown to induce cycling quiescence and chemoresistance of BCCs [98, 150]. Furthermore, MSC exosomes have also been implicated in the differentiation of myeloid-derived suppressor cells into M2 macrophages, supporting tumor growth [151]. TGF-β can act as mediator in MSC-induced tolerance of BCCs in the BMM through suppression of CD8+ T cells and NK function with concomitant increase of Tregs [152].

6.3 Macrophages

Depending on the microenvironmental cues, macrophages can promote or suppress BC development in the BM niche. A recent study indicated that BCC-derived exosomes educate macrophages to release pro-inflammatory cytokines that potentially recruit other immune cells, and ultimately, enhance metastasis [153]. Interestingly, BCC-derived exosomes activated toll-like receptor (TLR)-2 to induce NF-kB signaling in macrophages, which resulted in the secretion of pro-inflammatory cytokines to increase tumor metastasis [153]. In addition, BCC-derived exosomes facilitate macrophage polarization into an M2 phenotype to promote metastasis from the primary site to lymph nodes [154].

Since the crosstalk between macrophages and BCCs is bidirectional, exosomes released from macrophages can reprogram cancer cells to facilitate survival or decrease tumor burden. For instance, apoptotic BCCs enhance the release of exosomes from macrophages that further the progress of the tumor by inducing IL-6 signaling and increasing Cyclin-D1 levels [155]. M1-derived exosomes have antitumor properties by stimulating caspase-3 signaling in BCCs and can serve as a carrier of therapeutic agents, such as paclitaxel, to reduce tumor growth [156]. Our previous studies demonstrated that M2 macrophages can form gap junctional intercellular communication (GJIC) with breast CSCs in the BM and this was important for maintaining dormancy [47]. An opposite effect was observed with M1 macrophages, which promoted BCC metastasis to distant organs via exosomes [47].

6.4 Osteoblasts

BCCs migrate from the perivascular niche of the BM toward the endosteum. Osteoblasts are bone-depositing cells critical for the maintenance of bone structure. An imbalance between bone removal and deposition can be advantageous for cancer cells to establish within the niche. Such impairment has been reported in rodents and humans with metastatic BCC in which lesions are often presented as a hallmark of bone metastasis. In the endosteal niche, osteoblasts become educated by BCCs which results in achievement of cellular dormancy and stemness in the latter [157]. Another study indicated that osteoblasts can support cellular dormancy in BCCs in a Notch2-dependent manner. Disruption of Notch signaling resulted in BCC migration, proliferation, and decreased stemness [158]. In addition, BCCs release miRNAs such as miR-218 within extracellular vesicles to target collagen type-I alpha-1 chain (Col1α1) to decrease collagen secretion and suppress bone remodeling [159]. BCC-derived exosomes carrying miR-940 contribute to differentiation of MSCs into osteoblasts by targeting *ARHGAP1* and *FAM134A* to induce bone lesions in vivo and facilitate metastasis to the niche [160]. Furthermore, osteoblasts treated with BCC-derived exosomes induced expression of pro-osteoclast factors and cytokine release involved in the regulation of osteoclastogenesis [161]. Overall, osteoblasts in the endosteal niche are critical for the establishment and stabilization of BCC dormancy in BM.

7 Therapeutic Strategies

7.1 Current Therapies

Cancer treatment mainly consists of chemotherapy and/or radiotherapy which targets rapidly dividing cancer cells as well as rapidly dividing healthy cells. As a result of this lack of specificity, many patients experience untoward effects like hair loss, gastrointestinal symptoms, and myelosuppression. In addition, these treatments inadvertently induce selection of treatment-resistant clones that are implicated in cancer resurgence and an associated increase in mortality rates. At present, chemotherapy continues to be the first-line treatment for liquid and solid cancers despite poor patient prognoses.

Treatment for hematologic malignancies can combine chemotherapy with HSC transplantation (HSCT), radiotherapy, or newly developed molecular-based targeted therapies. HSCT is considered to be an adjuvant therapy option for patients resistant to chemotherapy and sometimes as post-remission therapy [162, 163]. HSCT involves transferring HSCs from the patient (autologous) or a donor (allogenic) into the patient following ablation of the patient's dysfunctional hematopoietic system. Although this procedure has undergone massive improvements over recent decades, major disadvantages of these therapies continue to include graft-versus-host disease (GvHD), drug toxicities, and risk of relapse due to presence of residual cancer cells [164, 165]. Altogether, HSCT has higher therapeutic benefit compared to standard chemotherapy and radiotherapy strategies, but its use is limited due to potential complications.

To minimize limitations of conventional therapies, many US Food and Drug Administration (FDA) clinical trials have been initiated for novel targeted therapies (most commonly monoclonal antibodies or molecular agents) that specifically interfere with molecular mechanisms that contribute to the growth and survival of cancer cells [166–168]. These targeted approaches aim to spare healthy cells, reducing adverse side effects experienced by patients. Remarkably, recent advances in high-throughput sequencing technologies have provided important insight into cancer initiation, progression, and heterogeneity. For instance, multi-omics investigations of genetic variants in liquid tumors have revealed over 120 genes that act as "drivers" for cancer cell survival [22]. Such genetic alterations can be utilized in precision medicine to improve the diagnosis of hematologic malignancies and identify targeted therapies to address the disease [169, 170].

Recently, several targeted therapies have been approved by the FDA to treat acute myeloid leukemia (AML) such as midostaurin (tyrosine kinase inhibitor) [171], gilteritinib (FLT3 inhibitor) [172], enasidenib and ivosidenib (isocitrate dehydrogenase inhibitors) [173, 174], glasdegib (hedgehog pathway inhibitor) [175], venetoclax (BCL2 inhibitor) [176], and gemtuzumab ozogamicin (monoclonal anti-CD33 conjugated antibody) [177]. Disadvantages of these approved strategies include inability to effectively address genetic heterogeneity and resistance developed by malignant cells either through alteration of the structure of the targeted molecule or the mechanistic pathway involved in cancer progression [178, 179].

7.2 Exosome-Based Therapies

Furthermore, as discussed in previous sections, increasing evidence suggests that the BMM is involved in the development of cancer through intercellular mediators, such as exosomes [180, 181]. Thus, it is theorized that current treatments lack clinical efficacy due to the role of the BMM [9, 10, 91, 182]. Hence, therapeutic strategies targeting exosome production, secretion, and uptake may be a viable avenue for improving therapeutic efficacy in patients with hematologic or BM-metastatic cancers. To address this need, numerous ongoing preclinical and clinical trials aim to identify targetable exosome-associated pathways involved in cancer progression and drug resistance. Inhibition of exosome formation by dimethyl amiloride resulted in reduced function of myeloid-derived suppressor cells that are implicated in cancer support by dampening the immune response [183]. Inhibiting B-cell lymphoma exosome production via indomethacin has also been shown to improve sensitivity of B-cell lymphoma to doxorubicin and pixantrone [184]. Similarly, MM cells show increased sensitivity to bortezomib when combined with administration of nSMase inhibitor GW4869 [142]. AML-derived exosomes have also been found to transfer chemoresistance from drug-resistant cells to sensitive cells, making targeting of exosome production and release a viable therapeutic route [185]. Along a similar vein, researchers have also attempted to develop technologies to remove pathogenic exosomes. Based on previously reported affinity hemodialysis technologies for other conditions [186–188], one group attempted to clear tumorigenesis-specific exosomes from bodily fluids which could act as a potential route for adjuvant therapy [189].

Targeting of specific exosome cargo has also been investigated for therapeutic uses. For example, intricate high-throughput microscopy studies revealed that PC12 cell-derived exosomes taken up by BM-MSCs elicit miR-21-dependent downregulation of TGF-β receptor II and tropomyosin-1 expression, two proteins implicated in cancer progression [190]. This study also identified that the PC12 cell-derived exosomes were endocytosed via clathrin-mediated endocytosis and micropinocytosis, allowing for several potential points of therapeutic intervention [190]. In addition, comparison of exosomes of imatinib-resistant and imatinib-sensitive CML cells proved that exosomes derived from imatinib-resistant CML cells contained a significantly higher abundance of miR-365, indicating that miR-365 may be a viable therapeutic target to increase imatinib sensitivity [191].

Furthermore, exosomes are attractive as drug delivery vehicles due to their nanoscale dimensions and ability to deliver their cargo to target cells [192]. An ideal drug delivery system enables controlled, site-specific delivery of therapeutic agent, avoids recognition, and prevents premature degradation by the immune system. Exosomes are less likely to be considered immunogenic or cytotoxic than synthetic delivery systems due to their endogenous origin. In addition, exosomes may protect encapsulated agents from rapid clearance in the blood, reducing systemic cytotoxicity. This is bolstered by the fact that exosomes show little long-term accumulation in any specific organ or tissue [193]. Therapeutic agents have successfully been loaded into exosomes. For example, paclitaxel was loaded into MSCs which subsequently released the drug via exosomes [194]. Treatment with paclitaxel-loaded exosomes led to decreased proliferation of pancreatic cancer cells compared to control exosomes, indicating successful packaging and delivery of active drug via exosomes [194]. Additionally, another group loaded exosomes with catalase, a potent antioxidant, for the treatment of Parkinson's disease [195]. Of the five drug loading processes trialed, sonication, extrusion, and permeabilization with saponin resulted in high catalase loading efficiency, sustained release, preservation of catalase against protease degradation, and satisfactory uptake of exosomes by neuronal cells [195].

The exosome-based therapeutic strategies described throughout this section are summarized in Fig. 2.

7.3 Limitations of Exosome-Based Therapies

Exosome-based drug delivery and therapeutic strategies appear promising, but there are several issues that must be addressed before safe and effective implementation in the clinical setting. First, ensuring the purity and abundance of exosomes is critical for development of exosome-based therapies. Therefore, exosome isolation and purification processes must be optimized and subsequently standardized in order to eliminate contaminants and improve reproducibility. Similarly, donor cells that provide a stable source of exosomes must be identified and their exosomes fully characterized. Culture conditions for these cells must be optimized and standardized to mitigate any effects on exosome production and encapsulated cargo. Moreover, more efficient processes to load drugs into exosomes must be developed to maximize efficiency of production

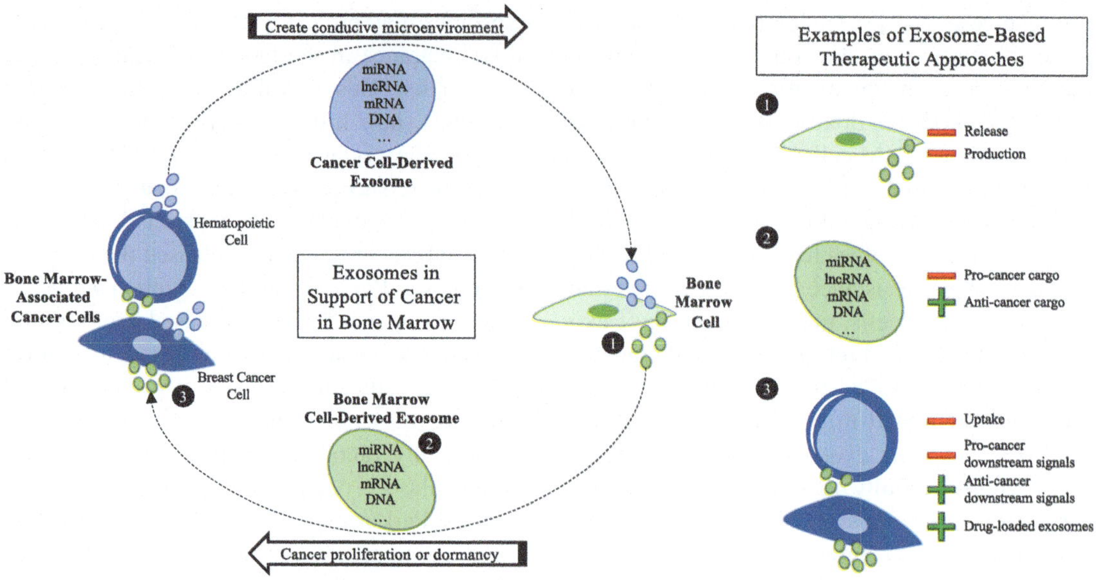

Fig. 2 **Strategies for leveraging exosomal communication for cancer therapeutics.** Exosomes are transferred bidirectionally between bone marrow (BM)-associated cancer cells and BM cells (left). Through this communication, the BM is made more conducive for cancer survival through supporting proliferation or dormancy of cancer cells. Exosomes can be used for therapeutics in several ways, for example (right), (1) blocking the release or production of exosomes, (2) inhibition of pro-cancer cargo or enhancement of anti-cancer cargo, and (3) interfering with uptake or downstream pro-cancer signaling, increasing anticancer downstream signals, or introducing releasing drugs carried via exosomes

and delivery of therapeutic agents. These processes must also be standardized to decrease inadvertent disruption of exosome integrity.

7.4 3D BMM: In Vitro Approaches to Improve Clinical Efficacy

Studies report FDA approval rates for drugs continually hovering around 10% [196, 197]. Of all drugs, cancer drugs have the lowest overall success rate, with only 5.1% of drugs that enter Phase 1 trials ultimately achieving FDA Approval [197]. Fifty-four percent of investigational drugs fail in late-stage clinical development (during or after Phase 3) [198]. Of these failed drugs, 57% failed due to "inadequate efficacy," indicating that research and development approaches must evolve in order to improve clinical efficacy [198]. One approach to reduce the drug clinical trial failure rate is incorporation of three-dimensional (3D) in vitro cell culture systems into preclinical biomedical research. It is well-understood that subjecting cells to a 3D landscape that mimics the nature of the desired native tissue elicits cellular responses that are more similar to that of cells in vivo than two-dimensional (2D) culture [199, 200]. As such, 3D culture provides a more physiologically relevant step in which potential drugs can be vetted preclinically, bridging tests in 2D systems and animal models, consequently lessening failures in the clinic. Thus, 3D models are vital for efficient drug development and improving understanding of the tissue in both health and disease.

Historically, BM has proven to be a complicated organ to study in vitro due to its pliant structure and complex cellular landscape. Although challenging, several groups have attempted to recapitulate the HSC niche in 3D in vitro models. Recent work has demonstrated increased maintenance of immature human and mouse hematopoietic cells when cultured in 3D scaffolds composed of polyurethane foam with stromal support cells [201], cancellous bone with MSC-derived osteoblasts as support cells [202], poly(D,L-lactide-co-glycolide) or polyurethane with collagen type-1 [203], and porous polyvinyl formal resin with stromal support cells [204]. Furthermore, maintenance and expansion of primitive human HSCs co-cultured with MSCs was demonstrated in 3D collagen-I and fibrin gel matrices [205, 206]. It was suggested in these studies that 3D scaffolds act as a stimulus and encourage the MSCs to mimic the BM microenvironment, indirectly providing critical cues to the HSCs. In terms of applicability for cancer pathophysiology and exosomes, silk scaffolds have been used to investigate the influence of exosomes from normal BM-MSCs and MM-exposed BM-MSCs on MM cells [124]. This study enabled the identification of several molecules that are distinct to MM-exposed BM-MSCs that may serve as candidate therapeutic targets. The 3D tissue-engineered BM model developed by de la Puente and colleagues allowed for physiologically relevant interactions between BMM cells and MM cells, including soluble gradients and induced drug resistance, as well as MM cell proliferation [207]. The group plans to utilize this model for the development of personalized therapies for MM patients, and this model is also ripe for use for the study of exosomes in the normal and malignant BMM, enabling identification of specific exosomal targets.

8 Conclusion

The BMM plays an undeniable role in maintenance of normal hematopoiesis. However, this mechanism through which HSCs depend on the BM is exploited by malignant cells. Through the exchange of exosomes among other factors, cells from hematologic malignancies and BM-metastatic BC derive support from distinct cell types in the BMM and, ultimately, promote their own survival. Current and future studies will gain a better understanding of exosomal heterotypic interactions in the tumor microenvironment. This will allow scientists to develop more effective therapies that take into account the role of the BMM. Exosome-based therapies are promising approaches to target intercellular communication that can serve also as an adjuvant to current approved therapies. The method by which to deliver develop exosomal treatment remain a challenge. By integrating 3D in in vitro modeling into the target identification and exosome therapy development paradigm, we can ensure higher rates of effective translation into preclinical and clinical settings.

References

1. Travlos, G. S. (2006). Normal structure, function, and histology of the bone marrow. *Toxicologic Pathology, 34*(5), 548–565.
2. Weissman, I. L. (2000). Stem cells: units of development, units of regeneration, and units in evolution. *Cell, 100*(1), 157–168.
3. He, S., Nakada, D., & Morrison, S. J. (2009). Mechanisms of stem cell self-renewal. *Annual Review of Cell and Developmental Biology, 25*, 377–406.
4. Pellin, D., Loperfido, M., Baricordi, C., Wolock, S. L., Montepeloso, A., Weinberg, O. K., Biffi, A., Klein, A. M., & Biasco, L. (2019). A comprehensive single cell transcriptional landscape of human hematopoietic progenitors. *Nature Communications, 10*(1), 2395.
5. Laurenti, E., & Gottgens, B. (2018). From haematopoietic stem cells to complex differentiation landscapes. *Nature, 553*(7689), 418–426.
6. Ye, F., Huang, W., & Guo, G. (2017). Studying hematopoiesis using single-cell technologies. *Journal of Hematology & Oncology, 10*(1), 27.
7. Buenrostro, J. D., Corces, M. R., Lareau, C. A., Wu, B., Schep, A. N., Aryee, M. J., Majeti, R., Chang, H. Y., & Greenleaf, W. J. (2018). Integrated Single-Cell Analysis Maps the Continuous Regulatory Landscape of Human Hematopoietic Differentiation. *Cell, 173*(6), 1535–1548. e16.
8. Hoggatt, J., Kfoury, Y., & Scadden, D. T. (2016). Hematopoietic Stem Cell Niche in Health and Disease. *Annual Review of Pathology, 11*, 555–581.
9. Omidi, Y., & Barar, J. (2014). Targeting tumor microenvironment: crossing tumor interstitial fluid by multifunctional nanomedicines. *BioImpacts: BI, 4*(2), 55–67.
10. Goulard, M., Dosquet, C., & Bonnet, D. (2018). Role of the microenvironment in myeloid malignancies. *Cellular and Molecular Life Sciences, 75*(8), 1377–1391.
11. Lee, M. W., Ryu, S., Kim, D. S., Lee, J. W., Sung, K. W., Koo, H. H., & Yoo, K. H. (2019). Mesenchymal stem cells in suppression or progression of hema-

tologic malignancy: current status and challenges. *Leukemia, 33*(3), 597–611.
12. Lord, B. I., Testa, N. G., & Hendry, J. H. (1975). The relative spatial distributions of CFUs and CFUc in the normal mouse femur. *Blood, 46*(1), 65–72.
13. Schofield, R. (1978). The relationship between the spleen colony-forming cell and the haemopoietic stem cell. *Blood Cells, 4*(1-2), 7–25.
14. Gong, J. K. (1978). Endosteal marrow: a rich source of hematopoietic stem cells. *Science, 199*(4336), 1443–1445.
15. Bradford, G. B., Williams, B., Rossi, R., & Bertoncello, I. (1997). Quiescence, cycling, and turnover in the primitive hematopoietic stem cell compartment. *Experimental Hematology, 25*(5), 445–453.
16. Cheshier, S. H., Morrison, S. J., Liao, X., & Weissman, I. L. (1999). In vivo proliferation and cell cycle kinetics of long-term self-renewing hematopoietic stem cells. *Proceedings of the National Academy of Sciences of the United States of America, 96*(6), 3120–3125.
17. Morrison, S. J., & Scadden, D. T. (2014). The bone marrow niche for haematopoietic stem cells. *Nature, 505*(7483), 327–334.
18. Wilson, A., & Trumpp, A. (2006). Bone-marrow haematopoietic-stem-cell niches. *Nature Reviews. Immunology, 6*(2), 93–106.
19. Kopp, H. G., Avecilla, S. T., Hooper, A. T., & Rafii, S. (2005). The bone marrow vascular niche: home of HSC differentiation and mobilization. *Physiology (Bethesda), 20*, 349–356.
20. Kunisaki, Y., Bruns, I., Scheiermann, C., Ahmed, J., Pinho, S., Zhang, D., Mizoguchi, T., Wei, Q., Lucas, D., Ito, K., Mar, J. C., Bergman, A., & Frenette, P. S. (2013). Arteriolar niches maintain haematopoietic stem cell quiescence. *Nature, 502*(7473), 637–643.
21. Kunisaki, Y., & Frenette, P. S. (2014). Influences of vascular niches on hematopoietic stem cell fate. *International Journal of Hematology, 99*(6), 699–705.
22. Di Meo, A., Bartlett, J., Cheng, Y., Pasic, M. D., & Yousef, G. M. (2017). Liquid biopsy: a step forward towards precision medicine in urologic malignancies. *Molecular Cancer, 16*(1), 80.
23. Kumar, B., Garcia, M., Weng, L., Jung, X., Murakami, J. L., Hu, X., McDonald, T., Lin, A., Kumar, A. R., DiGiusto, D. L., Stein, A. S., Pullarkat, V. A., Hui, S. K., Carlesso, N., Kuo, Y. H., Bhatia, R., Marcucci, G., & Chen, C. C. (2018). Acute myeloid leukemia transforms the bone marrow niche into a leukemia-permissive microenvironment through exosome secretion. *Leukemia, 32*(3), 575–587.
24. Agas, D., Lacava, G., & Sabbieti, M. G. (2018). Bone and bone marrow disruption by endocrine-active substances. *Journal of Cellular Physiology, 234*(1), 192–213.
25. Raposo, G., & Stoorvogel, W. (2013). Extracellular vesicles: exosomes, microvesicles, and friends. *The Journal of Cell Biology, 200*(4), 373–383.
26. Bobrie, A., Colombo, M., Krumeich, S., Raposo, G., & Thery, C. (2012). Diverse subpopulations of vesicles secreted by different intracellular mechanisms are present in exosome preparations obtained by differential ultracentrifugation. *Journal of Extracellular Vesicles, 1.*
27. Zhang, H., Freitas, D., Kim, H. S., Fabijanic, K., Li, Z., Chen, H., Mark, M. T., Molina, H., Martin, A. B., Bojmar, L., Fang, J., Rampersaud, S., Hoshino, A., Matei, I., Kenific, C. M., Nakajima, M., Mutvei, A. P., Sansone, P., Buehring, W., ... Lyden, D. (2018). Identification of distinct nanoparticles and subsets of extracellular vesicles by asymmetric flow field-flow fractionation. *Nature Cell Biology, 20*(3), 332–343.
28. Xu, R., Rai, A., Chen, M., Suwakulsiri, W., Greening, D. W., & Simpson, R. J. (2018). Extracellular vesicles in cancer - implications for future improvements in cancer care. *Nature Reviews. Clinical Oncology, 15*(10), 617–638.
29. Babst, M. (2011). MVB vesicle formation: ESCRT-dependent, ESCRT-independent and everything in between. *Current Opinion in Cell Biology, 23*(4), 452–457.
30. Henne, W. M., Stenmark, H., & Emr, S. D. (2013). Molecular mechanisms of the membrane sculpting ESCRT pathway. *Cold Spring Harbor Perspectives in Biology, 5*(9).
31. Katzmann, D. J., Odorizzi, G., & Emr, S. D. (2002). Receptor downregulation and multivesicular-body sorting. *Nature Reviews. Molecular Cell Biology, 3*(12), 893–905.
32. Raiborg, C., Rusten, T. E., & Stenmark, H. (2003). Protein sorting into multivesicular endosomes. *Current Opinion in Cell Biology, 15*(4), 446–455.
33. Piper, R. C., & Katzmann, D. J. (2007). Biogenesis and function of multivesicular bodies. *Annual Review of Cell and Developmental Biology, 23*, 519–547.
34. Stuffers, S., Sem Wegner, C., Stenmark, H., & Brech, A. (2009). Multivesicular endosome biogenesis in the absence of ESCRTs. *Traffic, 10*(7), 925–937.
35. Escola, J. M., Kleijmeer, M. J., Stoorvogel, W., Griffith, J. M., Yoshie, O., & Geuze, H. J. (1998). Selective enrichment of tetraspan proteins on the internal vesicles of multivesicular endosomes and on exosomes secreted by human B-lymphocytes. *The Journal of Biological Chemistry, 273*(32), 20121–20127.
36. Nazarenko, I., Rana, S., Baumann, A., McAlear, J., Hellwig, A., Trendelenburg, M., Lochnit, G., Preissner, K. T., & Zoller, M. (2010). Cell surface tetraspanin Tspan8 contributes to molecular pathways of exosome-induced endothelial cell activation. *Cancer Research, 70*(4), 1668–1678.
37. Hurwitz, S. N., Nkosi, D., Conlon, M. M., York, S. B., Liu, X., Tremblay, D. C., & Meckes, D. G., Jr. (2017). CD63 regulates epstein-barr virus LMP1 exosomal packaging, enhancement of vesicle

production, and noncanonical NF-kappaB signaling. *Journal of Virology, 91*(5).
38. Zhu, H., Guariglia, S., Yu, R. Y., Li, W., Brancho, D., Peinado, H., Lyden, D., Salzer, J., Bennett, C., & Chow, C. W. (2013). Mutation of SIMPLE in Charcot-Marie-Tooth 1C alters production of exosomes. *Molecular Biology of the Cell, 24*(11), 1619-37, S1-3.
39. Trajkovic, K., Hsu, C., Chiantia, S., Rajendran, L., Wenzel, D., Wieland, F., Schwille, P., Brugger, B., & Simons, M. (2008). Ceramide triggers budding of exosome vesicles into multivesicular endosomes. *Science, 319*(5867), 1244–1247.
40. Matsuo, H., Chevallier, J., Mayran, N., Le Blanc, I., Ferguson, C., Faure, J., Blanc, N. S., Matile, S., Dubochet, J., Sadoul, R., Parton, R. G., Vilbois, F., & Gruenberg, J. (2004). Role of LBPA and Alix in multivesicular liposome formation and endosome organization. *Science, 303*(5657), 531–534.
41. Phuyal, S., Hessvik, N. P., Skotland, T., Sandvig, K., & Llorente, A. (2014). Regulation of exosome release by glycosphingolipids and flotillins. *The FEBS Journal, 281*(9), 2214–2227.
42. Laulagnier, K., Grand, D., Dujardin, A., Hamdi, S., Vincent-Schneider, H., Lankar, D., Salles, J. P., Bonnerot, C., Perret, B., & Record, M. (2004). PLD2 is enriched on exosomes and its activity is correlated to the release of exosomes. *FEBS Letters, 572*(1-3), 11–14.
43. Ghossoub, R., Lembo, F., Rubio, A., Gaillard, C. B., Bouchet, J., Vitale, N., Slavik, J., Machala, M., & Zimmermann, P. (2014). Syntenin-ALIX exosome biogenesis and budding into multivesicular bodies are controlled by ARF6 and PLD2. *Nature Communications, 5*, 3477.
44. Johnstone, R. M., Adam, M., Hammond, J. R., Orr, L., & Turbide, C. (1987). Vesicle formation during reticulocyte maturation. Association of plasma membrane activities with released vesicles (exosomes). *The Journal of Biological Chemistry, 262*(19), 9412–9420.
45. Raposo, G., Nijman, H. W., Stoorvogel, W., Liejendekker, R., Harding, C. V., Melief, C. J., & Geuze, H. J. (1996). B lymphocytes secrete antigen-presenting vesicles. *The Journal of Experimental Medicine, 183*(3), 1161–1172.
46. Gutwein, P., Stoeck, A., Riedle, S., Gast, D., Runz, S., Condon, T. P., Marme, A., Phong, M. C., Linderkamp, O., Skorokhod, A., & Altevogt, P. (2005). Cleavage of L1 in exosomes and apoptotic membrane vesicles released from ovarian carcinoma cells. *Clinical Cancer Research, 11*(7), 2492–2501.
47. Walker, N. D., Elias, M., Guiro, K., Bhatia, R., Greco, S. J., Bryan, M., Gergues, M., Sandiford, O. A., Ponzio, N. M., Leibovich, S. J., & Rameshwar, P. (2019). Exosomes from differentially activated macrophages influence dormancy or resurgence of breast cancer cells within bone marrow stroma. *Cell Death & Disease, 10*(2), 59.
48. Valadi, H., Ekstrom, K., Bossios, A., Sjostrand, M., Lee, J. J., & Lotvall, J. O. (2007). Exosome-mediated transfer of mRNAs and microRNAs is a novel mechanism of genetic exchange between cells. *Nature Cell Biology, 9*(6), 654–659.
49. Thakur, B. K., Zhang, H., Becker, A., Matei, I., Huang, Y., Costa-Silva, B., Zheng, Y., Hoshino, A., Brazier, H., Xiang, J., Williams, C., Rodriguez-Barrueco, R., Silva, J. M., Zhang, W., Hearn, S., Elemento, O., Paknejad, N., Manova-Todorova, K., Welte, K., … Lyden, D. (2014). Double-stranded DNA in exosomes: a novel biomarker in cancer detection. *Cell Research, 24*(6), 766–769.
50. Kowal, J., Arras, G., Colombo, M., Jouve, M., Morath, J. P., Primdal-Bengtson, B., Dingli, F., Loew, D., Tkach, M., & Thery, C. (2016). Proteomic comparison defines novel markers to characterize heterogeneous populations of extracellular vesicle subtypes. *Proceedings of the National Academy of Sciences of the United States of America, 113*(8), E968–E977.
51. Villarroya-Beltri, C., Gutierrez-Vazquez, C., Sanchez-Cabo, F., Perez-Hernandez, D., Vazquez, J., Martin-Cofreces, N., Martinez-Herrera, D. J., Pascual-Montano, A., Mittelbrunn, M., & Sanchez-Madrid, F. (2013). Sumoylated hnRNPA2B1 controls the sorting of miRNAs into exosomes through binding to specific motifs. *Nature Communications, 4*, 2980.
52. Cha, D. J., Franklin, J. L., Dou, Y., Liu, Q., Higginbotham, J. N., Demory Beckler, M., Weaver, A. M., Vickers, K., Prasad, N., Levy, S., Zhang, B., Coffey, R. J., & Patton, J. G. (2015). KRAS-dependent sorting of miRNA to exosomes. *eLife, 4*, e07197.
53. McKenzie, A. J., Hoshino, D., Hong, N. H., Cha, D. J., Franklin, J. L., Coffey, R. J., Patton, J. G., & Weaver, A. M. (2016). KRAS-MEK Signaling Controls Ago2 Sorting into Exosomes. *Cell Reports, 15*(5), 978–987.
54. Batagov, A. O., & Kurochkin, I. V. (2013). Exosomes secreted by human cells transport largely mRNA fragments that are enriched in the 3'-untranslated regions. *Biology Direct, 8*, 12.
55. Buschow, S. I., Liefhebber, J. M., Wubbolts, R., & Stoorvogel, W. (2005). Exosomes contain ubiquitinated proteins. *Blood Cells, Molecules & Diseases, 35*(3), 398–403.
56. Smith, V. L., Jackson, L., & Schorey, J. S. (2015). Ubiquitination as a mechanism to transport soluble mycobacterial and eukaryotic proteins to exosomes. *Journal of Immunology, 195*(6), 2722–2730.
57. Hoshino, D., Kirkbride, K. C., Costello, K., Clark, E. S., Sinha, S., Grega-Larson, N., Tyska, M. J., & Weaver, A. M. (2013). Exosome secretion is enhanced by invadopodia and drives invasive behavior. *Cell Reports, 5*(5), 1159–1168.
58. Sinha, S., Hoshino, D., Hong, N. H., Kirkbride, K. C., Grega-Larson, N. E., Seiki, M., Tyska, M. J., & Weaver, A. M. (2016). Cortactin promotes exosome

secretion by controlling branched actin dynamics. *The Journal of Cell Biology, 214*(2), 197–213.
59. Bonifacino, J. S., & Glick, B. S. (2004). The mechanisms of vesicle budding and fusion. *Cell, 116*(2), 153–166.
60. Koles, K., Nunnari, J., Korkut, C., Barria, R., Brewer, C., Li, Y., Leszyk, J., Zhang, B., & Budnik, V. (2012). Mechanism of evenness interrupted (Evi)-exosome release at synaptic boutons. *The Journal of Biological Chemistry, 287*(20), 16820–16834.
61. Fader, C. M., Sanchez, D. G., Mestre, M. B., & Colombo, M. I. (2009). TI-VAMP/VAMP7 and VAMP3/cellubrevin: two v-SNARE proteins involved in specific steps of the autophagy/multivesicular body pathways. *Biochimica et Biophysica Acta, 1793*(12), 1901–1916.
62. Gross, J. C., Chaudhary, V., Bartscherer, K., & Boutros, M. (2012). Active Wnt proteins are secreted on exosomes. *Nature Cell Biology, 14*(10), 1036–1045.
63. Ruiz-Martinez, M., Navarro, A., Marrades, R. M., Vinolas, N., Santasusagna, S., Munoz, C., Ramirez, J., Molins, L., & Monzo, M. (2016). YKT6 expression, exosome release, and survival in non-small cell lung cancer. *Oncotarget, 7*(32), 51515–51524.
64. Stenmark, H. (2009). Rab GTPases as coordinators of vesicle traffic. *Nature Reviews. Molecular Cell Biology, 10*(8), 513–525.
65. Ostrowski, M., Carmo, N. B., Krumeich, S., Fanget, I., Raposo, G., Savina, A., Moita, C. F., Schauer, K., Hume, A. N., Freitas, R. P., Goud, B., Benaroch, P., Hacohen, N., Fukuda, M., Desnos, C., Seabra, M. C., Darchen, F., Amigorena, S., Moita, L. F., & Thery, C. (2010). Rab27a and Rab27b control different steps of the exosome secretion pathway. *Nature Cell Biology, 12*(1), 19–30.
66. Savina, A., Vidal, M., & Colombo, M. I. (2002). The exosome pathway in K562 cells is regulated by Rab11. *Journal of Cell Science, 115*(Pt 12), 2505–2515.
67. Mobius, W., Ohno-Iwashita, Y., van Donselaar, E. G., Oorschot, V. M., Shimada, Y., Fujimoto, T., Heijnen, H. F., Geuze, H. J., & Slot, J. W. (2002). Immunoelectron microscopic localization of cholesterol using biotinylated and non-cytolytic perfringolysin O. *The Journal of Histochemistry and Cytochemistry, 50*(1), 43–55.
68. Tauro, B. J., Greening, D. W., Mathias, R. A., Mathivanan, S., Ji, H., & Simpson, R. J. (2013). Two distinct populations of exosomes are released from LIM1863 colon carcinoma cell-derived organoids. *Molecular & Cellular Proteomics, 12*(3), 587–598.
69. van Niel, G., Raposo, G., Candalh, C., Boussac, M., Hershberg, R., Cerf-Bensussan, N., & Heyman, M. (2001). Intestinal epithelial cells secrete exosome-like vesicles. *Gastroenterology, 121*(2), 337–349.
70. Chen, Q., Takada, R., Noda, C., Kobayashi, S., & Takada, S. (2016). Different populations of Wnt-containing vesicles are individually released from polarized epithelial cells. *Scientific Reports, 6*, 35562.
71. Feng, D., Zhao, W. L., Ye, Y. Y., Bai, X. C., Liu, R. Q., Chang, L. F., Zhou, Q., & Sui, S. F. (2010). Cellular internalization of exosomes occurs through phagocytosis. *Traffic, 11*(5), 675–687.
72. Doherty, G. J., & McMahon, H. T. (2009). Mechanisms of endocytosis. *Annual Review of Biochemistry, 78*, 857–902.
73. Mulcahy, L. A., Pink, R. C., & Carter, D. R. (2014). Routes and mechanisms of extracellular vesicle uptake. *Journal of Extracellular Vesicles, 3*.
74. Rana, S., Yue, S., Stadel, D., & Zoller, M. (2012). Toward tailored exosomes: the exosomal tetraspanin web contributes to target cell selection. *The International Journal of Biochemistry & Cell Biology, 44*(9), 1574–1584.
75. Morelli, A. E., Larregina, A. T., Shufesky, W. J., Sullivan, M. L., Stolz, D. B., Papworth, G. D., Zahorchak, A. F., Logar, A. J., Wang, Z., Watkins, S. C., Falo, L. D., Jr., & Thomson, A. W. (2004). Endocytosis, intracellular sorting, and processing of exosomes by dendritic cells. *Blood, 104*(10), 3257–3266.
76. Parolini, I., Federici, C., Raggi, C., Lugini, L., Palleschi, S., De Milito, A., Coscia, C., Iessi, E., Logozzi, M., Molinari, A., Colone, M., Tatti, M., Sargiacomo, M., & Fais, S. (2009). Microenvironmental pH is a key factor for exosome traffic in tumor cells. *The Journal of Biological Chemistry, 284*(49), 34211–34222.
77. Jahn, R., & Sudhof, T. C. (1999). Membrane fusion and exocytosis. *Annual Review of Biochemistry, 68*, 863–911.
78. Zhang, L., & Yu, D. (2019). Exosomes in cancer development, metastasis, and immunity. *Biochimica Et Biophysica Acta. Reviews on Cancer, 1871*(2), 455–468.
79. Becker, A., Thakur, B. K., Weiss, J. M., Kim, H. S., Peinado, H., & Lyden, D. (2016). Extracellular Vesicles in Cancer: Cell-to-Cell Mediators of Metastasis. *Cancer Cell, 30*(6), 836–848.
80. Al-Nedawi, K., Meehan, B., Micallef, J., Lhotak, V., May, L., Guha, A., & Rak, J. (2008). Intercellular transfer of the oncogenic receptor EGFRvIII by microvesicles derived from tumour cells. *Nature Cell Biology, 10*(5), 619–624.
81. Bobrie, A., Colombo, M., Raposo, G., & Thery, C. (2011). Exosome secretion: molecular mechanisms and roles in immune responses. *Traffic, 12*(12), 1659–1668.
82. Ramteke, A., Ting, H., Agarwal, C., Mateen, S., Somasagara, R., Hussain, A., Graner, M., Frederick, B., Agarwal, R., & Deep, G. (2015). Exosomes secreted under hypoxia enhance invasiveness and stemness of prostate cancer cells by targeting adherens junction molecules. *Molecular Carcinogenesis, 54*(7), 554–565.
83. Global Burden of Disease Cancer, C., Fitzmaurice, C., Akinyemiju, T. F., Al Lami, F. H., Alam, T.,

Alizadeh-Navaei, R., Allen, C., Alsharif, U., Alvis-Guzman, N., Amini, E., Anderson, B. O., Aremu, O., Artaman, A., Asgedom, S. W., Assadi, R., Atey, T. M., Avila-Burgos, L., Awasthi, A., Ba Saleem, H. O., … Naghavi, M. (2018). Global, regional, and National cancer incidence, mortality, years of life lost, years lived with disability, and disability-adjusted life-years for 29 cancer groups, 1990 to 2016: A systematic analysis for the global burden of disease study. *JAMA Oncology, 4*(11), 1553–1568.
84. Mehdi, S. R., & Bhatt, M. L. (2011). Metastasis of solid tumors in bone marrow: A study from northern India. *Indian Journal of Hematology and Blood Transfusion, 27*(2), 93–95.
85. Society, A. C. (2019). *Cancer facts & figures 2019*. American Cancer Society.
86. Society, A. C. *Breast cancer facts & figures 2019–2020* (Vol. 2019). American Cancer Society, Inc..
87. Braun, S., & Pantel, K. (2001). Clinical significance of occult metastatic cells in bone marrow of breast cancer patients. *The Oncologist, 6*(2), 125–132.
88. Braun, S., Pantel, K., Muller, P., Janni, W., Hepp, F., Kentenich, C. R., Gastroph, S., Wischnik, A., Dimpfl, T., Kindermann, G., Riethmuller, G., & Schlimok, G. (2000). Cytokeratin-positive cells in the bone marrow and survival of patients with stage I, II, or III breast cancer. *The New England Journal of Medicine, 342*(8), 525–533.
89. Bliss, S. A., Paul, S., Pobiarzyn, P. W., Ayer, S., Sinha, G., Pant, S., Hilton, H., Sharma, N., Cunha, M. F., Engelberth, D. J., Greco, S. J., Bryan, M., Kucia, M. J., Kakar, S. S., Ratajczak, M. Z., & Rameshwar, P. (2018). Evaluation of a developmental hierarchy for breast cancer cells to assess risk-based patient selection for targeted treatment. *Scientific Reports, 8*(1), 367.
90. Ayala, F., Dewar, R., Kieran, M., & Kalluri, R. (2009). Contribution of bone microenvironment to leukemogenesis and leukemia progression. *Leukemia, 23*(12), 2233–2241.
91. Cheung, L. C., Tickner, J., Hughes, A. M., Skut, P., Howlett, M., Foley, B., Oommen, J., Wells, J. E., He, B., Singh, S., Chua, G. A., Ford, J., Mullighan, C. G., Kotecha, R. S., & Kees, U. R. (2018). New therapeutic opportunities from dissecting the pre-B leukemia bone marrow microenvironment. *Leukemia, 32*(11), 2326–2338.
92. Ergen, A. V., Boles, N. C., & Goodell, M. A. (2012). Rantes/Ccl5 influences hematopoietic stem cell subtypes and causes myeloid skewing. *Blood, 119*(11), 2500–2509.
93. Kusumbe, A. P., Ramasamy, S. K., Itkin, T., Mae, M. A., Langen, U. H., Betsholtz, C., Lapidot, T., & Adams, R. H. (2016). Age-dependent modulation of vascular niches for haematopoietic stem cells. *Nature, 532*(7599), 380–384.
94. Moudra, A., Hubackova, S., Machalova, V., Vancurova, M., Bartek, J., Reinis, M., Hodny, Z., & Jonasova, A. (2016). Dynamic alterations of bone marrow cytokine landscape of myelodysplastic syndromes patients treated with 5-azacytidine. *Oncoimmunology, 5*(10), e1183860.
95. Haas, S., Hansson, J., Klimmeck, D., Loeffler, D., Velten, L., Uckelmann, H., Wurzer, S., Prendergast, A. M., Schnell, A., Hexel, K., Santarella-Mellwig, R., Blaszkiewicz, S., Kuck, A., Geiger, H., Milsom, M. D., Steinmetz, L. M., Schroeder, T., Trumpp, A., Krijgsveld, J., & Essers, M. A. (2015). Inflammation-Induced Emergency Megakaryopoiesis Driven by Hematopoietic Stem Cell-like Megakaryocyte Progenitors. *Cell Stem Cell, 17*(4), 422–434.
96. Lucas, D., Scheiermann, C., Chow, A., Kunisaki, Y., Bruns, I., Barrick, C., Tessarollo, L., & Frenette, P. S. (2013). Chemotherapy-induced bone marrow nerve injury impairs hematopoietic regeneration. *Nature Medicine, 19*(6), 695–703.
97. Ganan-Gomez, I., Wei, Y., Starczynowski, D. T., Colla, S., Yang, H., Cabrero-Calvo, M., Bohannan, Z. S., Verma, A., Steidl, U., & Garcia-Manero, G. (2015). Deregulation of innate immune and inflammatory signaling in myelodysplastic syndromes. *Leukemia, 29*(7), 1458–1469.
98. Bliss, S. A., Sinha, G., Sandiford, O. A., Williams, L. M., Engelberth, D. J., Guiro, K., Isenalumhe, L. L., Greco, S. J., Ayer, S., Bryan, M., Kumar, R., Ponzio, N. M., & Rameshwar, P. (2016). Mesenchymal Stem Cell-Derived Exosomes Stimulate Cycling Quiescence and Early Breast Cancer Dormancy in Bone Marrow. *Cancer Research, 76*(19), 5832–5844.
99. Eltoukhy, H. S., Sinha, G., Moore, C. A., Gergues, M., & Rameshwar, P. (2018). Secretome within the bone marrow microenvironment: A basis for mesenchymal stem cell treatment and role in cancer dormancy. *Biochimie, 155*, 92–103.
100. Lim, P. K., Bliss, S. A., Patel, S. A., Taborga, M., Dave, M. A., Gregory, L. A., Greco, S. J., Bryan, M., Patel, P. S., & Rameshwar, P. (2011). Gap junction-mediated import of microRNA from bone marrow stromal cells can elicit cell cycle quiescence in breast cancer cells. *Cancer Research, 71*(5), 1550–1560.
101. Walker, N. D., Patel, J., Munoz, J. L., Hu, M., Guiro, K., Sinha, G., & Rameshwar, P. (2016). The bone marrow niche in support of breast cancer dormancy. *Cancer Letters, 380*(1), 263–271.
102. Patel, S. A., Ramkissoon, S. H., Bryan, M., Pliner, L. F., Dontu, G., Patel, P. S., Amiri, S., Pine, S. R., & Rameshwar, P. (2012). Delineation of breast cancer cell hierarchy identifies the subset responsible for dormancy. *Scientific Reports, 2*, 906.
103. Li, W., Johnson, S. A., Shelley, W. C., & Yoder, M. C. (2004). Hematopoietic stem cell repopulating ability can be maintained in vitro by some primary endothelial cells. *Experimental Hematology, 32*(12), 1226–1237.
104. Butler, J. M., Nolan, D. J., Vertes, E. L., Varnum-Finney, B., Kobayashi, H., Hooper, A. T., Seandel, M., Shido, K., White, I. A., Kobayashi, M., Witte, L., May, C., Shawber, C., Kimura, Y., Kitajewski, J., Rosenwaks, Z., Bernstein, I. D., & Rafii, S. (2010). Endothelial cells are essential for the self-renewal

and repopulation of Notch-dependent hematopoietic stem cells. *Cell Stem Cell, 6*(3), 251–264.
105. Kobayashi, H., Butler, J. M., O'Donnell, R., Kobayashi, M., Ding, B. S., Bonner, B., Chiu, V. K., Nolan, D. J., Shido, K., Benjamin, L., & Rafii, S. (2010). Angiocrine factors from Akt-activated endothelial cells balance self-renewal and differentiation of haematopoietic stem cells. *Nature Cell Biology, 12*(11), 1046–1056.
106. Winkler, I. G., Barbier, V., Nowlan, B., Jacobsen, R. N., Forristal, C. E., Patton, J. T., Magnani, J. L., & Levesque, J. P. (2012). Vascular niche E-selectin regulates hematopoietic stem cell dormancy, self renewal and chemoresistance. *Nature Medicine, 18*(11), 1651–1657.
107. Yao, L., Yokota, T., Xia, L., Kincade, P. W., & McEver, R. P. (2005). Bone marrow dysfunction in mice lacking the cytokine receptor gp130 in endothelial cells. *Blood, 106*(13), 4093–4101.
108. Chute, J. P., Muramoto, G. G., Fung, J., & Oxford, C. (2005). Soluble factors elaborated by human brain endothelial cells induce the concomitant expansion of purified human BM CD34+CD38- cells and SCID-repopulating cells. *Blood, 105*(2), 576–583.
109. Himburg, H. A., Muramoto, G. G., Daher, P., Meadows, S. K., Russell, J. L., Doan, P., Chi, J. T., Salter, A. B., Lento, W. E., Reya, T., Chao, N. J., & Chute, J. P. (2010). Pleiotrophin regulates the expansion and regeneration of hematopoietic stem cells. *Nature Medicine, 16*(4), 475–482.
110. Kiel, M. J., Yilmaz, O. H., Iwashita, T., Yilmaz, O. H., Terhorst, C., & Morrison, S. J. (2005). SLAM family receptors distinguish hematopoietic stem and progenitor cells and reveal endothelial niches for stem cells. *Cell, 121*(7), 1109–1121.
111. Mineo, M., Garfield, S. H., Taverna, S., Flugy, A., De Leo, G., Alessandro, R., & Kohn, E. C. (2012). Exosomes released by K562 chronic myeloid leukemia cells promote angiogenesis in a Src-dependent fashion. *Angiogenesis, 15*(1), 33–45.
112. Umezu, T., Tadokoro, H., Azuma, K., Yoshizawa, S., Ohyashiki, K., & Ohyashiki, J. H. (2014). Exosomal miR-135b shed from hypoxic multiple myeloma cells enhances angiogenesis by targeting factor-inhibiting HIF-1. *Blood, 124*(25), 3748–3757.
113. Li, S. (2008). Src-family kinases in the development and therapy of Philadelphia chromosome-positive chronic myeloid leukemia and acute lymphoblastic leukemia. *Leukemia & Lymphoma, 49*(1), 19–26.
114. Tadokoro, H., Umezu, T., Ohyashiki, K., Hirano, T., & Ohyashiki, J. H. (2013). Exosomes derived from hypoxic leukemia cells enhance tube formation in endothelial cells. *The Journal of Biological Chemistry, 288*(48), 34343–34351.
115. Doebele, C., Bonauer, A., Fischer, A., Scholz, A., Reiss, Y., Urbich, C., Hofmann, W. K., Zeiher, A. M., & Dimmeler, S. (2010). Members of the microRNA-17-92 cluster exhibit a cell-intrinsic antiangiogenic function in endothelial cells. *Blood, 115*(23), 4944–4950.
116. Zhang, B., Nguyen, L. X. T., Li, L., Zhao, D., Kumar, B., Wu, H., Lin, A., Pellicano, F., Hopcroft, L., Su, Y. L., Copland, M., Holyoake, T. L., Kuo, C. J., Bhatia, R., Snyder, D. S., Ali, H., Stein, A. S., Brewer, C., Wang, H., ... Marcucci, G. (2018). Bone marrow niche trafficking of miR-126 controls the self-renewal of leukemia stem cells in chronic myelogenous leukemia. *Nature Medicine, 24*(4), 450–462.
117. Paggetti, J., Haderk, F., Seiffert, M., Janji, B., Distler, U., Ammerlaan, W., Kim, Y. J., Adam, J., Lichter, P., Solary, E., Berchem, G., & Moussay, E. (2015). Exosomes released by chronic lymphocytic leukemia cells induce the transition of stromal cells into cancer-associated fibroblasts. *Blood, 126*(9), 1106–1117.
118. Mendez-Ferrer, S., Michurina, T. V., Ferraro, F., Mazloom, A. R., Macarthur, B. D., Lira, S. A., Scadden, D. T., Ma'ayan, A., Enikolopov, G. N., & Frenette, P. S. (2010). Mesenchymal and haematopoietic stem cells form a unique bone marrow niche. *Nature, 466*(7308), 829–834.
119. Sacchetti, B., Funari, A., Michienzi, S., Di Cesare, S., Piersanti, S., Saggio, I., Tagliafico, E., Ferrari, S., Robey, P. G., Riminucci, M., & Bianco, P. (2007). Self-renewing osteoprogenitors in bone marrow sinusoids can organize a hematopoietic microenvironment. *Cell, 131*(2), 324–336.
120. Sugiyama, T., Kohara, H., Noda, M., & Nagasawa, T. (2006). Maintenance of the hematopoietic stem cell pool by CXCL12-CXCR4 chemokine signaling in bone marrow stromal cell niches. *Immunity, 25*(6), 977–988.
121. Omatsu, Y., Sugiyama, T., Kohara, H., Kondoh, G., Fujii, N., Kohno, K., & Nagasawa, T. (2010). The essential functions of adipo-osteogenic progenitors as the hematopoietic stem and progenitor cell niche. *Immunity, 33*(3), 387–399.
122. Huan, J., Hornick, N. I., Shurtleff, M. J., Skinner, A. M., Goloviznina, N. A., Roberts, C. T., Jr., & Kurre, P. (2013). RNA trafficking by acute myelogenous leukemia exosomes. *Cancer Research, 73*(2), 918–929.
123. Burger, J. A., & Peled, A. (2009). CXCR4 antagonists: targeting the microenvironment in leukemia and other cancers. *Leukemia, 23*(1), 43–52.
124. Roccaro, A. M., Sacco, A., Maiso, P., Azab, A. K., Tai, Y. T., Reagan, M., Azab, F., Flores, L. M., Campigotto, F., Weller, E., Anderson, K. C., Scadden, D. T., & Ghobrial, I. M. (2013). BM mesenchymal stromal cell-derived exosomes facilitate multiple myeloma progression. *The Journal of Clinical Investigation, 123*(4), 1542–1555.
125. Wang, J., Hendrix, A., Hernot, S., Lemaire, M., De Bruyne, E., Van Valckenborgh, E., Lahoutte, T., De Wever, O., Vanderkerken, K., & Menu, E. (2014). Bone marrow stromal cell-derived exosomes as communicators in drug resistance in multiple myeloma cells. *Blood, 124*(4), 555–566.

126. Yeo, R. W., Lai, R. C., Zhang, B., Tan, S. S., Yin, Y., Teh, B. J., & Lim, S. K. (2013). Mesenchymal stem cell: an efficient mass producer of exosomes for drug delivery. *Advanced Drug Delivery Reviews, 65*(3), 336–341.
127. Garin, M. I., Chu, C. C., Golshayan, D., Cernuda-Morollon, E., Wait, R., & Lechler, R. I. (2007). Galectin-1: a key effector of regulation mediated by CD4+CD25+ T cells. *Blood, 109*(5), 2058–2065.
128. Kilpinen, L., Impola, U., Sankkila, L., Ritamo, I., Aatonen, M., Kilpinen, S., Tuimala, J., Valmu, L., Levijoki, J., Finckenberg, P., Siljander, P., Kankuri, E., Mervaala, E., & Laitinen, S. (2013). Extracellular membrane vesicles from umbilical cord blood-derived MSC protect against ischemic acute kidney injury, a feature that is lost after inflammatory conditioning. *Journal of Extracellular Vesicles, 2*.
129. Rabinovich, G. A., Alonso, C. R., Sotomayor, C. E., Durand, S., Bocco, J. L., & Riera, C. M. (2000). Molecular mechanisms implicated in galectin-1-induced apoptosis: activation of the AP-1 transcription factor and downregulation of Bcl-2. *Cell Death and Differentiation, 7*(8), 747–753.
130. Blois, S. M., Ilarregui, J. M., Tometten, M., Garcia, M., Orsal, A. S., Cordo-Russo, R., Toscano, M. A., Bianco, G. A., Kobelt, P., Handjiski, B., Tirado, I., Markert, U. R., Klapp, B. F., Poirier, F., Szekeres-Bartho, J., Rabinovich, G. A., & Arck, P. C. (2007). A pivotal role for galectin-1 in fetomaternal tolerance. *Nature Medicine, 13*(12), 1450–1457.
131. Guleria, I., Khosroshahi, A., Ansari, M. J., Habicht, A., Azuma, M., Yagita, H., Noelle, R. J., Coyle, A., Mellor, A. L., Khoury, S. J., & Sayegh, M. H. (2005). A critical role for the programmed death ligand 1 in fetomaternal tolerance. *The Journal of Experimental Medicine, 202*(2), 231–237.
132. Freeman, G. J., Long, A. J., Iwai, Y., Bourque, K., Chernova, T., Nishimura, H., Fitz, L. J., Malenkovich, N., Okazaki, T., Byrne, M. C., Horton, H. F., Fouser, L., Carter, L., Ling, V., Bowman, M. R., Carreno, B. M., Collins, M., Wood, C. R., & Honjo, T. (2000). Engagement of the PD-1 immunoinhibitory receptor by a novel B7 family member leads to negative regulation of lymphocyte activation. *The Journal of Experimental Medicine, 192*(7), 1027–1034.
133. Chen, W., Jin, W., Hardegen, N., Lei, K. J., Li, L., Marinos, N., McGrady, G., & Wahl, S. M. (2003). Conversion of peripheral CD4+CD25- naive T cells to CD4+CD25+ regulatory T cells by TGF-beta induction of transcription factor Foxp3. *The Journal of Experimental Medicine, 198*(12), 1875–1886.
134. Fantini, M. C., Becker, C., Monteleone, G., Pallone, F., Galle, P. R., & Neurath, M. F. (2004). Cutting edge: TGF-beta induces a regulatory phenotype in CD4+CD25- T cells through Foxp3 induction and down-regulation of Smad7. *Journal of Immunology, 172*(9), 5149–5153.
135. Winkler, I. G., Sims, N. A., Pettit, A. R., Barbier, V., Nowlan, B., Helwani, F., Poulton, I. J., van Rooijen, N., Alexander, K. A., Raggatt, L. J., & Levesque, J. P. (2010). Bone marrow macrophages maintain hematopoietic stem cell (HSC) niches and their depletion mobilizes HSCs. *Blood, 116*(23), 4815–4828.
136. Jafarzadeh, N., Safari, Z., Pornour, M., Amirizadeh, N., Forouzandeh Moghadam, M., & Sadeghizadeh, M. (2019). Alteration of cellular and immune-related properties of bone marrow mesenchymal stem cells and macrophages by K562 chronic myeloid leukemia cell derived exosomes. *Journal of Cellular Physiology, 234*(4), 3697–3710.
137. Taichman, R. S., Reilly, M. J., & Emerson, S. G. (1996). Human osteoblasts support human hematopoietic progenitor cells in vitro bone marrow cultures. *Blood, 87*(2), 518–524.
138. Visnjic, D., Kalajzic, Z., Rowe, D. W., Katavic, V., Lorenzo, J., & Aguila, H. L. (2004). Hematopoiesis is severely altered in mice with an induced osteoblast deficiency. *Blood, 103*(9), 3258–3264.
139. Calvi, L. M., Adams, G. B., Weibrecht, K. W., Weber, J. M., Olson, D. P., Knight, M. C., Martin, R. P., Schipani, E., Divieti, P., Bringhurst, F. R., Milner, L. A., Kronenberg, H. M., & Scadden, D. T. (2003). Osteoblastic cells regulate the haematopoietic stem cell niche. *Nature, 425*(6960), 841–846.
140. Zhang, J., Niu, C., Ye, L., Huang, H., He, X., Tong, W. G., Ross, J., Haug, J., Johnson, T., Feng, J. Q., Harris, S., Wiedemann, L. M., Mishina, Y., & Li, L. (2003). Identification of the haematopoietic stem cell niche and control of the niche size. *Nature, 425*(6960), 836–841.
141. Liu, Z., Liu, H., Li, Y., Shao, Q., Chen, J., Song, J., & Fu, R. (2019). Multiple myeloma-derived exosomes inhibit osteoblastic differentiation and improve IL-6 secretion of BMSCs from multiple myeloma. *Journal of Investigative Medicine*.
142. Faict, S., Muller, J., De Veirman, K., De Bruyne, E., Maes, K., Vrancken, L., Heusschen, R., De Raeve, H., Schots, R., Vanderkerken, K., Caers, J., & Menu, E. (2018). Exosomes play a role in multiple myeloma bone disease and tumor development by targeting osteoclasts and osteoblasts. *Blood Cancer Journal, 8*(11), 105.
143. Zhou, W., Fong, M. Y., Min, Y., Somlo, G., Liu, L., Palomares, M. R., Yu, Y., Chow, A., O'Connor, S. T., Chin, A. R., Yen, Y., Wang, Y., Marcusson, E. G., Chu, P., Wu, J., Wu, X., Li, A. X., Li, Z., Gao, H., … Wang, S. E. (2014). Cancer-secreted miR-105 destroys vascular endothelial barriers to promote metastasis. *Cancer Cell, 25*(4), 501–515.
144. Chavez-Macgregor, M., Aviles-Salas, A., Green, D., Fuentes-Alburo, A., Gomez-Ruiz, C., & Aguayo, A. (2005). Angiogenesis in the bone marrow of patients with breast cancer. *Clinical Cancer Research, 11*(15), 5396–5400.
145. Feng, Q., Zhang, C., Lum, D., Druso, J. E., Blank, B., Wilson, K. F., Welm, A., Antonyak, M. A., & Cerione, R. A. (2017). A class of extracellular vesicles from breast cancer cells activates VEGF receptors and tumour angiogenesis. *Nature Communications, 8*, 14450.

146. Lee, J. K., Park, S. R., Jung, B. K., Jeon, Y. K., Lee, Y. S., Kim, M. K., Kim, Y. G., Jang, J. Y., & Kim, C. W. (2013). Exosomes derived from mesenchymal stem cells suppress angiogenesis by down-regulating VEGF expression in breast cancer cells. *PLoS One, 8*(12), e84256.
147. Lin, R., Wang, S., & Zhao, R. C. (2013). Exosomes from human adipose-derived mesenchymal stem cells promote migration through Wnt signaling pathway in a breast cancer cell model. *Molecular and Cellular Biochemistry, 383*(1-2), 13–20.
148. Corcoran, K. E., Trzaska, K. A., Fernandes, H., Bryan, M., Taborga, M., Srinivas, V., Packman, K., Patel, P. S., & Rameshwar, P. (2008). Mesenchymal stem cells in early entry of breast cancer into bone marrow. *PLoS One, 3*(6), e2563.
149. Greco, S. J., Patel, S. A., Bryan, M., Pliner, L. F., Banerjee, D., & Rameshwar, P. (2011). AMD3100-mediated production of interleukin-1 from mesenchymal stem cells is key to chemosensitivity of breast cancer cells. *American Journal of Cancer Research, 1*(6), 701–715.
150. Ono, M., Kosaka, N., Tominaga, N., Yoshioka, Y., Takeshita, F., Takahashi, R. U., Yoshida, M., Tsuda, H., Tamura, K., & Ochiya, T. (2014). Exosomes from bone marrow mesenchymal stem cells contain a microRNA that promotes dormancy in metastatic breast cancer cells. *Science Signaling, 7*(332), ra63.
151. Ge, Y., Bohm, H. H., Rathinasamy, A., Xydia, M., Hu, X., Pincha, M., Umansky, L., Breyer, C., Hillier, M., Bonertz, A., Sevko, A., Domschke, C., Schuetz, F., Frebel, H., Dettling, S., Herold-Mende, C., Reissfelder, C., Weitz, J., Umansky, V., & Beckhove, P. (2019). Tumor-specific regulatory T cells from the bone marrow orchestrate antitumor immunity in breast cancer. *Cancer Immunology Research, 7*(12), 1998–2012.
152. Patel, S. A., Meyer, J. R., Greco, S. J., Corcoran, K. E., Bryan, M., & Rameshwar, P. (2010). Mesenchymal stem cells protect breast cancer cells through regulatory T cells: role of mesenchymal stem cell-derived TGF-beta. *Journal of Immunology, 184*(10), 5885–5894.
153. Chow, A., Zhou, W., Liu, L., Fong, M. Y., Champer, J., Van Haute, D., Chin, A. R., Ren, X., Gugiu, B. G., Meng, Z., Huang, W., Ngo, V., Kortylewski, M., & Wang, S. E. (2014). Macrophage immunomodulation by breast cancer-derived exosomes requires Toll-like receptor 2-mediated activation of NF-kappaB. *Scientific Reports, 4*, 5750.
154. Piao, Y. J., Kim, H. S., Hwang, E. H., Woo, J., Zhang, M., & Moon, W. K. (2018). Breast cancer cell-derived exosomes and macrophage polarization are associated with lymph node metastasis. *Oncotarget, 9*(7), 7398–7410.
155. Yu, X., Zhang, Q., Zhang, X., Han, Q., Li, H., Mao, Y., Wang, X., Guo, H., Irwin, D. M., Niu, G., & Tan, H. (2019). Exosomes from macrophages exposed to apoptotic breast cancer cells promote breast cancer proliferation and metastasis. *Journal of Cancer, 10*(13), 2892–2906.
156. Wang, P., Wang, H., Huang, Q., Peng, C., Yao, L., Chen, H., Qiu, Z., Wu, Y., Wang, L., & Chen, W. (2019). Exosomes from M1-polarized macrophages enhance paclitaxel antitumor activity by activating macrophages-mediated inflammation. *Theranostics, 9*(6), 1714–1727.
157. Kolb, A. D., Shupp, A. B., Mukhopadhyay, D., Marini, F. C., & Bussard, K. M. (2019). Osteoblasts are "educated" by crosstalk with metastatic breast cancer cells in the bone tumor microenvironment. *Breast Cancer Research, 21*(1), 31.
158. Capulli, M., Hristova, D., Valbret, Z., Carys, K., Arjan, R., Maurizi, A., Masedu, F., Cappariello, A., Rucci, N., & Teti, A. (2019). Notch2 pathway mediates breast cancer cellular dormancy and mobilisation in bone and contributes to haematopoietic stem cell mimicry. *British Journal of Cancer, 121*(2), 157–171.
159. Liu, X., Cao, M., Palomares, M., Wu, X., Li, A., Yan, W., Fong, M. Y., Chan, W. C., & Wang, S. E. (2018). Metastatic breast cancer cells overexpress and secrete miR-218 to regulate type I collagen deposition by osteoblasts. *Breast Cancer Research, 20*(1), 127.
160. Hashimoto, K., Ochi, H., Sunamura, S., Kosaka, N., Mabuchi, Y., Fukuda, T., Yao, K., Kanda, H., Ae, K., Okawa, A., Akazawa, C., Ochiya, T., Futakuchi, M., Takeda, S., & Sato, S. (2018). Cancer-secreted hsa-miR-940 induces an osteoblastic phenotype in the bone metastatic microenvironment via targeting ARHGAP1 and FAM134A. *Proceedings of the National Academy of Sciences of the United States of America, 115*(9), 2204–2209.
161. Loftus, A., Cappariello, A., George, C., Ucci, A., Shefferd, K., Green, A., Paone, R., Ponzetti, M., Delle Monache, S., Muraca, M., Teti, A., & Rucci, N. (2019). Extracellular vesicles from osteotropic breast cancer cells affect bone resident cells. *Journal of Bone and Mineral Research.*
162. Yanada, M., Matsuo, K., Suzuki, T., & Naoe, T. (2006). Allogeneic hematopoietic stem cell transplantation as part of postremission therapy improves survival for adult patients with high-risk acute lymphoblastic leukemia: A metaanalysis. *Cancer, 106*(12), 2657–2663.
163. Othus, M., Appelbaum, F. R., Petersdorf, S. H., Kopecky, K. J., Slovak, M., Nevill, T., Brandwein, J., Larson, R. A., Stiff, P. J., Walter, R. B., Tallman, M. S., Stenke, L., & Erba, H. P. (2015). Fate of patients with newly diagnosed acute myeloid leukemia who fail primary induction therapy. *Biology of Blood and Marrow Transplantation, 21*(3), 559–564.
164. Bruserud, O., Foss, B., Abrahamsen, J. F., Gjertsen, B. T., & Ernst, P. (2000). Autologous stem cell transplantation as post-remission therapy in adult acute myelogenous leukemia: Does platelet contamination of peripheral blood mobilized stem cell grafts influence the risk of leukemia relapse? *Journal*

of Hematotherapy & Stem Cell Research, 9(4), 433–443.
165. Kambham, N., Higgins, J. P., Sundram, U., & Troxell, M. L. (2014). Hematopoietic stem cell transplantation: Graft versus host disease and pathology of gastrointestinal tract, liver, and lung. *Advances in Anatomic Pathology, 21*(5), 301–320.
166. Kayser, S., & Levis, M. J. (2018). Advances in targeted therapy for acute myeloid leukaemia. *British Journal of Haematology, 180*(4), 484–500.
167. Gill, H., Leung, A. Y., & Kwong, Y. L. (2016). Molecularly targeted therapy in acute myeloid leukemia. *Future Oncology, 12*(6), 827–838.
168. Wouters, B. J., & Delwel, R. (2016). Epigenetics and approaches to targeted epigenetic therapy in acute myeloid leukemia. *Blood, 127*(1), 42–52.
169. Kuo, F. C., Mar, B. G., Lindsley, R. C., & Lindeman, N. I. (2017). The relative utilities of genome-wide, gene panel, and individual gene sequencing in clinical practice. *Blood, 130*(4), 433–439.
170. Scherer, F., Kurtz, D. M., Diehn, M., & Alizadeh, A. A. (2017). High-throughput sequencing for non-invasive disease detection in hematologic malignancies. *Blood, 130*(4), 440–452.
171. Stone, R. M., Mandrekar, S. J., Sanford, B. L., Laumann, K., Geyer, S., Bloomfield, C. D., Thiede, C., Prior, T. W., Dohner, K., Marcucci, G., Lo-Coco, F., Klisovic, R. B., Wei, A., Sierra, J., Sanz, M. A., Brandwein, J. M., de Witte, T., Niederwieser, D., Appelbaum, F. R., … Dohner, H. (2017). Midostaurin plus chemotherapy for acute myeloid leukemia with a FLT3 mutation. *The New England Journal of Medicine, 377*(5), 454–464.
172. Perl, A. E., Altman, J. K., Cortes, J., Smith, C., Litzow, M., Baer, M. R., Claxton, D., Erba, H. P., Gill, S., Goldberg, S., Jurcic, J. G., Larson, R. A., Liu, C., Ritchie, E., Schiller, G., Spira, A. I., Strickland, S. A., Tibes, R., Ustun, C., … Levis, M. (2017). Selective inhibition of FLT3 by gilteritinib in relapsed or refractory acute myeloid leukaemia: a multicentre, first-in-human, open-label, phase 1-2 study. *The Lancet Oncology, 18*(8), 1061–1075.
173. Stein, E. M., DiNardo, C. D., Fathi, A. T., Pollyea, D. A., Stone, R. M., Altman, J. K., Roboz, G. J., Patel, M. R., Collins, R., Flinn, I. W., Sekeres, M. A., Stein, A. S., Kantarjian, H. M., Levine, R. L., Vyas, P., MacBeth, K. J., Tosolini, A., VanOostendorp, J., Xu, Q., … de Botton, S. (2019). Molecular remission and response patterns in patients with mutant-IDH2 acute myeloid leukemia treated with enasidenib. *Blood, 133*(7), 676–687.
174. DiNardo, C. D., Stein, E. M., de Botton, S., Roboz, G. J., Altman, J. K., Mims, A. S., Swords, R., Collins, R. H., Mannis, G. N., Pollyea, D. A., Donnellan, W., Fathi, A. T., Pigneux, A., Erba, H. P., Prince, G. T., Stein, A. S., Uy, G. L., Foran, J. M., Traer, E., … Kantarjian, H. M. (2018). Durable remissions with ivosidenib in IDH1-mutated relapsed or refractory AML. *The New England Journal of Medicine, 378*(25), 2386–2398.
175. Cortes, J. E., Heidel, F. H., Hellmann, A., Fiedler, W., Smith, B. D., Robak, T., Montesinos, P., Pollyea, D. A., DesJardins, P., Ottmann, O., Ma, W. W., Shaik, M. N., Laird, A. D., Zeremski, M., O'Connell, A., Chan, G., & Heuser, M. (2019). Randomized comparison of low dose cytarabine with or without glasdegib in patients with newly diagnosed acute myeloid leukemia or high-risk myelodysplastic syndrome. *Leukemia, 33*(2), 379–389.
176. Roberts, A. W., Davids, M. S., Pagel, J. M., Kahl, B. S., Puvvada, S. D., Gerecitano, J. F., Kipps, T. J., Anderson, M. A., Brown, J. R., Gressick, L., Wong, S., Dunbar, M., Zhu, M., Desai, M. B., Cerri, E., Heitner Enschede, S., Humerickhouse, R. A., Wierda, W. G., & Seymour, J. F. (2016). Targeting BCL2 with Venetoclax in Relapsed Chronic Lymphocytic Leukemia. *The New England Journal of Medicine, 374*(4), 311–322.
177. Amadori, S., Suciu, S., Selleslag, D., Aversa, F., Gaidano, G., Musso, M., Annino, L., Venditti, A., Voso, M. T., Mazzone, C., Magro, D., De Fabritiis, P., Muus, P., Alimena, G., Mancini, M., Hagemeijer, A., Paoloni, F., Vignetti, M., Fazi, P., … Baron, F. (2016). Gemtuzumab ozogamicin versus best supportive care in older patients with newly diagnosed acute myeloid leukemia unsuitable for intensive chemotherapy: Results of the randomized phase III EORTC-GIMEMA AML-19 trial. *Journal of Clinical Oncology, 34*(9), 972–979.
178. Lee, Y. T., Tan, Y. J., & Oon, C. E. (2018). Molecular targeted therapy: Treating cancer with specificity. *European Journal of Pharmacology, 834*, 188–196.
179. Estey, E., Levine, R. L., & Lowenberg, B. (2015). Current challenges in clinical development of "targeted therapies": The case of acute myeloid leukemia. *Blood, 125*(16), 2461–2466.
180. Ge, R., Tan, E., Sharghi-Namini, S., & Asada, H. H. (2012). Exosomes in cancer microenvironment and beyond: Have we overlooked these extracellular messengers? *Cancer Microenvironment, 5*(3), 323–332.
181. Azmi, A. S., Bao, B., & Sarkar, F. H. (2013). Exosomes in cancer development, metastasis, and drug resistance: A comprehensive review. *Cancer Metastasis Reviews, 32*(3-4), 623–642.
182. Allan, D. S., & De Lisio, M. (2018). Reversing pathological remodelling of the bone marrow microenvironment in acute myeloid leukemia. *Stem Cell Investigation, 5*, 29.
183. Chalmin, F., Ladoire, S., Mignot, G., Vincent, J., Bruchard, M., Remy-Martin, J. P., Boireau, W., Rouleau, A., Simon, B., Lanneau, D., De Thonel, A., Multhoff, G., Hamman, A., Martin, F., Chauffert, B., Solary, E., Zitvogel, L., Garrido, C., Ryffel, B., … Ghiringhelli, F. (2010). Membrane-associated Hsp72 from tumor-derived exosomes mediates STAT3-dependent immunosuppressive function of mouse and human myeloid-derived suppressor cells. *The Journal of Clinical Investigation, 120*(2), 457–471.

184. Koch, R., Aung, T., Vogel, D., Chapuy, B., Wenzel, D., Becker, S., Sinzig, U., Venkataramani, V., von Mach, T., Jacob, R., Truemper, L., & Wulf, G. G. (2016). Nuclear Trapping through Inhibition of Exosomal Export by Indomethacin Increases Cytostatic Efficacy of Doxorubicin and Pixantrone. *Clinical Cancer Research, 22*(2), 395–404.
185. Bouvy, C., Wannez, A., Laloy, J., Chatelain, C., & Dogne, J. M. (2017). Transfer of multidrug resistance among acute myeloid leukemia cells via extracellular vesicles and their microRNA cargo. *Leukemia Research, 62*, 70–76.
186. Tullis, R. H., Duffin, R. P., Zech, M., & Ambrus, J. L., Jr. (2002). Affinity hemodialysis for antiviral therapy. I. Removal of HIV-1 from cell culture supernatants, plasma, and blood. *Therapeutic Apheresis, 6*(3), 213–220.
187. Lentz, M. R. (1989). Continuous whole blood UltraPheresis procedure in patients with metastatic cancer. *Journal of Biological Response Modifiers, 8*(5), 511–527.
188. Tullis, R. H., Duffin, R. P., Handley, H. H., Sodhi, P., Menon, J., Joyce, J. A., & Kher, V. (2009). Reduction of hepatitis C virus using lectin affinity plasmapheresis in dialysis patients. *Blood Purification, 27*(1), 64–69.
189. Marleau, A. M., Chen, C. S., Joyce, J. A., & Tullis, R. H. (2012). Exosome removal as a therapeutic adjuvant in cancer. *Journal of Translational Medicine, 10*, 134.
190. Tian, T., Zhu, Y. L., Zhou, Y. Y., Liang, G. F., Wang, Y. Y., Hu, F. H., & Xiao, Z. D. (2014). Exosome uptake through clathrin-mediated endocytosis and macropinocytosis and mediating miR-21 delivery. *The Journal of Biological Chemistry, 289*(32), 22258–22267.
191. Min, Q. H., Wang, X. Z., Zhang, J., Chen, Q. G., Li, S. Q., Liu, X. Q., Li, J., Liu, J., Yang, W. M., Jiang, Y. H., Xu, Y. M., Lin, J., Gao, Q. F., Sun, F., Zhang, L., & Huang, B. (2018). Exosomes derived from imatinib-resistant chronic myeloid leukemia cells mediate a horizontal transfer of drug-resistant trait by delivering miR-365. *Experimental Cell Research, 362*(2), 386–393.
192. Luan, X., Sansanaphongpricha, K., Myers, I., Chen, H., Yuan, H., & Sun, D. (2017). Engineering exosomes as refined biological nanoplatforms for drug delivery. *Acta Pharmacologica Sinica, 38*(6), 754–763.
193. Goh, W. J., Zou, S., Ong, W. Y., Torta, F., Alexandra, A. F., Schiffelers, R. M., Storm, G., Wang, J. W., Czarny, B., & Pastorin, G. (2017). Bioinspired cell-derived nanovesicles versus exosomes as drug delivery systems: A cost-effective alternative. *Scientific Reports, 7*(1), 14322.
194. Pascucci, L., Cocce, V., Bonomi, A., Ami, D., Ceccarelli, P., Ciusani, E., Vigano, L., Locatelli, A., Sisto, F., Doglia, S. M., Parati, E., Bernardo, M. E., Muraca, M., Alessandri, G., Bondiolotti, G., & Pessina, A. (2014). Paclitaxel is incorporated by mesenchymal stromal cells and released in exosomes that inhibit in vitro tumor growth: a new approach for drug delivery. *Journal of Controlled Release, 192*, 262–270.
195. Haney, M. J., Klyachko, N. L., Zhao, Y., Gupta, R., Plotnikova, E. G., He, Z., Patel, T., Piroyan, A., Sokolsky, M., Kabanov, A. V., & Batrakova, E. V. (2015). Exosomes as drug delivery vehicles for Parkinson's disease therapy. *Journal of Controlled Release, 207*, 18–30.
196. DiMasi, J. A., Grabowski, H. G., & Hansen, R. W. (2016). Innovation in the pharmaceutical industry: New estimates of R&D costs. *Journal of Health Economics, 47*, 20–33.
197. Thomas, D. W., Burns, J., Audette, J., Carroll, A., Dow-Hygelund, C., Hay, M. (2016). *Clinical development success rates 2006–2015*. BIO, Biomedtracker, Amplion.
198. Hwang, T. J., Carpenter, D., Lauffenburger, J. C., Wang, B., Franklin, J. M., & Kesselheim, A. S. (2016). Failure of investigational drugs in late-stage clinical development and publication of trial results. *JAMA Internal Medicine, 176*(12), 1826–1833.
199. Baker, B. M., & Chen, C. S. (2012). Deconstructing the third dimension: how 3D culture microenvironments alter cellular cues. *Journal of Cell Science, 125*(Pt 13), 3015–3024.
200. Magin, C. M., Alge, D. L., & Anseth, K. S. (2016). Bio-inspired 3D microenvironments: a new dimension in tissue engineering. *Biomedical Materials, 11*(2), 022001.
201. Jozaki, T., Aoki, K., Mizumoto, H., & Kajiwara, T. (2010). In vitro reconstruction of a three-dimensional mouse hematopoietic microenvironment in the pore of polyurethane foam. *Cytotechnology, 62*(6), 531–537.
202. Tan, J., Liu, T., Hou, L., Meng, W., Wang, Y., Zhi, W., & Deng, L. (2010). Maintenance and expansion of hematopoietic stem/progenitor cells in biomimetic osteoblast niche. *Cytotechnology, 62*(5), 439–448.
203. Mortera-Blanco, T., Mantalaris, A., Bismarck, A., Aqel, N., & Panoskaltsis, N. (2011). Long-term cytokine-free expansion of cord blood mononuclear cells in three-dimensional scaffolds. *Biomaterials, 32*(35), 9263–9270.
204. Miyoshi, H., Murao, M., Ohshima, N., & Tun, T. (2011). Three-dimensional culture of mouse bone marrow cells within a porous polymer scaffold: effects of oxygen concentration and stromal layer on expansion of haematopoietic progenitor cells. *Journal of Tissue Engineering and Regenerative Medicine, 5*(2), 112–118.
205. Leisten, I., Kramann, R., Ventura Ferreira, M. S., Bovi, M., Neuss, S., Ziegler, P., Wagner, W., Knuchel, R., & Schneider, R. K. (2012). 3D co-culture of hematopoietic stem and progenitor cells and mesenchymal stem cells in collagen scaffolds as a model of the hematopoietic niche. *Biomaterials, 33*(6), 1736–1747.

206. Ferreira, M. S., Jahnen-Dechent, W., Labude, N., Bovi, M., Hieronymus, T., Zenke, M., Schneider, R. K., & Neuss, S. (2012). Cord blood-hematopoietic stem cell expansion in 3D fibrin scaffolds with stromal support. *Biomaterials, 33*(29), 6987–6997.

207. de la Puente, P., Muz, B., Gilson, R. C., Azab, F., Luderer, M., King, J., Achilefu, S., Vij, R., & Azab, A. K. (2015). 3D tissue-engineered bone marrow as a novel model to study pathophysiology and drug resistance in multiple myeloma. *Biomaterials, 73*, 70–84.

Structural Biology of the Tumor Microenvironment

Joseph W. Freeman

1 Structural Biology of the TME

Cancers can be described as "rogue organs" [1] because they are composed of multiple cell types and tissues. The transformed cells can recruit and alter healthy cells from surrounding tissues for their own benefit. It is these interactions that create the tumor microenvironment (TME). The TME describes the cells, factors, and extracellular matrix proteins that make up the tumor and the area around it; the biology of the TME influences tumor progression. Changes in the TME can lead to the growth and development of the tumor, the death of the tumor, or tumor metastasis. Metastasis is the process by which cancer spreads from its initial site to a different part of the body. Metastasis occurs when cancer cells enter the circulatory system or lymphatic system after they break away from a tumor. Once the cells leave, they can travel to a different part of the body and form new tumors. Therefore, understanding the TME is critical to fully understand cancer and find a way to successfully combat it. Knowledge of the TME can better inform researchers of the ability of potential therapies to reach tumor cells. It can also give researchers potential targets to kill the tumor. Instead of directly killing the cancer cells, therapies can target an aspect of the TME which could then halt tumor development or lead to tumor death. In other cases, targeting another aspect of the TME could make it easier for another therapy to kill the cancer cells, for example, using nanoparticles with collagenases to target the collagen in the surrounding environment to expose the cancer cells to drugs [2].

The TME can be split simply into cells and the structural matrix. Within these groups are fibroblasts, structural proteins, immune cells, lymphocytes, bone marrow-derived inflammatory cells, blood vessels, and signaling molecules [3–5]. From structure to providing nutrients for growth, each of these components plays a critical role in tumor maintenance. Together these components impact cancer growth, development, and resistance to therapies [6]. In this chapter, we will describe the TME and express the importance of the cellular and structural elements of the TME.

2 Cellular Elements

2.1 Fibroblasts

Fibroblasts are an important part of the TME [7–9]. Fibroblasts include endothelial cells which are responsible for tumor structure and protection

J. W. Freeman (✉)
Department of Biomedical Engineering, Rutgers University, New Brunswick, NJ, USA
e-mail: jfreeman@soe.rutgers.edu

D. Banerjee, R. K. Tiwari (eds.), *Tumor Microenvironment: Cellular, Metabolic and Immunologic Interactions*, Advances in Experimental Medicine and Biology 1350,
https://doi.org/10.1007/978-3-030-83282-7_4

from immune cells [5]. Cancer-associated fibroblasts (CAFs), also called myofibroblasts, make up the majority of the cells in the stroma [1, 10]. After injury fibroblasts in the tissue respond to paracrine signals by becoming CAFs [1, 11]. The creation of myofibroblasts can create fibrosis in organs, which increases cancer risk [12, 13]. The CAFs maintain and modify the ECM within the tumor [14]. CAFs come from several different cells including smooth muscle cells, endothelial cells, mesenchymal stem cells, and myoepithelial cells [1, 15–18]. Early tumor development is characterized by changes in the composition and mechanical properties of the ECM [19–21]. CARs can increase the tumor mass by producing more collagen [22]. As more collagen is produced, it is cross-linked with other ECM molecules like elastin using lysyl oxidase (LOX) [19, 21–23].

The presence of CAFs is also important for angiogenesis. When fibroblast growth factor-2 (FGF-2) secretion from CAFs is inhibited, there is a reduction in angiogenesis [19, 24]. Along with controlling angiogenesis locally, fibroblasts express stromal cell-derived factor-1 (SDF-1/CXCL12) which is a signal for circulating immature endothelial cells. This leads to cancer vascularization and metastasis [25].

CAFs secrete mitogenic growth factors for malignant cells; these include hepatocyte growth factor (HGF), fibroblast growth factor (FGF), and insulin-like growth factor 1 (IGF1) [15–18]. CAFs also support tumor growth through attracting immune cells and enhancing neovascularization [25]. The arrangement of CAFs differs depending on the cancer. CAFs can be arranged into fibrovascular cores that extend throughout the body of the tumor [21]. In other cancers, the CAFs are around the malignant cells housed within dense supportive tissue that fills the space in the tumor increasing its density [21].

2.2 Adipocytes

In intra-abdominal tumors that metastasize into the omentum, adipocytes recruit malignant cells and promote their growth. The malignant cells use fatty acids for energy [1, 26].

2.3 Vascular Endothelial Cells

Vascular endothelial cells are important for the TME because they provide the vasculature which allows the tumor to receive necessary nutrients and waste transport to increase in size. This arises from an exchange of factors between malignant cells and the vascular endothelial cells. These factors include platelet-derived growth factors (PDGFs), vascular endothelial growth factors (VEGFs), and fibroblast growth factors (FGFs) [1, 27]. This communication is typically stimulated by hypoxic conditions in the TME; hypoxia causes malignant cells and inflammatory cells to secrete these factors which then stimulate new vessels to sprout from existing ones toward the TME [1, 27].

2.4 Pericytes

Pericytes, or perivascular stromal cells, provide structure to the blood vessels [1, 28]. In clinical studies, it has been shown that a low amount of pericyte coverage in the blood vessels is linked to a higher degree of metastasis and poor prognosis [29, 30]. In mouse models, low pericyte levels were linked to suppressed tumor growth and increased hypoxia, epithelial-mesenchymal transition (EMT), and mesenchymal-epithelial transition (MET) [1, 31].

2.5 Lymphatic Endothelial Cells

Just as blood vessels can grow into and within the TME lymphatic vessels can also be drawn into and developed within the TME, this occurs through the production of VEGFC or VEGFD [1, 32]. Malignant cells can invade existing lymphatic vessels. Malignant cells and macrophages can also sponsor lymphatic sprouting through the secretion of VEGFC and VEGFD. Along with lymphatic sprouting, this can also lead to the enlargement of lymphatic vessels and lymph nodes. Lymphatic tissues within the TME (cells and vessels) are involved in the movement of malignant cells and changing the host immune response to the tumor [33].

2.6 Immune Cells

Immune cells also play an important role in the TME. Granulocytes, lymphocytes, and macrophages are found in the TME [5]. Most adult solid tumors contain leukocytes (including both myeloid- and lymphoid-lineage cells) [6, 34]. These immune cells are involved in different immune responses such as inflammatory reactions orchestrated by the tumor that lead to promote survival. The most prominent immune cell type in the TME is the macrophage [35, 36]. These tumor-associated macrophages (TAMs) are plentiful in most cancers and are typically tumorigenic [1, 37]. They aid in the migration, invasion, and metastases of malignant cells [38]. The presence of a large population of TAMs has been linked to poor cancer prognoses [39].

Macrophages can suppress antitumor immune responses and promote metastasis by aiding in the release of tumor cells into the vasculature [35]. Metastasis is the primary cause of mortality and morbidity due to cancer [40]; it is estimated that approximately 90% of cancer deaths are due to metastasis [40, 41]. Studies have shown that macrophages help circulating cancer cells leave blood vessels from areas far from the initial tumor site [3, 4, 42]. Immune cells in this space can express proteolytic enzymes to remodel and change the properties of the surrounding ECM. The effects of the enzymes can also alter the function of the ECM as well, leading to changes in cellular proliferation, altering cellular differentiation, and releasing bioactive agents [43].These enzymes include metallo, serine, and cysteine proteases [6, 43]. These immune cells can also create growth mediators that stimulate the proliferation of cancer cells and nearby stromal cells [6, 44]. These mediators include growth factors (such as fibroblast growth factors (FGFs), epidermal growth factor (EGF), transforming growth factor-β (TGF-β), and tumor necrosis factor-α (TNF-α)), interleukins (ILs), chemokines, histamine, and heparins [6, 44]. As this chapter focuses on the structural biology of the TME, it will only focus on macrophages that exhibit behavior that affects aspects of the TME structure (ECM, vasculature, lymphatic system).

There are several different types of T cells that are found within the TME. CD8+ memory T cells (CD8 + CD45RO+) are typically found in patients with a good prognosis [1, 45]. These cells are supported by helper T cells, CD4 + T helper 1 (TH1) cells. Other cells include TH2, TH17, and immunosuppressive T regulatory cells (Tregs), which aid in tumor growth [1, 45]. Tregs inhibit the recognition and removal of tumor cells by the immune system [1, 46]. In some cases, Tregs can also suppress tumor development [1, 47–49].

Similar to fibroblasts, macrophages are also involved in TME angiogenesis [1, 50, 51]. Oligonucleotide arrays of TAMs indicate that they are highly encoded for angiogenic molecules [52]. The behavior of the macrophages is modulated by the nature of the TME. As the density of the TME increases, the level of hypoxia within the TME increases. As with fibroblasts, the angiogenic behavior of the TAMs is stimulated by hypoxia. TAMs amass in TMEs that are necrotic or hypoxic. TAMs are attracted to these areas by the release of VEGF, endothelial-monocyte-activating polypeptide 2 (EMAP2), and endothelins [53]. In fact, researchers have identified a hypoxia-induced pro-angiogenic macrophage phenotype in humans [1, 54, 55].

Along with macrophages, neutrophils may also involve with development of the TME. Several studies have shown that tumor-associated neutrophils (TANs) promote tumor growth and development and tumor angiogenesis [56–58]. Additional studies have shown that TANs can suppress the immune system and degrade the existing ECM [59, 60]. On the other hand, other studies have shown that neutrophils possess antitumor abilities after cytokine/immunological activation or through the inhibition of TGF-β [61–64].

3 Structural Elements

3.1 Vasculature

Vasculature within the TME is unlike "normal" vasculature, the vessels are abnormal in several aspects [1, 65]. Blood vessels in the TME are not homogenous; they are highly branched and tortuous with uneven vessel lumen. These vessels are also leaky; this leakiness increases interstitial fluid pressure leading to unevenness of blood flow, oxygenation, and nutrient distribution in the TME. These less than ideal conditions lead to more hypoxia in the TME which can lead to metastasis [27].

Vascular cells (vascular endothelial cells and pericytes) are responsible for bringing the vasculature to the cancer cells, providing nutrients and getting rid of waste [66]. Tumor vasculature arises from preexisting blood vessels that branch toward the tumor or from endothelial progenitor cells [5, 36].

As stated earlier, the tumor vascular network is disorganized and leaky. This would be a disadvantage in normal tissues. Disorganization increases the surface area but does not efficiently oxygenate tissues or remove waste. Leaky vessels steal nutrients away from needy cells and prevent waste from efficiently flowing out of the tissues. In tumors however these characteristics are major advantages. This leakiness increases the permeability of the vessels which drives further tumor-induced angiogenesis, disturbs blood flow, allows for the infiltration of inflammatory cell, and creates opportunities for tumor cell extravasation and metastasis [67]. Disorganization allows for longer vessels inside of the tumors to create more opportunities for angiogenesis and metastasis.

Tumor vasculature is composed of a series of vessels, composed of endothelial cells surrounded by pericytes. In normal, healthy vessels, the endothelial cells form the inner lining of the vessel, the portion that contacts the blood; the pericytes surround the surface of the vessel [68]. The absence of pericytes leads to vessels that are leaky or extremely dilated [68]. There are several important differences between normal blood vessels and tumor blood vessels.

As in every tissue/organ, increasing access to blood leads to increased access to nutrients and increased proliferation. This should be seen in tumors. In mouse models, increasing angiogenesis increases cancer cell proliferation, while inhibiting angiogenesis reduces the amount of hyperproliferation [6, 69–72]. In microvascular endothelial cell (HMEC-1) and breast cancer cell (MDA-MB-231) co-cultures, there is a significant cross talk between the two populations, creating chemical cues that make angiogenesis more favorable [73]. MDA-MB-231 significantly increased expression of ANG2 mRNA (20-fold relative to monoculture). In addition, MDA-MB-231 and HMEC-1 co-cultures produced increased levels of ANG2 and VEGF protein coupled with decreased expression of ANG1 compared to the cells in monoculture. This shifts the ANG1/ANG2 ratio toward ANG2, which correlates with vessel destabilization and sprouting in vivo. These behaviors are indicators of neovascularization. In another experiment, a functional angiogenesis assay showed well-defined microvascular endothelial cell (TIME) tube formation when cultured in media collected from MDA-MB-231/HMEC-1 co-cultures [73]. This behavior was seen in bilayered collagen I tumor model where TIME cells co-cultured with the MDA-MB-231 cells showed an increase in cell number, elongated morphology, and invasive sprouted into the underlying acellular collagen I layer [74]. In both studies, co-culture with less aggressive cancer cells did not create a robust angiogenic response [73, 74]. This connection to angiogenesis links fibroblast cancer cell migration from the primary tumor locations leading to metastasis [5].

3.2 Extracellular Matrix

The ECM is defined as a system of macromolecules such as collagens, enzymes, and glycoproteins that provide biomechanical strength and structure in the body [36, 42, 75, 76]. Along with providing physical structure, the ECM also has a dynamic role in the growth, development, and spread of cancers [1, 75]. The ECM also influences cellular behaviors such as proliferation, adhesion, migration, invasion, and communication between cells [8, 75, 77, 78]. This is done through the modulation of cellular adhesion and presence of a variety of growth factors including angiogenic factors and chemokines that interact with cell surface receptors and cause cells to secrete new structural proteins and cross-link them to alter tensile and compressive strength and elasticity [75, 79].

Cell-ECM adhesion is accomplished largely through interactions of integrin receptors with various motifs present in the matrix such as RGD in collagen [80]. Integrins are heterodimeric transmembrane proteins composed of one alpha and one beta subunit; with 18 different alpha units and 8 different beta units, there are a total of 24 identified integrins in the human body [81]. This heterogeneity of integrin receptors is further modified by alternative splicing and intercellular signaling which can regulate integrin binding affinity [80, 81]. In addition to integrin binding to collagen through RGD, many integrins have shown binding to other motifs allowing binding of other extracellular matrix proteins: laminin, fibronectin, vitronectin, ICAM-1, ICAM-2, C3b, fibrinogen, VCAM-1, factor X, thrombospondin, and osteopontin [80] (maybe do a table showing which integrins bind which ECM molecules).

Integrins set up the formation of focal adhesions which structurally secure the cell to the matrix and sense forces in the matrix, the type of the matrix, and topology of the matrix. Integrins often act in concert with growth factor receptors, which are activated by sequestered growth factors either released or presented to the receptors due to interactions with molecules present on the surface of the cell membrane [76]. This information is transmitted to the cell through recruitment of intracellular kinases linked to integrin and growth factor receptors or directly through mechanically transmitting forces to the nucleus through mechanosomes altering transcription [76, 82]. These signals drive many cellular programs involved in cell proliferation, differentiation, and migration depending on many factors: integrin type, matrix type, matrix forces, presence of matrix-bound growth factors, and cell type.

Due to their involvement in signaling responsible for proliferation, adhesion, and migration, overexpression of many integrin types has been found to be correlated with worse prognosis in cancer, such as $\alpha v\beta 3$, $\alpha v\beta 5$, $\alpha v\beta 6$, $\alpha 4\beta 1$, $\alpha 5\beta 1$, and $\alpha 6\beta 4$ [83–94]. Additionally, some of these receptors should be absent in fully developed adult epithelial tissues, specifically $\alpha v\beta 3$, $\alpha v\beta 6$, and $\alpha 5\beta 1$ integrins. This has led to the targeting of these receptors and downstream effectors with antibodies or other small molecules to inhibit their action. On the other hand, some integrin types have been found to inhibit cancer metastasis such as $\alpha 2\beta 1$, whose expression is often lost in breast cancer. It is found that re-expression of $\alpha 2\beta 1$ has reversed the malignant phenotype of breast cancer and prevents metastasis to other tissues [95]. A more complete review of integrins and their involvement in cancer was conducted previously by Desgrosellier et al. [81].

3.3 ECM Structural Proteins

Collagens are a family of structural proteins and represent the main component of extracellular matrix present within many epithelial tissues. There are several types of collagen with varying abundance depending on the tissue. Collagens form triple helical strands of varying lengths that self-assemble into fibrils, fibers, and/or bundles of varying geometry and microstructure depending on the type [96]. Type I collagens, for instance, make up the skin, bone, tendons, and ligaments serving functional roles in each of the tissues. In bone collagen provides a scaffold for calcium deposition creating a composite material that resists both compression and tension. Within tendons and ligaments, it forms fiber bundles which tether muscle to bone or bone to bone, respectively. Another type of collagen, type III, forms the reticulum a mesh of fine collagen fibers that acts to organize the tissue above the basement membrane, while yet another type collagen IV forms the actual basement membrane.

Usually, the ECM of tumors is stiffer than surrounding tissues; this is created my modifications from CAFs. Within the TME, CAFs rearrange collagen and elastin while cross-linking them together using lysyl oxidase and transglutaminase [23, 97]. This process increases the stiffness of the tumor. In order to remodel the ECM malignant cells, TAMs and CAFs secrete matrix metalloproteinases (MMPs) that degrade ECM proteins. Their degradation releases chemokines, growth factors, and angiogenic factors that lead to further growth of the tumor. These changes also enable migration of cancer cells, while adhesion gradients within the ECM and ECM concentration alter cancer cell migration within the tumor [98, 99]. There is also an upregulation of cathepsins which process and activate heparinases that aid in metastasis, angiogenesis, and inflammation [100, 101].

Laminins are structural proteins often found in the basement membrane of tissues and have been shown to act as ligands for several integrin receptors. Laminins are heterotrimeric ecm proteins consisting of combinations of α-, β-, and γ-chains that come in various combinations. LamB1 laminin contains an internal ribosomal entry site (IRES) implicated in cancer development. Specifically, LamB1 has been found to translate at increased levels through IRES sites on its transcript following binding of La protein during EMT of cancer cells [102]. Laminin5 is a marker of invading human cancer cells and is coexpressed with urokinase plasminogen activator on budding colon adenocarcinoma. 67 kDa laminin receptor is a marker for cancer.

Fibronectin is yet another protein component of the ECM. It contains binding domains for integrin, collagen, fibrin, and heparan sulfate proteoglycans often serving as a link between cellular integrin receptors and the ECM. In addition to being present in the ECM, fibronectin exists within the plasma portion of blood as a soluble inactive form; here it helps with clotting upon vascular injury. Fibronectin is a dimer that consists of two identical subunits connected through a pair of disulfide bonds.

Proteoglycans are proteins modified with polysaccharide chains which serve structural and signaling purposes. ECM environments rich in glycosaminoglycan (GAG) hyaluronan (HA) trigger EMT through activating cellular CD44 receptors [103–106]. Tenascin C a glycoprotein has also been shown to be increased in expression in late-stage mammary invasive ductal carcinomas around the border of the tumor. It then contributes to metastasis by regulating tyrosine-protein kinase src and focal adhesion kinase signaling within cancer cells enabling EMT [107, 108]. The heparan sulfate proteoglycan (HSPG) syndecan-1 is also involved as CAF can begin to express it in addition to the cancerous cells in a tumor; cancer cells can sense this shift in expression and this triggers EMT [109]. However not all ECM proteins help tumor growth and metastasis as illustrated by an ecm protein tubulointerstitial nephritis antigen-like 1 (TINALG1). TINALG competitively binds to alpha5beta1, alphaVbeta1, and epidermal growth factor receptor (EGFR) to inhibiting tumors driven by FAK/EGFR signaling [110].

References

1. Balkwill, F. R., Capasso, M., & Hagemann, T. (2012). The tumor microenvironment at a glance. *Journal of Cell Science, 125*(Pt 23), 5591–5596.
2. Zinger, A., et al. (2019). Collagenase nanoparticles enhance the penetration of drugs into pancreatic tumors. *ACS Nano, 13*(10), 11008–11021.
3. Spill, F., et al. (2016). Impact of the physical microenvironment on tumor progression and metastasis. *Current Opinion in Biotechnology, 40*, 41–48.
4. Del Prete, A., et al. (2017). Leukocyte trafficking in tumor microenvironment. *Current Opinion in Pharmacology, 35*, 40–47.
5. Arneth, B. (2019). Tumor microenvironment. *Medicina (Kaunas, Lithuania), 56*(1).
6. Hanahan, D., & Coussens, L. M. (2012). Accessories to the crime: Functions of cells recruited to the tumor microenvironment. *Cancer Cell, 21*(3), 309–322.
7. Pattabiraman, D. R., & Weinberg, R. A. (2014). Tackling the cancer stem cells – What challenges do they pose? *Nature Reviews Drug Discovery, 13*(7), 497–512.
8. Korneev, K. V., et al. (2017). TLR-signaling and proinflammatory cytokines as drivers of tumorigenesis. *Cytokine, 89*, 127–135.
9. LeBleu, V. (2015). Imaging the tumor microenvironment. *Cancer Journal, 21*, 174–178.

10. Sugimoto, H., et al. (2006). Identification of fibroblast heterogeneity in the tumor microenvironment. *Cancer Biology & Therapy, 5*, 1640–1646.
11. Li, B., & Wang, J. H. (2011). Fibroblasts and myofibroblasts in wound healing: Force generation and measurement. *Journal of Tissue Viability, 20*, 108–120.
12. Desmoulière, A., Guyot, C., & Gabbiani, G. (2004). The stroma reaction myofibroblast: A key player in the control of tumor cell behavior. *The International Journal of Developmental Biology, 48*, 509–517.
13. Radisky, D. C., Kenny, P. A., & Bissell, M. J. (2007). Fibrosis and cancer: Do myofibroblasts come also from epithelial cells via EMT? *Journal of Cellular Biochemistry, 101*, 830–839.
14. Kalluri, R., & Zeisberg, M. (2006). Fibroblasts in cancer. *Nature Reviews. Cancer, 6*(5), 392–401.
15. Willis, B. C., duBois, R. M., & Borok, Z. (2006). Epithelial origin of myofibroblasts during fibrosis in the lung. *Proceedings of the American Thoracic Society, 3*, 377–382.
16. Tomasek, J. J., et al. (2002). Myofibroblasts and mechano-regulation of connective tissue remodelling. *Nature Reviews Molecular Cell Biology, 3*, 349–363.
17. Spaeth, E. L., et al. (2009). Mesenchymal stem cell transition to tumor-associated fibroblasts contributes to fibrovascular network expansion and tumor progression. *PLoS One, 4*, e4992.
18. Brittan, M., et al. (2002). Bone marrow derivation of pericryptal myofibroblasts in the mouse and human small intestine and colon. *Gut, 50*, 752–757.
19. Bhome, R., et al. (2015). A top-down view of the tumor microenvironment: structure, cells and signaling. *Frontiers in Cell and Developmental Biology, 3*(33).
20. Bonnans, C., Chou, J., & Werb, Z. (2014). Remodelling the extracellular matrix in development and disease. *Nature Reviews. Molecular Cell Biology, 15*(12), 786–801.
21. Erez, N., et al. (2010). Cancer-associated fibroblasts are activated in incipient neoplasia to orchestrate tumor-promoting inflammation in an NF-kappaB-dependent manner. *Cancer Cell, 17*, 135–147.
22. Erler, J. T., et al. (2006). Lysyl oxidase is essential for hypoxia-induced metastasis. *Nature, 440*(7088), 1222–1226.
23. Levental, K. R., et al. (2009). Matrix crosslinking forces tumor progression by enhancing integrin signaling. *Cell, 139*(5), 891–906.
24. Pietras, K., et al. (2008). Functions of paracrine PDGF signaling in the proangiogenic tumor stroma revealed by pharmacological targeting. *PLoS Medicine, 5*(1), e19.
25. Orimo, A., et al. (2005). Stromal fibroblasts present in invasive human breast carcinomas promote tumor growth and angiogenesis through elevated SDF-1/CXCL12 secretion. *Cell, 12*(3), 335–348.
26. Nieman, K. M., et al. (2011). Adipocytes promote ovarian cancer metastasis and provide energy for rapid tumor growth. *Nature Medicine, 17*(11), 1498–1503.
27. Carmeliet, P., & Jain, R. K. (2011). Molecular mechanisms and clinical applications of angiogenesis. *Nature, 473*, 298–307.
28. Armulik, A., Genové, G., & Betsholtz, C. (2011). Pericytes: Developmental, physiological, and pathological perspectives, problems, and promises. *Developmental Cell, 21*, 193–215.
29. O'Keeffe, M. B., et al. (2008). Investigation of pericytes, hypoxia, and vascularity in bladder tumors: Association with clinical outcomes. *Oncology Research, 17*, 93–101.
30. Yonenaga, Y., et al. (2005). Absence of smooth muscle actin-positive pericyte coverage of tumor vessels correlates with hematogenous metastasis and prognosis of colorectal cancer patients. *Oncology, 69*, 159–166.
31. Cooke, V. G., et al. (2012). Pericyte depletion results in hypoxia-associated epithelial-to-mesenchymal transition and metastasis mediated by met signaling pathway. *Cancer Cell, 21*(1), 66–81.
32. Alitalo, K. (2011). The lymphatic vasculature in disease. *Nature Medicine, 17*, 1371–1380.
33. Swartz, M. A., & Lund, A. W. (2012). Lymphatic and interstitial flow in the tumour microenvironment: Linking mechanobiology with immunity. *Nature Reviews Cancer, 12*, 210–219.
34. Tlsty, T. D., & Coussens, L. M. (2006). Tumor stroma and regulation of cancer development. *Annual Review of Pathology, 1*, 119–150.
35. Mantovani, A., et al. (2008). Cancer-related inflammation. *Nature, 454*(7203), 436–444.
36. Hanahan, D., & Weinberg, R. A. (2011). Hallmarks of cancer: The next generation. *Cell, 144*(5), 646–674.
37. Qian, B. Z., & Pollard, J. W. (2010). Macrophage diversity enhances tumor progression and metastasis. *Cell, 141*, 39–51.
38. Condeelis, J., & Pollard, J. W. (2006). Macrophages: Obligate partners for tumor cell migration, invasion, and metastasis. *Cell, 124*, 263–266.
39. Bingle, L., Brown, N. J., & Lewis, C. E. (2002). The role of tumour-associated macrophages in tumour progression: Implications for new anticancer therapies. *Journal of Pathology, 196*, 254–265.
40. Seyfried, T. N., & Huysentruyt, L. C. (2013). On the origin of cancer metastasis. *Critical Reviews in Oncogenesis, 18*(1–2), 43–73.
41. Chaffer, C., & Weinberg, R. (2011). A perspective on cancer cell metastasis. *Science, 331*(6024), 1559–1564.
42. Grivennikov, S. I., Greten, F. R., & Karin, M. (2010). Immunity, inflammation, and cancer. *Cell, 140*(6), 883–899.
43. Lu, P., et al. (2011). Extracellular matrix degradation and remodeling in development and disease. *Cold Spring Harbor Perspectives in Biology, 3*(12).
44. Balkwill, F., Charles, K. A., & Mantovani, A. (2005). Smoldering and polarized inflammation in the ini-

tiation and promotion of malignant disease. *Cancer Cell, 7*(3), 211–217.
45. Fridman, W. H., et al. (2012). The immune contexture in human tumours: Impact on clinical outcome. *Nature Reviews Cancer, 12*, 298–306.
46. Campbell, D. J., & Koch, M. A. (2011). Treg cells: Patrolling a dangerous neighborhood. *Nature Medicine, 17*(8), 929–930.
47. Tzankov, A., et al. (2008). Correlation of high numbers of intratumoral FOXP3+ regulatory T cells with improved survival in germinal center-like diffuse large B-cell lymphoma, follicular lymphoma and classical Hodgkin's lymphoma. *Haematologica, 93*, 193–200.
48. Koreishi, A. F., et al. (2010). The role of cytotoxic and regulatory T cells in relapsed/refractory Hodgkin lymphoma. *Applied Immunohistochemistry & Molecular Morphology, 18*, 206–211.
49. Fozza, C., & Longinotti, M. (2011). T-cell traffic jam in Hodgkin's lymphoma: Pathogenetic and therapeutic implications. *Advanced Hematology*.
50. Lin, E. Y., et al. (2006). Macrophages regulate the angiogenic switch in a mouse model of breast cancer. *Cancer Research, 66*, 11238–11246.
51. Zumsteg, A., & Christofori, G. (2009). Corrupt policemen: Inflammatory cells promote tumor angiogenesis. *Current Opinion in Oncology, 21*, 60–70.
52. Ojalvo, L. S., et al. (2010). Gene expression analysis of macrophages that facilitate tumor invasion supports a role for Wnt-signaling in mediating their activity in primary mammary tumors. *Journal of Immunology, 184*, 702–712.
53. Murdoch, C., Giannoudis, A., & Lewis, C. E. (2004). Mechanisms regulating the recruitment of macrophages into hypoxic areas of tumors and other ischemic tissues. *Blood, 104*, 2224–2234.
54. Burke, B., et al. (2002). Expression of HIF-1alpha by human macrophages: Implications for the use of macrophages in hypoxia-regulated cancer gene therapy. *Journal of Pathology, 196*, 204–212.
55. White, J. R., et al. (2004). Genetic amplification of the transcriptional response to hypoxia as a novel means of identifying regulators of angiogenesis. *Genomics, 83*, 1–8.
56. Pekarek, L. A., et al. (1995). Inhibition of tumor growth by elimination of granulocytes. *Journal of Experimental Medicine, 181*, 435–440.
57. Shojaei, F., et al. (2008). Role of Bv8 in neutrophil-dependent angiogenesis in a transgenic model of cancer progression. *Proceedings of the National Academy of Sciences of the United States of America, 105*, 2640–2645.
58. Nozawa, H., Chiu, C., & Hanahan, D. (2006). Infiltrating neutrophils mediate the initial angiogenic switch in a mouse model of multistage carcinogenesis. *Proceedings of the National Academy of Sciences of the United States of America, 103*, 12493–12498.
59. DeLarco, J. E., Wuertz, B. R., & Furcht, L. T. (2004). The potential role of neutrophils in promoting the metastatic phenotype of tumors releasing interleukin-8. *Clinical Cancer Research, 10*, 4895–4900.
60. Youn, J. I., & Gabrilovich, D. I. (2010). The biology of myeloid-derived suppressor cells: The blessing and the curse of morphological and functional heterogeneity. *European Journal of Immunology, 40*, 2969–2975.
61. Colombo, M. P., et al. (1992). Local cytokine availability elicits tumor rejection and systemic immunity through granulocyte-T-lymphocyte cross-talk. *Cancer Research, 52*, 4853–4857.
62. Fridlender, Z. G., et al. (2009). Polarization of tumor-associated neutrophil phenotype by TGF-beta: "N1" versus "N2" TAN. *Cancer Cell, 16*, 183–194.
63. Granot, Z., et al. (2011). Tumor entrained neutrophils inhibit seeding in the premetastatic lung. *Cancer Cell, 20*, 300–311.
64. Hicks, A. M., et al. (2006). Transferable anticancer innate immunity in spontaneous regression/complete resistance mice. *Proceedings of the National Academy of Sciences of the United States of America, 103*(20), 7753–7758.
65. Jain, R. K. (2005). Normalization of tumor vasculature: An emerging concept in antiangiogenic therapy. *Science, 307*, 58–62.
66. Armulik, A., Abramsson, A., & Betsholtz, C. (2005). Endothelial/pericyte interactions. *Circulation Research, 97*(6), 512–523.
67. Azzi, S., Hebda, J. K., & Gavard, J. (2013). Vascular permeability and drug delivery in cancers. *Frontiers in Oncology, 3*, 211.
68. Bergers, G., & Song, S. (2005). The role of pericytes in blood-vessel formation and maintenance. *Neuro-Oncology, 7*(4), 452–464.
69. Parangi, S., et al. (1996). Antiangiogenic therapy of transgenic mice impairs de novo tumor growth. *Proceedings of the National Academy of Sciences of the United States of America, 93*(5), 2002–2007.
70. Brem, H., et al. (1993). The combination of anti-angiogenic agents to inhibit primary tumor growth and metastasis. *Journal of Pediatric Surgery, 28*(10), 1253–1125.
71. Hanahan, D., & Folkman, J. (1996). Patterns and emerging mechanisms of the angiogenic switch during tumorigenesis. *Cell, 86*(3), 353–364.
72. Bergers, G., et al. (1999). Effects of angiogenesis inhibitors on multistage carcinogenesis in mice. *Science, 284*(5415), 808–812.
73. Buchanan, C. F., et al. (2012). Cross-talk between endothelial and breast cancer cells regulates reciprocal expression of angiogenic factors in vitro. *Journal of Cellular Biochemistry, 113*(4), 1142–1151.
74. Szot, C. S., et al. (2013). In vitro angiogenesis induced by tumor-endothelial cell co-culture in bilayered, collagen I hydrogel bioengineered tumors. *Tissue Engineering. Part C, Methods, 19*(11), 864–874.

75. Lu, P., Weaver, V. M., & Werb, Z. (2012). The extracellular matrix: A dynamic niche in cancer progression. *Journal of Cell Biology, 196*(4), 395–406.
76. Hynes, R. O. (2009). The extracellular matrix: Not just pretty fibrils. *Science, 326*(5957), 1216–1219.
77. Feig, C., et al. (2013). Targeting CXCL12 from FAP-expressing carcinoma-associated fibroblasts synergizes with anti-PD-L1 immunotherapy in pancreatic cancer. *Proceedings of the National Academy of Sciences of the United States of America, 110*, 20212–20217.
78. Anderson, B. O., et al. (2011). Optimisation of breast cancer management in low-resource and middle-resource countries: Executive summary of the Breast Health Global Initiative consensus, 2010. *Lancet Oncology, 12*(4), 387–398.
79. Frantz, C., Stewart, K. M., & Weaver, V. M. (2010). The extracellular matrix at a glance. *Journal of Cell Science, 123*, 4195–4200.
80. Hynes, R. O. (1992). Integrins – Versatility, modulation, and signaling in cell-adhesion. *Cell, 69*(1), 11–25.
81. Desgrosellier, J. S., & Cheresh, D. A. (2010). Integrins in cancer: Biological implications and therapeutic opportunities. *Nature Reviews Cancer, 10*(1), 9–22.
82. Huang, C. Y., & Ogawa, R. (2010). Mechanotransduction in bone repair and regeneration. *FASEB Journal, 24*(10), 3625–3632.
83. Takayama, S., et al. (2005). The relationship between bone metastasis from human breast cancer and integrin αvβ3 expression. *Anticancer Research, 25*(1A), 79–83.
84. Bates, R. C., et al. (2005). Transcriptional activation of integrin β6 during the epithelial-mesenchymal transition defines a novel prognostic indicator of aggressive colon carcinoma. *The Journal of Clinical Investigation, 115*(2), 339–347.
85. Elayadi, A. N., et al. (2007). A peptide selected by biopanning identifies the integrin αvβ6 as a prognostic biomarker for nonsmall cell lung cancer. *Cancer Research, 67*(12), 5889–5895.
86. Taylor, S. T., Hickman, J. A., & Dive, C. (2000). Epigenetic determinants of resistance to etoposide regulation of Bcl-xL and Bax by tumor microenvironmental factors. *JNCI: Journal of the National Cancer Institute, 92*(1), 18–23.
87. Slack-Davis, J. K., et al. (2009). Vascular cell adhesion Molecule-1 is a regulator of ovarian cancer peritoneal metastasis. *Cancer Research, 69*(4), 1469–1476.
88. Nista, A., et al. (1997). Functional role of α4β1 and α5β1 integrin fibronectin receptors expressed on adriamycin-resistant MCF-7 human mammary carcinoma cells. *International Journal of Cancer, 72*(1), 133–141.
89. Stewart, R. L., & O'Connor, K. L. (2015). Clinical significance of the integrin α6β4 in human malignancies. *Laboratory Investigation, 95*(9), 976–986.
90. Chao, C., et al. (1996). A function for the integrin α6β4 in the invasive properties of colorectal carcinoma cells. *Cancer Research, 56*(20), 4811–4819.
91. Bello, L., et al. (2001). αvβ3 and αvβ5 integrin expression in glioma periphery. *Neurosurgery, 49*(2), 380–390.
92. Sung, V., et al. (1998). Bone sialoprotein supports breast cancer cell adhesion proliferation and migration through differential usage of the αvβ3 and αvβ5 integrins. *Journal of Cellular Physiology, 176*(3), 482–494.
93. Montgomery, A. M., Reisfeld, R. A., & Cheresh, D. A. (1994). Integrin alpha v beta 3 rescues melanoma cells from apoptosis in three-dimensional dermal collagen. *Proceedings of the National Academy of Sciences, 91*(19), 8856.
94. Max, R., et al. (1997). Immunohistochemical analysis of integrin αvβ3 expression on tumor-associated vessels of human carcinomas. *International Journal of Cancer, 71*(3), 320–324.
95. Zutter, M. M., et al. (1995). Re-expression of the alpha 2 beta 1 integrin abrogates the malignant phenotype of breast carcinoma cells. *Proceedings of the National Academy of Sciences, 92*(16), 7411.
96. Balasubramanian, P., et al. (2013). Collagen in human tissues: Structure, function, and biomedical implications from a tissue engineering perspective. In A. Abe et al. (Eds.), *Polymer composites – Polyolefin fractionation – Polymeric peptidomimetics – Collagens* (pp. 173–206). Springer.
97. Weigelt, B., & Bissell, M. J. (2008). Unraveling the microenvironmental influences on the normal mammary gland and breast cancer. *Seminars in Cancer Biology, 18*, 311–321.
98. Arneth, B. (2020). Tumor microenvironment. *Medicina (Kaunas), 56*(1), 15.
99. Walker, C., Mojares, E., & Del Río Hernández, A. (2018). Role of extracellular matrix in development and cancer progression. *International Journal of Molecular Sciences, 19*, 3028.
100. Lerner, I., et al. (2011). Heparanase powers a chronic inflammatory circuit that promotes colitis-associated tumorigenesis in mice. *The Journal of Clinical Investigation, 121*(5), 1709–1721.
101. Edovitsky, E., et al. (2004). Heparanase gene silencing, tumor invasiveness, angiogenesis, and metastasis. *Journal of the National Cancer Institute, 96*, 1219–1230.
102. Petz, M., et al. (2012). La enhances IRES-mediated translation of laminin B1 during malignant epithelial to mesenchymal transition. *Nucleic Acids Research, 40*(1), 290–302.
103. Boyle, S. T., et al. (2020). Acute compressive stress activates RHO/ROCK-mediated cellular processes. *Small GTPases, 11*(5), 354–370.
104. El-Haibi, C. P., et al. (2012). Critical role for lysyl oxidase in mesenchymal stem cell-driven breast cancer malignancy. *Proceedings of the National Academy of Sciences of the United States of America, 109*(43), 17460–17465.

105. Heldin, P., et al. (2013). Deregulation of hyaluronan synthesis, degradation and binding promotes breast cancer. *Journal of Biochemistry, 154*(5), 395–408.
106. Venning, F. A., Wullkopf, L., & Erler, J. T. (2015). Targeting ECM disrupts cancer progression. *Frontiers in Oncology, 5*.
107. Nagaharu, K., et al. (2011). Tenascin C induces epithelial-mesenchymal transition-like change accompanied by SRC activation and focal adhesion kinase phosphorylation in human breast cancer cells. *American Journal of Pathology, 178*(2), 754–763.
108. Yoshida, T., et al. (1997). Co-expression of tenascin and fibronectin in epithelial and stromal cells of benign lesions and ductal carcinomas in the human breast. *Journal of Pathology, 182*(4), 421–428.
109. Mennerich, D., et al. (2004). Shift of syndecan-1 expression from epithelial to stromal cells during progression of solid tumours. *European Journal of Cancer, 40*(9), 1373–1382.
110. Shen, M., et al. (2019). Tinagl1 suppresses triple-negative breast cancer progression and metastasis by simultaneously inhibiting integrin/FAK and EGFR signaling. *Cancer Cell, 35*(1), 64.

Metabolic Interactions Between Tumor and Stromal Cells in the Tumor Microenvironment

Deepshikha Mishra and Debabrata Banerjee

1 Introduction

Tumor and its microenvironment are highly complex and heterogeneous. Tumor microenvironment (TME) contains stromal cell of different types including fibroblasts, immune cells, as well as endothelial cells having varied influence on the local metabolic activity. Recent advances in our understanding of complexity of the TME have revealed that a multifaceted interaction between tumor cells with their neighboring stroma is essential for tumor growth and metastasis. The tumor stroma responds to various signals present in the microenvironment and helps to establish cancer-associated fibroblasts (CAFs). The tumor stroma also helps in recruitment of other host cells via tumor cell-derived signals. Molecular interactions in the tumor microenvironment are dynamic, and allow reciprocal exchange of nutrients, secretory molecules, and other signals between tumor and stromal cells. These interactions between tumor cells and nonmalignant stromal cells in the tumor microenvironment not only promote tumor development and progression, but largely control most of the characteristic hallmarks of tumorigenesis and stimulate chemotherapeutic drug resistance. Shared interactions between tumor and stromal cells facilitated either directly by cell-to-cell contact or via the release of secretory molecules, including cytokines, chemokines, and extracellular matrix (ECM) remodeling proteins activate signaling pathways that encourage cell growth, survival, and overall development. The secretory molecules reciprocally shared among tumor cells and neighboring cells instigate epithelial-mesenchymal transition (EMT), tumor cell migration, invasion, and dissemination to secondary sites.

The multidimensional interactions between tumor and stromal cells also allow enhanced access to nutrients and other factors in the local environment and lead to a metabolic reprogramming. The metabolic activities in the microenvironment are prone to get altered by the influence of both tumor and stromal factors present in the microenvironment. Metabolic reprogramming allows in the fulfillment of demands associated with the cancerous growth of cells. Tumor-stroma interactions further fuel this process and help in satisfying elevated demands within a complex microenvironment. Different stromal components in the tumor microenvironment provide additional nutrients that supplement local nutrient pool. Stromal cells present in the immediate proximity of tumor cells are inevitably affected by the meta-

D. Mishra (✉) · D. Banerjee (✉)
Department of Pharmacology, Robert Wood Johnson Medical School, Rutgers University, New Brunswick, NJ, USA
e-mail: banerjed@rutgers.edu

D. Banerjee, R. K. Tiwari (eds.), *Tumor Microenvironment: Cellular, Metabolic and Immunologic Interactions*, Advances in Experimental Medicine and Biology 1350,
https://doi.org/10.1007/978-3-030-83282-7_5

bolic alterations caused by neighbor cancerous cells. Stromal fibroblasts present in the tumor microenvironment also known as cancer-associated fibroblasts (CAFs) have a key role in metabolic reprogramming. CAFs are predominantly resident mesenchymal cells in origin that get activated and reprogrammed in response to signals from cancer cells. The metabolic reprogramming of CAFs in the tumor microenvironment alters multiple signaling pathways that allow enhanced tumor-stroma interactions, which further accelerate growth and development of cancer. Tumor cells display heightened glucose uptake, and even under normoxic conditions display increased generation of lactate through pyruvate conversion by aerobic glycolysis, also known as the Warburg effect. This adaptation not only allows generation of biosynthetic precursors for added nutritional demands of tumor cells but also directs the metabolic reprograming of neighboring stromal cells. Lactate generated as a result of metabolic reprograming of tumor cells and stromal cells plays diverse role in the tumor microenvironment. Both tumor and stromal CAFs consume and secrete lactate differently which makes it an integral modulating factor in tumor microenvironment. Molecular evidences collected over the last several years have directed toward a deeper examination of interactions between tumor cells and stromal cells in diverse microenvironments.

In this chapter, we provide information about metabolic reprogramming in cancer cells, molecular interactions between tumor and stromal cells, focusing primarily on CAFs and tumor cell interaction. We have covered the role of cytokines, chemokines, and lactate in driving tumor-stroma interactions in the microenvironment. Here, we have discussed the pro-tumorigenic molecular interactions in between tumor cells and CAFs mediated via altered signaling pathways, cytokines, chemokines, and lactate in the tumor vicinity. A better understanding of the complex cancer cell-CAF interactions will help in designing successful therapeutic strategies targeting the stromal-rich tumors in the clinic.

2 Metabolic Alterations in Cancer Cells

Cancer cells alter the metabolism for their own need. Cells acquire energy and accumulate the building blocks necessary for their growth and proliferation through breaking down nutrients by means of metabolic pathways. The energy generated within cells by these metabolic pathways is stored in the form of adenosine triphosphate (ATP) molecules. Normal or quiescent cells depend primarily on aerobic respiration/oxidative phosphorylation to fulfill their energy demands; however, cancer cells grow rapidly and hence have increased demands for energy which they meet quite differently. To maintain the constant pools of ATP, cancer cells make an effort to increase the import of nutrients from their cellular environment and additionally procure carbon intermediates that fulfill the elevated demands of building blocks necessary for DNA, protein, and lipid synthesis for biomass generation [88]. Otto Warburg made the first groundbreaking observation in the 1920s in the field of cancer metabolism and discovered that tumors took up strikingly higher levels of glucose compared to normal tissues [86]. He further showed that, even in the presence of sufficient oxygen, cancer cells produced drastically more lactate than normal tissues signifying the glycolytic fermentation [85]. Seminal findings by Warburg established that altered metabolism was exclusive to cancer cells; however, his hypothesis that altered metabolism was a result of mitochondrial defects was later found to be not correct as mitochondria in most of the tumor are not defective in terms of performing oxidative phosphorylation. Instead, further studies made it evident that proliferating cancer cells have reprogrammed mitochondrial metabolism to meet the demands of macromolecular synthesis, a possibility never thought-out by Warburg [87].

Resting cells maintain basal levels of nutrients including glucose and amino acids by lineage-specific growth factor signaling, which allows optimal level of macromolecular synthesis and ATP production, required to maintain cellular homeostasis. Cells in the absence of extrinsic signals often employ autophagic degradation of organelles and macromolecules, which ultimately results in cell death. However, cancerous cells, in contrast, show heightened ligand signaling that instigates cells to take up nutrients at higher rate and divert them into metabolic pathways that support enhanced ATP and macromolecule synthesis including nucleic acids, proteins, and lipids. Glycolysis in resting cells allows conversion of glucose to pyruvate at basal rate, which is further oxidized in the TCA cycle. However, cancer cells with high glycolytic flux subsequently convert pyruvate to lactate with the help of lactate dehydrogenase enzyme, which restores NAD+ from NADH. The regenerated NAD+ permits glycolysis to continue, and the resultant lactate is secreted by the cell [25]. Work done by Hanahan and Weinberg established the groundwork behind cancer reprograming by deciphering the remarkable abilities shared by almost all of human cancer types. They showed that cancer cells display six essential alterations in normal cellular physiology that collectively drive toward malignant cellular growth. Cancer cells adapt themselves and display self-sufficiency in growth signals, become insensitive to antigrowth signals, evade apoptosis, and acquire limitless replicative potential, interminable angiogenesis, tissue invasion, and metastasis. Acquisition of these physiologic capabilities not only results in tumor development but also allows successful breaching of various anticancer signaling and control mechanisms present in the cells [33].

In the last few decades, accumulating evidence in the field of cancer metabolism have provided valuable insights and have enhanced our understanding of aerobic glycolysis and other metabolic adaptations observed in cancer cells, which help to keep up the anabolic requirements related with cell growth and proliferation [87]. Recent advances have highlighted the remarkable metabolic differences between proliferative and quiescent cells by active metabolic reprogramming led by proto-oncogenes and tumor suppressors. This altered metabolism serves as a prime feature driving tumorigenesis [87]. Tumor development is dependent on the metabolic reprogramming and is a common feature. Oncogenic mutations driving this process directly or indirectly help accelerated growth of the tumor. Metabolic reprogramming in the cancer cell helps in acquisition of necessary nutrients from an often nutrient-poor environment. The cancer cell exploits opportunities to acquire these nutrients to support viability and build new biomass. The metabolic reprogramming results in altered intracellular and extracellular levels of metabolites which have significant effects on level of gene expression, cellular differentiation, and eventually the entire tumor microenvironment. These cancer-associated metabolic changes primarily cause a deregulated uptake of glucose and amino acids, practicing opportunistic modes of nutrient acquirement, using glycolysis/TCA cycle intermediates for biomass generation and NADPH production, elevated demand for nitrogen, and modifications in metabolite-driven gene regulation. Most tumors display several of the abovementioned hallmark changes, while a few tumors display all of them [65]. The metabolic reprogramming or altered tumor cellular bioenergetics drives malignant transformation, tumor development, invasion, and metastasis. The whole complex and dynamic process of metabolic reprogramming reflects robustness of tumor cells even under unfavorable conditions [92].

3 Signaling Pathways Promoting Metabolic Alterations in Tumor

It has been previously established that, to fulfill the elevated demands of growth and proliferation, cancer cells rewire their cellular metabolism or metabolic reprogramming and the diversity of the metabolic alterations of a cancer cell then dictates heterogeneity in the metabolic needs of the cell. This heterogeneity is influenced by genetic and nongenetic factors, which allow metabolic flexibility in terms of nutrient utilization by tumor cell and facilitate its growth. Apart from pathways of aerobic glycolysis, other pathways including glutamine-dependent anaplerosis, de novo lipid biosynthesis, and cellular mediators of gene expression pathways such as phosphatidylinositol 3-kinase (PI3K)/Akt/mTOR signaling, Myc, and hypoxia-inducible factor 1 (HIF1) also play a major role in this reorganization of metabolic activities that helps in maintaining cellular bioenergetics, macromolecular synthesis, and cell division [25]. One of the ways of metabolic reprogramming is also a result of mutations in enzymes or a changed enzyme isoform expression that can force different metabolic pathways. These altered metabolic enzymes may provide oncogenic signals and may impact specific pathways and alter overall metabolic regulation [34]. One of the metabolic enzymes playing a vital role in metabolic reprogramming is lactate dehydrogenase (LDH). It is the primary enzyme that allows interconversion of pyruvate to lactate and helps in exchange of metabolic fuel by tumor-stroma interaction [56].

Cancer cells display deregulations in signaling pathways, and transcription factors including PI3K, mTOR, MYC, and hypoxia-inducible factor can drive metabolic alterations or metabolic transformation and hence serve as important targets in cancer metabolism-based therapeutics. Further, isoforms of metabolic enzymes highly expressed in specific cancers may also serve as novel druggable targets with improved therapeutic potential [78]. Aerobic glycolysis in tumor cells is influenced by multiple signaling pathways. Oncogenic stimulation of signaling pathways activated by the loss of p53 tumor suppressor or activation of PI3K oncoprotein alters signaling pathways that further modifies cellular metabolism. PI3K activated AKT stimulates glycolysis by activating mTOR and by regulating glycolytic enzymes. mTOR changes metabolism in broader ways, and it influences glycolytic phenotype by augmenting activity of hypoxia-inducible factor 1 (HIF1), which modulates hypoxia-adaptive transcriptional profile. HIF1 increases expression of glycolytic enzymes, glucose transporters (GLUT), and pyruvate dehydrogenase kinase isozyme 1 (PDK1), limiting entry of pyruvate into tricarboxylic acid (TCA) cycle. MYC, in a HIF-mediated manner, also helps in activating several other genes of the glycolytic pathway. Deregulated signaling pathways elicit responses from tumor cells, further modulating metabolic adaptations. These adaptations help in tumor proliferation by providing sufficient levels of energy, macromolecular biosynthetic ability, and a balanced maintenance of the redox status. Metabolic adaptations are a necessity for proliferating tumor cells, so that they can effectively respond to the signals put out by oncogenic signaling pathways [16]. Another metabolic adaptation in some of the proliferative cancer cell is the preferential expression of the pyruvate kinase (PKM2) lesser active M2 isoform. With the use of alternative pathways, the less active PKM2 consequently results in an accumulation of 3-phosphoglycerate (3PG), which is diverted into serine biosynthetic pathway. Together, these metabolic adaptations promote distinct metabolic phenotypes among proliferating cells [83].

4 Signaling Pathway Alterations in Tumor-Associated Stroma

Apart from cancer cells, stromal cells also display deregulated signaling pathways to promote tumor growth, development, and response to therapy. Highly abundant cancer-associated fibroblasts particularly influence this process by interacting with different cells, including endothelial and immune cells and other components of TME, such as collagens, fibronectin, and elastin. CAFs benefit by receiving both physical and chemical signals produced in the TME, and accordingly change their phenotype from being quiescent fibroblasts to a more proliferative and secretory phenotype. CAFs have gained more clinical interest in driving disease progression and have emerged as a prominent molecular target in designing future clinical therapeutic strategies [22]. Gene expression profiling is highly advantageous in identifying stromal gene signatures associated with cases with advanced tumor grade and metastasis and may suggest the role of microenvironment in influencing cancer initiation, and metastatic progression [81]. Some of the tumor-associated genes that are significantly upregulated in the stroma include components of extracellular matrix and matrix metalloproteinases. Tumor-associated stroma continuously undergoes gene expression changes during the process of cancer progression, allowing transition from preinvasive to invasive tumor growth. This transition to high-grade tumors with aggressive invasive growth is often dependent upon the increased expression of different matrix metalloproteinases, such as MMP2, MMP11, and MMP14 [49]. Molecular components of the microenvironment such as matrix metalloproteinases and factors including transforming growth factor-beta1, platelet-derived growth factor, and hepatocyte growth factor are the important mediators of tumor cells-CAF interaction, and can hence be exploited as possible molecular targets for anticancer therapy [55].

Transcriptomic analysis in colorectal cancer (CRC) patient-derived CAFs identified deregulated genes related to Wnt signaling and TGFβ signaling [1]. Further, CAFs were found as the primary source of WNT2, and organotypic coculture assay shows that WNT2 facilitated fibroblast motility, promoted extracellular matrix remodeling, and enhanced CRC cell invasion. This finding highlights stromal-derived WNT2 and its receptor as favorable stromal targets [43]. Single-cell RNA and protein technologies revealed a deeper role of stromal CAFs in regulating heterogeneity in pancreatic cancer. It was found that progression toward proliferative phenotype with invasive epithelial-to-mesenchymal transition is associated with deregulated MAPK-STAT3 signaling (mitogen-activated protein kinase and signal transducer and activator of transcription 3). Stromal abundance not only leads to intratumoral heterogeneity but is also associated with varied clinical outcomes in human pancreatic ductal carcinoma [45].

As the brain is one of the primary sites of relapse for different cancers, understanding the mechanisms behind brain metastasis is a necessity. The complexity of the microenvironment in brain tumor makes it challenging to investigate. Recently, it was found that malignant cells in the brain shift to epithelial and neuronal-like lineage programs to adapt in the brain TME, and different regions of the brain have specific transcriptional hallmarks of metastasis. Further, it was revealed that tumor stroma undergoes coadaptation in the brain [89]. Resident fibroblasts coming in contact with tumor epithelial cells (TEC) can get activated and irreversibly convert to cancer-associated fibroblasts that instigate oncogenic signaling in TEC. Transcriptomic study done in pancreatic cancer using KPC mice model (KRAS/mut p53-induced pancreatic cancer) showed that treatment with Minnelide, an anticancer compound, deregulated TGFβ signaling in CAF resulting in reversal of activated state to a non-proliferative quiescent state. Further, TEC treated with conditioned media from drug-treated CAFs demonstrated reduced oncogenic signaling, expressed through downregulated transcription factor Sp1. Through early clinical findings, this study encourages the use of Minnelide to target cross talk between TEC and CAFs. Using Minnelide may help in actively reducing the reactive stromal fibroblasts underscoring the importance of stromal-based anticancer strategies for effective treatment of the disease [23].

In lung cancer, it was found that stromal cells activate expression of genes that support oncogenesis. It was shown that expression of genes of mammalian target of rapamycin (mTOR) pathway and extracellular matrix (ECM) was primarily involved in driving this process. Further, expression of two distinct genes, IL-6 and BMP1, in lung cancer-associated stroma was found to be activated in lung cancer patients [74]. Similarly, the reactive stroma in the TME of prostate cancer also displays upregulated expression of genes associated with ECM remodeling and immune functions. Also, the reactive stroma displayed significant metabolic alterations, which makes prostate cancer more prone to biochemical recurrence [4].

5 Stromal Heterogeneity in the Tumor Microenvironment

Tumor cells engage in active cross talk with the non-transformed cells in the tumor vicinity, and as a result of this cross talk, metabolic adaptations not only are restricted to tumor cells but also affect proximal nontumor cells. Solid tumors can be considered as abnormal organs that are composed of different cell types and extracellular matrix. The stromal components of the tumor organ can be divided into different components, including the stromal cells, and the ECM which is composed of fibrous proteins (collagen, fibronectin, and laminin), proteoglycans, and hyaluronic acid. The stromal cells include mesenchymal supporting cells such as fibroblasts and adipocytes. The other types of stromal cells include the cells of immune and vascular system. Tumor-promoting or tumor-inhibiting role of some of the non-transformed cells including normal epithelial cells, myoepithelial cells, mesenchymal stem cells, fibroblasts, adipocytes, endothelial cells, perivascular cells, bone marrow-derived cells, dendritic cells, etc. is reviewed elsewhere [28]. Accumulating evidence over the years have built the basis for the tumor-promoting role of metabolic reprogramming, and its direct association with tumorigenesis is now being more and more appreciated as is the importance of tumor microenvironment in directly supporting cell growth and metastasis. Tumor stroma is an active player in cancer and is comprised of multiple supporting players including stromal fibroblasts, immune cells, vascular networks, and the extracellular matrix. Cancer cells can alter behavior of normal cells (non-transformed cells) for their development, so that they can benefit from growth factors and chemokines that support tumor growth, and matrix-degrading enzymes that increase invasion and metastasis of tumor. In addition, these non-transformed cells can act as support system by controlling environmental conditions caused by stromal changes like increased interstitial pressure and flow within the tumor [36].

Not all tumors behave in a similar manner by exhibiting identical metabolic phenotype; rather, they may display differential nutrient uptake and metabolism. Unraveling metabolic heterogeneity may provide beneficial information regarding metabolic signatures that could be investigated for their therapeutic potential [17]. In the past, most of the investigations into dysregulated genes and their functional consequences in cancer biology have been focused on cancer cells. However, recent investigations have started looking at tumors as complex tissues, with an intricate collection of cancer cells along with subverted normal cell populations. The cancer cells and the supposedly normal stromal cells work in active collaboration promoting neoplastic growth. Molecular interactions between malignant cells and supporting stromal cells promote heightened tumor growth, development, and escape from antitumor therapies [33]. The different types of stromal cells, including the resident fibroblasts, pericytes, endothelial cells, and immune cells, make the microenvironment rich and diverse. Stromal components of tumor stroma may be of prognostic value, and deeper understanding tumor stroma molecular interactions within the tumor microenvironment particularly between tumor cells and cancer-associated fibroblasts will allow development of complementary stroma-targeted therapies in addition to conventional tumor cell directed therapies for cancer control in the future [67].

Tumor development encompasses the coevolution of transformed cells together with the stroma, and the successful outgrowth of tumors is dependent upon the tumor-promoting adaptations in the stromal cells which can be grouped into three broad classes including cancer-associated fibroblastic (CAF) cells, infiltrating immune cells (IICs), and angiogenic vascular cells (AVCs). The stromal cells present in the tumor microenvironment impact almost all of the hallmarks or characteristics of cancer cells [31–32]. Among the wide variety of cells including T lymphocytes, B lymphocytes, NK cells, tumor-associated macrophages (TAMs), myeloid-derived suppressor cells (MDSCs), dendritic cells, adipocytes, and vascular endothelial cells in the tumor microenvironment, the CAFs are receiving special attention for their tumor-promoting role [10]. A recent study carried out on mouse and human pancreatic ductal adenocarcinoma (PDAC) using single-cell transcriptomics analysis identified three subsets of CAF, specifically myofibroblastic (myCAFs), inflammatory (iCAFs), and antigen-presenting CAFs (apCAFs) along with their putative roles in various aspects of tumor progression [29].

The role of non-transformed cells in the complex tumor microenvironment in supporting and satisfying metabolic demands of cancer cells is less well studied. Nonmalignant stromal cells in the immediate proximity, also called tumor-associated stromal cells, are unavoidably affected by the changes happening in the cancerous neighborhood. Tumor-associated stromal cells can augment the tumor growth by serving as additional nutrient support that can supplement nutrient pool provided by the local vasculature. They secrete a wide variety of metabolites that support biosynthetic and bioenergetics pathways of cancer cells. Recently, it was proposed by Schwörer et al. that metabolites released and consumed by tumor cells act as paracrine factors and drive regenerative response in stromal cells by controlling the non-malignant cellular composition of a developing tumor [75]. Normal cells can support growth and survival of cancer cells by releasing nutrients in a nutrient limiting environment. Cancer cells benefit by forming a symbiotic association with non-transformed cells via metabolic activities not active in cancer cells including utilization of fatty acids released by adipocytes, astrocyte-mediated de novo glutamine synthesis, bone marrow stromal cell-mediated cysteine release, and amino acids generated by degradation of intracellular proteins which can serve as bioenergetic fuel and nutrients sources for cancer cells [63]. The metabolic alteration in cancer cells creates predictable gradients of extracellular metabolites that drive the phenotypic diversity of cells within the tumor milieu. These gradients might act as tumor morphogens and convey spatial information in tumors to organize embryonic tissues, imposing a certain hierarchical order within the microenvironment [18]. Genetic alterations as well as environmental factors impact the metabolic heterogeneity across a variety of tumors. Availability of nutrients in the cellular vicinity of tumor is varied because of abnormal tumor vasculature. This leads to a differential availability of oxygen and nutrients, and affects pH. The altered gradient and availability levels of substrates of metabolic pathways including glucose, amino acids, and lipids are also sensed by signaling mechanisms which in turn affect overall tumor metabolism [84].

6 CAFs as Mediators of Tumor-Stroma Interaction

The normal stroma differs profoundly from the stroma associated with a carcinoma, in which fibroblasts play a well-recognized role. They directly play role in the synthesis, deposition, and remodeling of the ECM in tumor stroma. They serve as a source of paracrine growth factors that influence the tumor growth [14]. Additionally, they support cancer cells through all stages of cancer progression, not only by supplying growth factors and chemokines but also by angiogenic recruitment of cells including endothelial cells and pericytes [38]. Neoplastic transformation causes initial insult that instigates the coevolution of the tumor niche comprising transformed and non-transformed cell types within the tumor environs.

Stromal mesenchymal stem cells (MSCs) are multipotent cells with the capacity to differentiate into a phenotype similar to CAFs. MSCs are known to participate in cancer progression and act in concert with CAFs in the inflammatory tumor microenvironment. Cancer-associated fibroblasts (CAFs) are one such mesenchyme-derived cell type of non-transformed cell that have significant plasticity and can diverge according to its origin, localization, activation status, and stress response. They are one of the major cellular components of the tumor microenvironment, and compared with normal fibroblasts, CAFs significantly promote tumorigenesis by exhibiting increased proliferation, distinctive cytokine secretion profile, and extracellular matrix (ECM) production [37]. Cancer-associated fibroblasts differ from normal fibroblasts (NFs) by specific differences in their gene expression pattern. Cooperative interaction between heterotypic fibroblasts and tumor cells supports tumor growth and invasion and may also confer therapeutic resistance [80]. Early stages of malignant tumor growth coordinates host stromal response leading to generation of CAFs from activated fibroblasts [44]. Cancer cells then signal CAFs to produce components of extracellular matrix, growth factors, tumor supporting cytokines, chemokines, enzymes, and metabolites to expedite their own survival and proliferation [39]. A diabolic interplay between CAFs and cancer cells activates epithelial-mesenchymal transition and acquisition of stem cell properties and stimulates the metabolic reprogramming of both cancer cells and stromal cells [20]. Pro-tumorigenic functions of CAFs may help to foster metabolic reprogramming and shaping of the tumor microenvironment of tumors [39].

Immunomodulation is one of the mechanisms through which CAFs encourage tumor growth and support metastasis. Regulating immune response in the TME plays a vital role in influencing disease outcome. Functional interactions between CAFs and immune cells regulate different signaling axis that disseminate immunosuppressive microenvironment. CAFs from stroma of human breast cancer and mammary tumors of transgenic mice show significantly upregulated Chi3L1. Genetic disruption of Chi3L1 led to a diminished tumor growth, macrophage recruitment, and differentiation to M2-like phenotype. It also resulted in an altered tumor immune microenvironment by increasing CD8+ and CD4+ T cell tumor infiltration, supporting a Th1 phenotype [21]. Targeting molecular interactions of stromal cells that promote immune suppression to expedite tumor progression and metastasis can be of clinical relevance in different cancers. As shown for lung squamous cell carcinoma, CAFs were found to foster tumor progression by encouraging immunosuppression through controlling the recruitment and differentiation of monocytes. It was further shown that CAFs caused differentiation of monocytes to a ROS-generating, myeloid-derived suppressor cell (MDSC) phenotype, highlighting the advantages of abolishing CAF-MDSC axis for a possible therapeutic approach to negate CAF-mediated immunosuppressive microenvironment [90]. It has also been shown that CAFs produce elevated levels of IL-33 that acts on the tumor-associated macrophages (TAMs) instigating them to undergo M1 to M2 transition. IL-33-stimulated TAMs exhibited greater than 200-fold surge of MMP9 that provoked the IL-33/ST2/NF-κB/MMP9/laminin pathway directed tumor stroma-mediated metastasis. Together, this data provides mechanistic insights pertaining to CAF-TAM association in cancer metastasis and specifies a promising therapeutic target for cancer treatment [5].

7 Chemokines in Driving Tumor-Stroma Interactions

Chemokines are soluble, small molecular, chemotactic cytokines that bind to their G-protein-coupled receptors (GPCRs) to provoke cellular response, primarily by stimulating migration of the cells [72]. These chemotactic cytokines are regulators of cell migration and can regulate growth of tumors by inducing cancer cell proliferation and inhibiting cell death. Chemokines also regulate tumor growth by indirectly controlling tumor stromal cells in the tumor microenvironment [19]. However, cancer cells do not always express receptors for chemokine. Often, they gain the expression of chemokine receptors either by gene mutation, fusion, or conditions in the native environment including hypoxia. Depending upon the local chemokine ligand concentration, cancer cells expressing chemokine receptor can migrate to distant sites in response to the chemokine gradient. Also, under certain conditions, acquisition of chemokine receptor by tumor cells makes them more prone to invade and spread. Chemokine ligand present at the tumor site can communicate proliferative, anti-apoptotic signals and induce a pro- inflammatory environment in the neighboring stroma [8, 9]. Chemokines, secreted by tumor as well as stromal cells, are one of the vital components of the TME and play a driving role in tumorigenesis. They can act either in an autocrine or paracrine way to support tumor cell growth by promoting tumor angiogenesis in the harsh acidic microenvironment. Further, growing evidence points to their involvement in tumor cell-CAF interactions. Tumor cells and CAFs display bidirectional cross talk which augment CAFs ability to secrete different tumor-promoting chemokines, which fosters tumor cell proliferation, migration, and invasion [57]. Of particular importance is the CXCL12-CXCR4 axis which aids metastasis to distant organs. Tumor cells in the generally hypoxic environments upregulate their CXCR4 expression which prepares them to migrate toward a CXCL12 gradient established by CAFs within a normoxic microenvironment [69]. A wide variety of human tumor cells originated from epithelial, mesenchymal, and hematopoietic cancers express CXCR4, although not all cancer cells are CXCR4 positive in the primary tumor site and may be associated with the more aggressive and metastatic phenotype [8, 9]. Molecular signals from the stromal cells from the microenvironment also have a significant influence on the progression of these cancers. Mesenchymal cells (marrow-derived nonneoplastic stromal cells) present in a large proportion in the tumor milieu secrete chemokine stromal cell-derived factor-1 (SDF-1/CXCL12) constitutively. CXCL12 secreted by stromal cells aids in attracting cancer cells through receptor CXCR4, which is expressed predominantly by cancer cells. CXCR4 supports tumor progression directly by promoting metastatic spread to distant cellular niches, allowing better tumor cell survival, and indirectly by a paracrine mechanism dependent on stromal-derived CXCL12 [15]. In breast cancer stroma, elevated CXCL1 expression correlates with bad patient prognosis. Further, CXCL1 expression is negatively controlled by TGF-β signaling and is specifically localized to α-SMA, FSP1 positive fibroblasts further highlighting that decreased TGF-β signaling in CAFs enhances CXCL1 expression [94].

In breast cancer, it was found CAFs and tumor-conditioned media (TCM)-exposed human bone marrow-derived MSCs stimulated TNF-α and IL-1β expression and further encouraged the release of chemokines, including CCL2, CXCL8 and CCL5. Release of chemokines was found to promote pro-cancerous environment in breast tumors [41]. Prolonged exposure to tumor-conditioned medium (TCM) results in a CAF-like myofibroblastic phenotype of mesenchymal stem cells (hMSCs) derived from human bone marrow. These phenotypically differentiated hMSCs cells also display functional properties of CAFs and exhibit myofibroblast marker expression including alpha-smooth muscle actin and sustained stromal cell-derived factor-1 (SDF-1) expression. Further, as revealed by gene expression profiling, TCM-exposed hMSCs and CAFs both show similarities in gene expression profile [58]. Gene expression analysis revealed a significant upregulation of stromal cell-derived factor-1 (SDF-1) in MSCs exposed to TCM. Exposure to TCM and recombinant SDF-1 both activated downstream STAT3/ERK signaling in human MSCs, and the treatment with MAPK/ERK kinase (MEK) inhibitor PD98059 led to a significant impairment in hMSC migration. Additionally, focal adhesion kinases (FAKs) and paxillin were also found to be activated after the exposure to TCM in the hMSCs, which were associated with F-actin filament reorganization in hMSCs [30]. CAFs display traits of myofibroblasts, promote tumor growth by secreting stromal cell-derived factor-1 (SDF-1, also called CXCL12), and mediate recruitment of endothelial progenitor cells (EPCs) at tumor sites [61]. SDF-1-CXCR4 signaling pathway plays significant tumor-promoting role in the microenvironment, as CAF-derived SDF-1 directly interacts with the CXCR4 receptor present on tumor cells and promotes neo-angiogenesis via the recruited endothelial progenitor cells (EPCs) at tumor sites [62].

MSCs are very similar to macrophages in terms of cell plasticity, as both can undergo phenotypic changes depending upon their local environment. Gene expression analysis carried out on macrophage-conditioned medium-exposed MSCs revealed pro-inflammatory phenotype-associated gene expression profile, with an increased expression of chemokines, including IL-8, CCL2, CCL5, CCL7, CCL20, and CXCL6. This finding helped in developing a better understanding of the influence of macrophage-rich microenvironment on MSCs in solid tumors [6]. Chemokine stromal cell-derived factor-1 (SDF-1)/CXCL12 required for MSC migration was found to be controlled by tumor suppressor p53. It was found that P53 inhibits MSC migration in response to tumor cells via a decrease in CXCL12 transcription, suggesting direct involvement of stromal p53 in the recruitment of MSCs to solid tumors [46]. It was found that breast cancer cells, which often grow under hypoxic conditions

(1.5% O_2), secrete elevated levels of IL-6 to activate and attract MSCs. The secreted IL-6 acts in a paracrine manner to enhance migratory ability and cell survival by activating MAPK and STAT3 signaling pathways [70]. IL-8 also plays a very important role in MSC migration, by stimulating increased expression of SDF-1 by MSCs, via activating protein kinase C (PKC) zeta isoform [66]. A knockdown of SDF-1 expression inhibited migration of MSCs toward CM from tumor cells, suggesting its requirement for migratory responses in the tumor microenvironment [54]. Apart from the abovementioned chemokines, proteins such as cyclophilin B and hepatoma-derived growth factor also promote MSC chemotaxis [47].

8 Lactate in Driving Tumor-Stroma Interactions

Lactate, in recent years, has emerged as a key regulator of cancer development and progression. The oncogenic hypoxic environment stimulates glycolytic metabolism in cancers, thus directing lactate production. Contrary to previous concepts, lactate is now known to do more than just being a by-product of glycolysis. It can act as a metabolic fuel as well as act as a signaling molecule in cancer cells. The lactate shuttles allowing exchange of lactate among cancerous cells are regulated by the enzyme lactate dehydrogenase (LDH), which allows interconversion of lactate to pyruvate and through monocarboxylate transporters (MCTs), which allow transport of lactate in and out of cells [27]. Lactate levels in many types of tumors are found to be directly correlated with enhanced metastasis, recurrence, and poor outcome. Lactate is not limited to influencing cancer cell metabolism but also affects neighboring stromal cells that support tumorigenesis. Lactate can be metabolized by tumor cells as energy source as well as can be shuttled to adjacent stromal cells for stimulating metabolic reprogramming. Lactate also promotes tumor inflammation that fuels tumor angiogenesis [26]. It has also been reported to stimulate the transcription of genes associated with stemness that promotes cancer recurrence and metastasis, contributing to a poor clinical outcome [50, 52].

Lactagenic (lactate-producing) cancer cells exhibit enhanced glucose uptake, increased activity and expression of glycolytic enzymes, reduced mitochondrial function, and amplified production, accumulation, and release of lactate with upregulated expression of monocarboxylate transporters for lactate exchange. Mutated oncogenes and tumor suppressors drive lactagenic cancer cells to display heightened aerobic glycolysis in a highly orchestrated manner. Apart from cancer cell metabolism, directly or indirectly, lactate is involved in all essential steps of carcinogenesis, fostering angiogenesis, migration, metastasis, and immune escape [73]. Role of lactate in the tumor microenvironment as a metabolic fuel and as a signaling molecule is currently being investigated with renewed enthusiasm given its emerging role in the TME. It has been found that lactate is a key player driving metabolic cross talk between tumor cells and adjacent stromal cells including CAFs, endothelial cells, and immune cells present in the tumor microenvironment. The metabolic symbiosis among these cells supports cancer aggressiveness and response to therapy. In the tumor microenvironment, lactate plays the role of a signaling oncometabolite that drives molecular interactions in between cancer-cancer cells and cancer-stromal cells [11]. As solid tumors are metabolically heterogeneous, the metabolic symbiosis between glycolytic and oxidative tumor cells countenances higher nutritional availability dependent upon the cellular location. MCTs are differentially expressed and are very important in this process; MCT4 transporter is preferentially expressed by glycolytic cancer cells (hypoxic) favoring lactate export, whereas MCT1 expressed by oxidative cells (normoxic) allows enhanced lactate import. The imported lactate is utilized as an energy source via conversion to pyruvate which then enters the TCA cycle in the mitochondria. Thus, lactate permits a metabolic symbiosis between glycolytic and oxidative cancer cells. Apart from glycolytic tumor cells, cancer-associated fibroblasts (CAFs) with a glycolytic phenotype may also be a major source of lactate production, although this may be a small portion of the CAFs present in the TME which are mainly oxidative. CAFs can exchange lactate with oxidative tumor cells; this cross talk fuels metabolic reprogramming of cancer as well as stromal cells in the TME [24]. Symbiotic association between tumor cells and CAFs drives metabolic reprogramming, which is dependent upon exchange of chemokines as well lactate in between both of these components. It was found that some of the breast cancer cells (MDA-MB-231) secrete higher levels of lactate, and this lactate specifically helps in the recruitment of hMSCs toward tumor, by activating pathways that enhance cell migration. Further, it was also shown that stromal hMSCs and CAFs in the tumor vicinity have the ability to take up the expelled lactate in the microenvironment and use it as an energy source. NMR spectroscopic analysis revealed that the lactate taken up by hMSCs and CAFs is converted to (13)C-alpha ketoglutarate confirming that stromal cells can utilize lactate produced by tumor cells [71]. Later, it was reported that lactate taken up by stromal CAFs is used for the fulfillment of energetic demands of their own and of tumor cells after recycling, which suggests a reciprocally supportive, lactate-pyruvate metabolic relationship in the tumor microenvironment (TME) [64] (Fig. 1).

Another example of cancer cell-induced CAFs reprogramming is observed in pancreatic ductal adenocarcinomas (PDACs) based on their distinct reliance on branched-chain α-ketoacid (BCKA) in stromal-rich tumors. These branched-chain amino acids (BCAAs) present in stromal-rich tumor milieu are utilized by a mutualistic metabolism [93]. The stromal cues in the PDAC milieu evoke a rapid adaptive response, causing a changed transcriptional profile along with an altered metabolome within the cancer cell. Stroma-induced changes cause increased histone acetylation that contribute toward accelerated tumor growth, suggesting indispensable stromal inputs [76]. PDAC is a lethal type of cancer and is typically composed of pancreatic malignant cells surrounded by stromal-rich tumor microenvironment consisting of CAFs, immune cells, endothelial cells, and ECM; cross talk between the tumor cells and stromal cells drive PDAC disease progression [77]. Targeting pathways associated with metabolic reprogramming of CAFs, including lactate transporter pathway, oxidative stress pathway, and autophagy, can result in disruption of the metabolic cross talk between cancer and stromal cells, and break the subservience to tumor cells of stromal fibroblasts [7].

9 Epigenetic Reprogramming in the Tumor Microenvironment

Role of cancer cells in the epigenetic reprogramming of fibroblasts has recently started garnering attention, and the molecular mechanisms driving this process are being investigated more closely. The significant findings about functional and mechanistic contributions of CAFs have been gleaned from studies carried out in breast cancers. CAFs are a heterogeneous population of cells and show diverse phenotypes that differ from their normal counterparts on the basis of different epigenetic modification with altered DNA methylation patterns [3]. The conversion of MSCs into CAFs is often associated with extensive epigenetic reprogramming and is usually manifested by extensive loss of DNA methylation with gain of cytosine hydroxymethylation at specific promoters. CAFs in breast cancer are specifically known to secrete various soluble growth factors, cytokines, and components responsible for remodeling extracellular matrix, which help in initiating and promoting tumor growth and metastasis and developing therapeutic resistance. These soluble factors play lead role in CAF reliant reprograming of cancer cells by affecting a large number of genes of multiple signaling pathways, including metabolism, inflammation, proliferation, and epigenetic modulation. This CAF-mediated reprograming of breast cancer cells is based upon cross talk between cancerous and stroma components and results in a changed gene expression pattern. It was revealed by RNAseq analysis that several genes were significantly upregulated in the presence CAF-secreted factors via change in DNA meth-

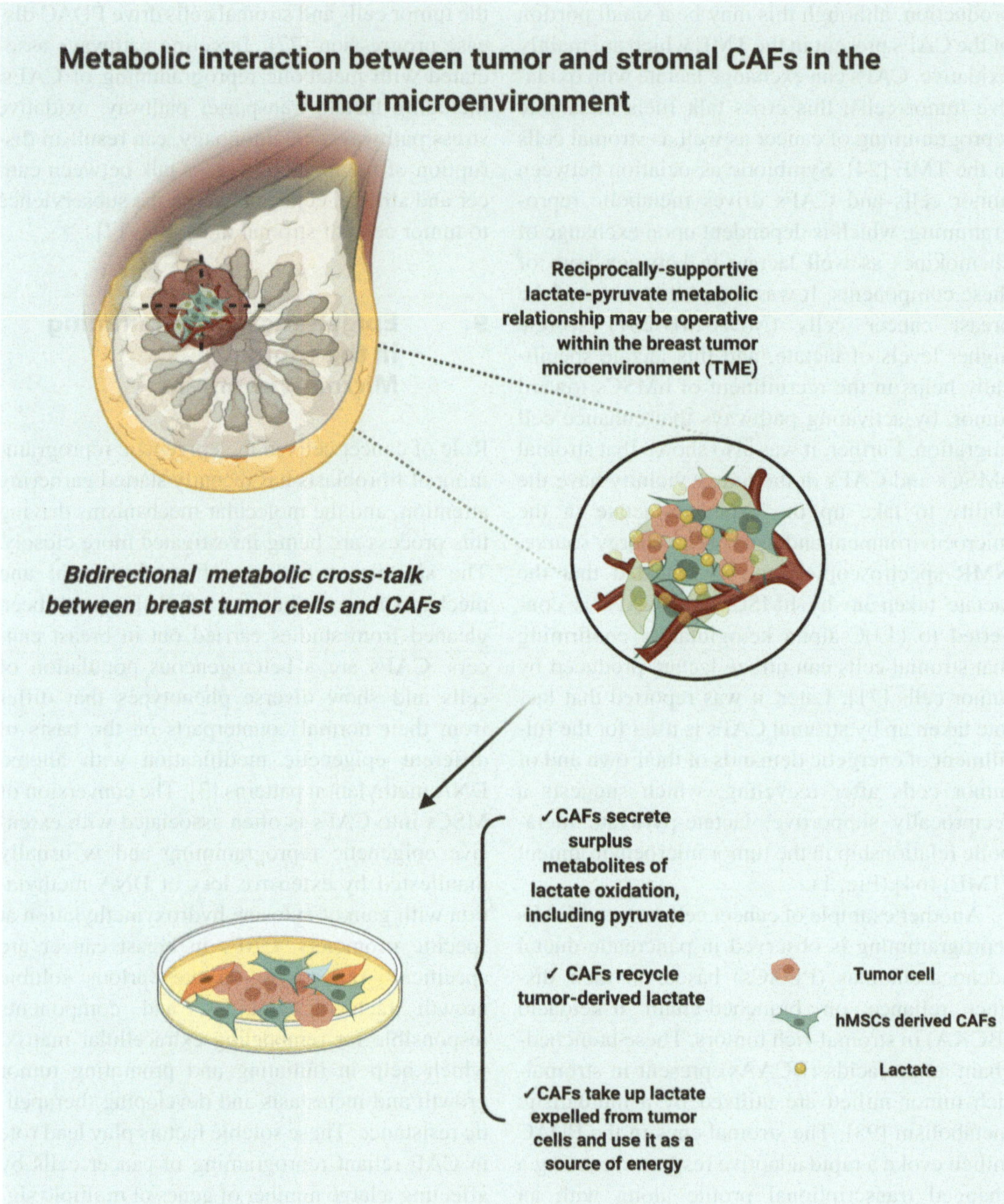

Fig. 1 In vitro model depicting tumor-stromal CAF-mediated interactions in the TME

ylation pattern, suggesting an epigenetic control of these genes [53] (Fig. 2).

Very recently, it was revealed that CAFs display a glycolytic phenotype with metabolic shift toward lactate production, and a depletion or suppression in its production alters metabolic profile of tumor and inhibits tumor growth. Hypoxia induces pro-glycolytic phenotype, with CAF-like transcriptome in normal fibroblast. Epigenetic reprogramming mediated via HIF-1α and glycolytic enzymes helps in sustaining glycolytic phenotype of the CAFs. The pro-glycolytic CAFs

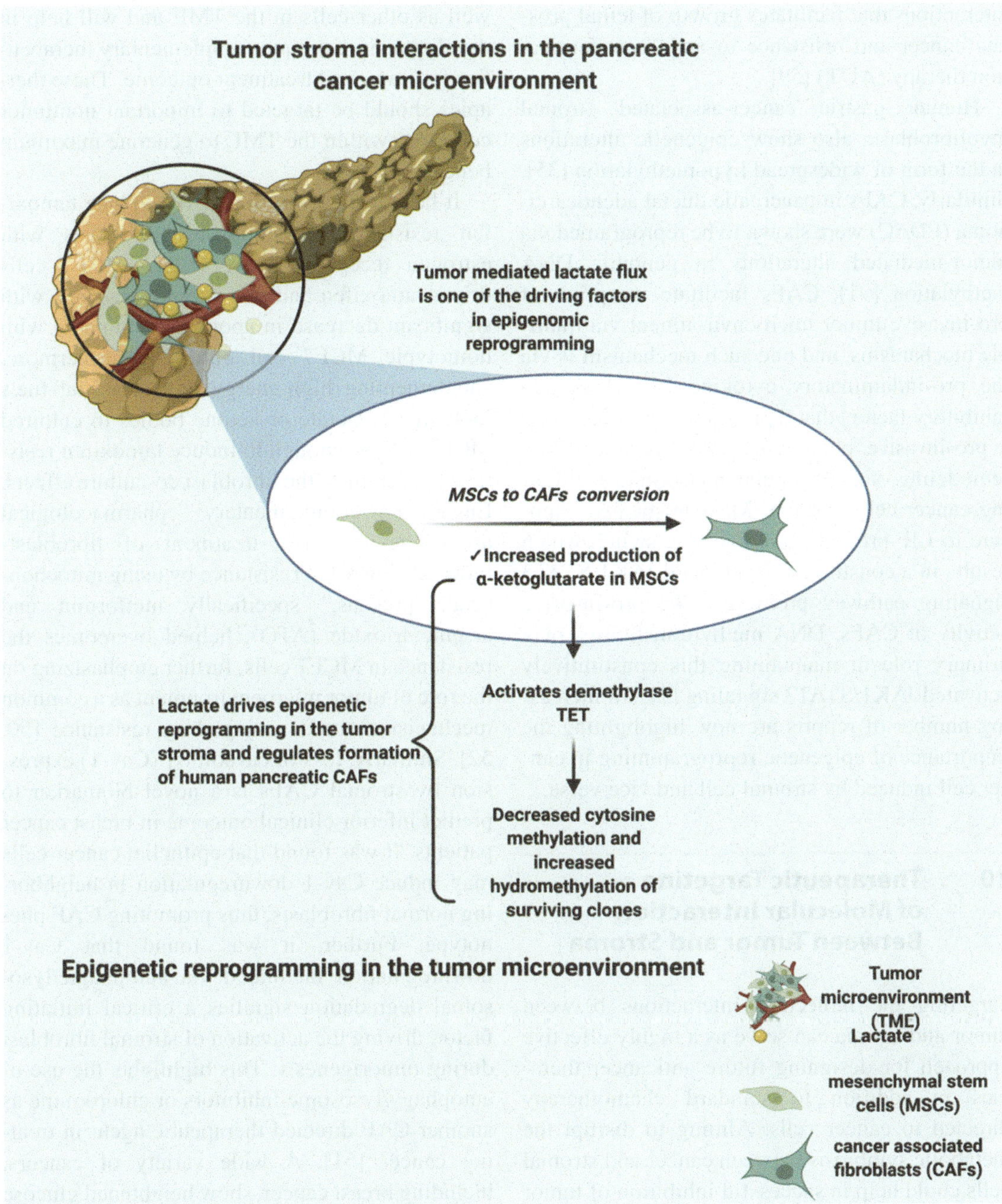

Fig. 2 Lactate-mediated epigenetic reprogramming in the TME

support breast tumor growth by attaining epigenetic control of glycolysis [12]. Secretory metabolites such as lactate released by cancer cell in the immediate milieu help in driving this conversion. Stromal cells in the immediate vicinity of tumor can incorporate lactate flux generated by tumor cells. Lactate flux in pancreatic CAFs leads to TET activation, alpha ketoglutarate production, and increased cytosine hydroxymethylation [13] (Fig. 2).

Similarly, epigenetic changes in prostatic CAFs instigate a series of stromal-epithelial interactions that facilitates growth of lethal prostate cancer and resistance to androgen deprivation therapy (ADT) [59].

Human gastric cancer-associated stromal myofibroblasts also show epigenetic alterations in the form of widespread hypomethylation [35]. Similarly, CAFs in pancreatic ductal adenocarcinoma (PDAC) were shown to be reprogramed via tumor-mediated alterations in genomic DNA methylation [91]. CAFs facilitate inception of pro-invasive tumor microenvironment via multiple mechanisms, and one such mechanism is via the pro-inflammatory cytokine LIF (leukemia inhibitory factor) that reprograms fibroblasts into a pro-invasive phenotype. This process allows remodeling of extracellular matrix and facilitating cancer cell invasion. Mechanistically, exposure to LIF prompts an epigenetic switch which results in a constitutively activated JAK1/STAT3 signaling pathway promoting the pro-invasive activity of CAFs. DNA methyltransferases play primary role in maintaining this constitutively activated JAK1/STAT3 signaling [2]. An increasing number of reports are now highlighting the importance of epigenetic reprogramming in cancer cell induced by stromal cell and vice versa.

10 Therapeutic Targeting of Molecular Interaction Between Tumor and Stroma

Targeting the molecular interactions between tumor and stroma can serve as a highly effective approach for designing future anticancer therapies in addition to standard chemotherapy directed to cancer cells. Aiming to disrupt the metabolic symbiosis between cancer and stromal cells could help in successful inhibition of tumor progression and metastasis. Metabolic reprogramming allows changes that are necessary for the synthesis of biomass and bioenergetics of tumor cells and contributes to activation of CAFs resulting in enhanced interaction between tumor cells and stromal cells. Designing innovative strategies that can target molecular interactions between tumor and stroma will lead to eradication of the pro-tumorigenic activity of CAFs as well as other cells in the TME and will help in development of unique complementary therapeutics for improved treatment outcome. These therapies should be targeted to important nontumor cell types within the TME to generate maximum benefit.

It has been shown that CAFs induce tamoxifen resistance. Co-culturing fibroblasts with estrogen receptor-positive (ER+) MCF7 cells drives tamoxifen and fulvestrant resistance with significant decrease in apoptosis compared with homotypic MCF7 cell cultures. Furthermore, supplementing high-energy mitochondrial fuels including L-lactate or ketone bodies to cultured MCF7 cells is enough to induce tamoxifen resistance and mimics the fibroblast co-culture effects. Engaging complementary pharmacological approaches for the treatment of fibroblast-induced tamoxifen resistance by using mitochondrial "poisons," specifically metformin and arsenic trioxide (ATO), helped overcomes the resistance in MCF7 cells, further emphasizing on the role of tumor microenvironment as a common mechanism for convening drug resistance [50, 52]. Similarly, loss of caveolin-1 (Cav-1) expression by stromal CAFs is a novel biomarker to predict inferior clinical outcome in breast cancer patients. It was found that epithelial cancer cells may induce Cav-1 downregulation in neighboring normal fibroblasts, thus promoting CAF phenotype. Further, it was found that Cav-1 downregulation facilitated via autophagic/lysosomal degradation signifies a critical initiating factor, driving the activation of stromal fibroblast during tumorigenesis. This highlights the use of autophagy/lysosome inhibitors or chloroquine as another CAF directed therapeutic agent in treating cancer [51]. A wide variety of cancers, including breast cancer, show heightened glucose consumption, with associated lactate production. Extruded lactate consequently causes acidification of the TME, which is associated with increased tendency for cell proliferation, invasion, migration, angiogenesis, and higher rate of cell survival. As breast carcinoma patients show upregulated MCT1 expression, inhibiting lactate transport can be a potential approach for breast cancer treatment. Knockdown of MCT1/

MCT4 in basal-like breast carcinoma via siRNA reduced cell proliferation, migration invasion, and tumor cell aggressiveness in vitro further emphasizing MCTs as promising targets in cancer therapy [60].

Metabolic coupling in mitochondria in cancer cells and catabolism in stromal CAFs fosters tumor growth, relapse, metastasis, and resistance to anticancer drugs. Catabolic-associated fibroblasts (CAFs) contribute the essential fuels including L-lactate, ketones, fatty acids, glutamine, and other amino acids to anabolic cancer cell metabolism. This catabolic metabolism allows glycolytic reprogramming in the TME. Oncogenes provide the momentum for inception of CAF phenotype in neighboring normal fibroblasts through the paracrine oxidative stress. This oncogene driven transition is associated with loss of caveolin-1 (Cav-1) expression and increased MCT4 expression in adjoining stromal fibroblasts, functionally reproducing an overall catabolic metabolism phenotype in the TME. Therapeutic strategies that allow metabolic uncoupling of oxidative cancer cells and their adjoining glycolytic stroma could be highly beneficial in targeting lethal subtype of cancers [48]. It is now well established that metabolic symbiosis besides promoting tumor growth and metastasis also promotes resistance to anticancer therapies. Targeting this metabolic association via combinatorial treatment using a glycolysis inhibitor (3PO) for efficiently inhibiting tumor growth and a complementary genetic ablation of MCT's expression may help in overcoming resistance and serve as an appealing possibility for development of anticancer therapy in patients [68].

Components of extracellular matrix and CAFs regulate tumor progression at every step of growth, development, and resistance to chemotherapies. Tumor growth is highly amplified in stromal-rich tumors including pancreatic, biliary, and breast cancers, certain types of hepatocellular cancer (HCC), and several other cancers. The molecular interaction between CAFs, ECM, and tumor cells involves a variety of mechanisms targeting ECM remodeling, enriched angiogenesis, and elevated secretion of pro-tumorigenic and immunosuppressive cytokines for better immunosuppression. As CAFs express α-smooth muscle actin (α-SMA) and fibroblast activation protein (FAP) and display upregulated expression of platelet-derived growth factor receptor β (PDGFRβ), they are similar to activated myofibroblasts/hepatic stellate cells (HSC). If a particle (nanoparticles) is designed with suitable size and zeta potential, it can be injected specifically at the tumor site. A few nanoparticles have been tested and found to be effective in delivering drugs specifically to target activated HSC/myofibroblasts in the liver. This is a promising approach and further development of nanocarriers will help in designing stroma-based cancer therapies to target stroma-rich cancers [40]. Stromal-targeting agent such as all-trans retinoic acid (ATRA) in combination with chemotherapy has been shown to be effective in suppression of tumor growth in stromal-rich tumors like pancreatic ductal adenocarcinoma. These encouraging results warrant repurposing of drugs/agents in clinical studies for effective stromal targeting in pancreatic cancer [42].

Tumor stroma can impact the action and efficacy of chemotherapeutic agents against their specific target tissues in different ways, such as by generating high interstitial pressure and fibrosis, as well as via degradation of drugs by stromal enzymes expediting resistance to anticancer therapy and disease recurrence. Impenetrable fibrosis makes access of therapeutic agents to cancer cells limited by generating a barrier of the extracellular matrix; it further promotes degradation of drugs via stromal cytochrome P450 (CYP); and increased interstitial pressure prevents the entry of therapeutic agents [82]. Currently, chemotherapies are designed to target tumor cells; however, for more effective therapies with better outcome, it is necessary to control the tumor stroma as well. Such approach should be designed keeping in mind that the source of stromal cells is normal cells in the host and can be unintentionally harmed [79]. Further, it should always be taken into consideration that stroma-targeting agents used to eliminate cancer cannot eradicate tumor growth completely, but can work effectively as a complementary approach.

11 Conclusion

Studies in the last few decades have begun exploring the role of the tumor microenvironment and its components in determining fate of tumor growth and metastasis. CAFs have surfaced as significant players among other stromal cells as they are highly abundant in a wide variety of solid tumors. The interaction between tumor cells and adjoining CAFs largely occurs by paracrine signals in the form of cytokines and metabolites or via the intricate components of the proximate extracellular matrix. Here, we have discussed some of the molecular mechanisms underlying tumor cells and stromal CAF-mediated regulation of tumor progression. Molecular interactions between tumor and stroma provide distinctive structural features that differ significantly from their corresponding normal tissue. Cancer cells respond to the molecular signals that promote cell migration by changes allowing reorganization of cytoskeletal shape, as well as adhesion by secretion of chemokines, cytokines, and proteolytic enzymes. Additionally, signals derived from tumor cell help in the activation and recruitment of host cells, including MSCs, fibroblasts, and monocytes present in the tumor microenvironment. Thus, the active reciprocal molecular interactions between tumor and stromal cells within the tumor microenvironment orchestrate events associated with tumor progression.

In the past few decades, efforts have been directed toward investigating diverse types of tumor-stromal cell interactions and identifying key players driving these interactions using different experimental model systems. Studies done in this field have highlighted the role of cellular components of the TME such as CAFs as well as the molecular components such as chemokines and other molecules such as lactate in driving tumor progression. Dissecting these molecular interactions will help in developing novel molecular targets for future drug discovery targeting cancer cell invasion, migration, and survival. In this chapter, we have provided an overview of the metabolic interactions in between tumor and stromal cells within the tumor microenvironment. We have highlighted on the role metabolic reprogramming mediated via tumor-stroma interactions in cancers and discussed some of the factors governing this process. Role of chemokines and lactate in driving the metabolic interactions in between tumor cells and CAFs emphasizes the influence of stromal factors on the growth and development of tumor. This is especially important as metabolic targets impacted via CAF can be proposed as potential secondary therapeutic strategies for cancer control. Additionally, we have also discussed the role of epigenetic factors underlying the tumor-stroma metabolic interaction. Addressing the reciprocal metabolic exchange of nutrients in between cancer and stromal CAFs will help in developing a better understanding of metabolic heterogeneity in the TME. Investigating the metabolic cross talk will be advantageous in identifying novel targets for therapeutic advances. It has been our sincere attempt to cite important studies in the field, and we regret the inadvertent and unintentional omission of studies that would have benefitted this section.

References

1. Aizawa, T., Karasawa, H., Funayama, R., Shirota, M., Suzuki, T., Maeda, S., Suzuki, H., Yamamura, A., Naitoh, T., Nakayama, K., & Unno, M. (2019, October). Cancer-associated fibroblasts secrete Wnt2 to promote cancer progression in colorectal cancer. *Cancer Medicine, 8*(14), 6370–6382. https://doi.org/10.1002/cam4.2523
2. Albrengues, J., Bertero, T., Grasset, E., Bonan, S., Maiel, M., Bourget, I., Philippe, C., Herraiz Serrano, C., Benamar, S., Croce, O., Sanz-Moreno, V., Meneguzzi, G., Feral, C. C., Cristofari, G., & Gaggioli, C. (2015, December 15). Epigenetic switch drives the conversion of fibroblasts into proinvasive cancer-associated fibroblasts. *Nature Communications, 6*, 10204. https://doi.org/10.1038/ncomms10204
3. Allen, M., & Louise, J. J. (2011). Jekyll and Hyde: The role of the microenvironment on the progression of cancer. *The Journal of Pathology, 223*(2), 162–176. https://doi.org/10.1002/path.2803
4. Andersen, M. K., Rise, K., Giskeødegård, G. F., Richardsen, E., Bertilsson, H., Størkersen, Ø., Bathen, T. F., Rye, M., & Tessem, M. B. (2018, September 24). Integrative metabolic and transcriptomic profiling of prostate cancer tissue containing reactive stroma. *Scientific Reports, 8*(1), 14269. https://doi.org/10.1038/s41598-018-32549-1

5. Andersson, P., Yang, Y., Hosaka, K., Zhang, Y., Fischer, C., Braun, H., Liu, S., Yu, G., Liu, S., Beyaert, R., Chang, M., Li, Q., & Cao, Y. (2018, October 18). Molecular mechanisms of IL-33-mediated stromal interactions in cancer metastasis. *JCI Insight, 3*(20), e122375. https://doi.org/10.1172/jci.insight.122375
6. Anton, K., Banerjee, D., & Glod, J. (2012). Macrophage-associated mesenchymal stem cells assume an activated, migratory, pro-inflammatory phenotype with increased IL-6 and CXCL10 secretion. *PLoS One, 7*(4), e35036. https://doi.org/10.1371/journal.pone.0035036
7. Avagliano, A., Granato, G., Ruocco, M. R., Romano, V., Belviso, I., Carfora, A., Montagnani, S., & Arcucci, A. (2018, June 5). Metabolic Reprogramming of Cancer Associated Fibroblasts: The Slavery of Stromal Fibroblasts. *BioMed Research International, 2018*, 6075403. https://doi.org/10.1155/2018/6075403
8. Balkwill, F. (2004a, July). Cancer and the chemokine network. *Nature Reviews. Cancer, 4*(7), 540–550. https://doi.org/10.1038/nrc1388
9. Balkwill, F. (2004b, June). The significance of cancer cell expression of the chemokine receptor CXCR4. *Seminars in Cancer Biology, 14*(3), 171–179. https://doi.org/10.1016/j.semcancer.2003.10.003
10. Balkwill, F. R., Capasso, M., & Hagemann, T. (2012). The tumor microenvironment at a glance. *Journal of Cell Science, 125*(Pt 23), 5591–5596. https://doi.org/10.1242/jcs.116392
11. Baltazar, F., Afonso, J., Costa, M., & Granja, S. (2020, March 18). Lactate beyond a waste metabolite: Metabolic affairs and signaling in malignancy. *Frontiers in Oncology, 10*, 231. https://doi.org/10.3389/fonc.2020.00231
12. Becker, L. M., O'Connell, J. T., Vo, A. P., Cain, M. P., Tampe, D., Bizarro, L., Sugimoto, H., McGow, A. K., Asara, J. M., Lovisa, S., McAndrews, K. M., Zielinski, R., Lorenzi, P. L., Zeisberg, M., Raza, S., LeBleu, V. S., & Kalluri, R. (2020, June 2). Epigenetic reprogramming of cancer-associated fibroblasts deregulates glucose metabolism and facilitates progression of breast cancer. *Cell Reports, 31*(9), 107701. https://doi.org/10.1016/j.celrep.2020.107701
13. Bhagat, T. D., Von Ahrens, D., Dawlaty, M., Zou, Y., Baddour, J., Achreja, A., Zhao, H., Yang, L., Patel, B., Kwak, C., Choudhary, G. S., Gordon-Mitchell, S., Aluri, S., Bhattacharyya, S., Sahu, S., Bhagat, P., Yu, Y., Bartenstein, M., Giricz, O., … Verma, A. (2019, November 1). Lactate-mediated epigenetic reprogramming regulates formation of human pancreatic cancer-associated fibroblasts. *Elife, 8*, e50663. https://doi.org/10.7554/eLife.50663
14. Bhowmick, N. A., Neilson, E. G., & Moses, H. L. (2004). Stromal fibroblasts in cancer initiation and progression. *Nature, 432*(7015), 332–337. https://doi.org/10.1038/nature03096
15. Burger, J. A., & Kipps, T. J. (2006, March 1). CXCR4: A key receptor in the crosstalk between tumor cells and their microenvironment. *Blood, 107*(5), 1761–1767. https://doi.org/10.1182/blood-2005-08-3182
16. Cairns, R. A., Harris, I. S., & Mak, T. W. (2011). Regulation of cancer cell metabolism. *Nature Reviews. Cancer, 11*(2), 85–95. https://doi.org/10.1038/nrc2981
17. Cantor, J. R., & Sabatini, D. M. (2012). Cancer cell metabolism: One hallmark, many faces. *Cancer Discovery, 2*(10), 881–898. https://doi.org/10.1158/2159-8290.CD-12-0345
18. Carmona-Fontaine, C., Deforet, M., Akkari, L., Thompson, C. B., Joyce, J. A., & Xavier, J. B. (2017). Metabolic origins of spatial organization in the tumor microenvironment. *Proceedings of the National Academy of Sciences of the United States of America, 114*(11), 2934–2939. https://doi.org/10.1073/pnas.1700600114
19. Chow, M. T., & Luster, A. D. (2014, December). Chemokines in cancer. *Cancer Immunology Research, 2*(12), 1125–1131. https://doi.org/10.1158/2326-6066.CIR-14-0160
20. Cirri, P., & Chiarugi, P. (2012). Cancer-associated-fibroblasts and tumour cells: A diabolic liaison driving cancer progression. *Cancer Metastasis Reviews, 31*(1–2), 195–208. https://doi.org/10.1007/s10555-011-9340-x
21. Cohen, N., Shani, O., Raz, Y., Sharon, Y., Hoffman, D., Abramovitz, L., & Erez, N. (2017, August). Fibroblasts drive an immunosuppressive and growth-promoting microenvironment in breast cancer via secretion of Chitinase 3-like 1. *Oncogene, 36*(31), 4457–4468. https://doi.org/10.1038/onc.2017.65
22. D'Arcangelo, E., Wu, N. C., Cadavid, J. L., & McGuigan, A. P. (2020, March). The life cycle of cancer-associated fibroblasts within the tumour stroma and its importance in disease outcome. *British Journal of Cancer, 122*(7), 931–942. https://doi.org/10.1038/s41416-019-0705-1
23. Dauer, P., Zhao, X., Gupta, V. K., Sharma, N., Kesh, K., Gnamlin, P., Dudeja, V., Vickers, S. M., Banerjee, S., & Saluja, A. (2018, March 1). Inactivation of cancer-associated-fibroblasts disrupts oncogenic signaling in pancreatic cancer cells and promotes its regression. *Cancer Research, 78*(5), 1321–1333. https://doi.org/10.1158/0008-5472.CAN-17-2320
24. de la Cruz-López, K. G., Castro-Muñoz, L. J., Reyes-Hernández, D. O., García-Carrancá, A., & Manzo-Merino, J. (2019, November 1). Lactate in the regulation of tumor microenvironment and therapeutic approaches. *Frontiers in Oncology, 9*, 1143. https://doi.org/10.3389/fonc.2019.01143
25. DeBerardinis, R. J., Lum, J. J., Hatzivassiliou, G., & Thompson, C. B. (2008, January). The biology of cancer: Metabolic reprogramming fuels cell growth and proliferation. *Cell Metabolism, 7*(1), 11–20. https://doi.org/10.1016/j.cmet.2007.10.002
26. Doherty, J. R., & Cleveland, J. L. (2013, September). Targeting lactate metabolism for cancer therapeutics. *The Journal of Clinical Investigation, 123*(9),

3685–3692. https://doi.org/10.1172/JCI69741. Epub 2013 Sep 3.
27. Draoui, N., & Feron, O. (2011, November). Lactate shuttles at a glance: From physiological paradigms to anti-cancer treatments. *Disease Models & Mechanisms, 4*(6), 727–732. https://doi.org/10.1242/dmm.007724
28. Egeblad, M., Nakasone, E. S., & Werb, Z. (2010). Tumors as organs: Complex tissues that interface with the entire organism. *Developmental Cell, 18*(6), 884–901. https://doi.org/10.1016/j.devcel.2010.05.012
29. Elyada, E., Bolisetty, M., Laise, P., Flynn, W. F., Courtois, E. T., Burkhart, R. A., Teinor, J. A., Belleau, P., Biffi, G., Lucito, M. S., Sivajothi, S., Armstrong, T. D., Engle, D. D., Yu, K. H., Hao, Y., Wolfgang, C. L., Park, Y., Preall, J., Jaffee, E. M., … Tuveson, D. A. (2019, August). Cross-species single-cell analysis of pancreatic ductal adenocarcinoma reveals antigen-presenting cancer-associated fibroblasts. *Cancer Discovery, 9*(8), 1102–1123. https://doi.org/10.1158/2159-8290.CD-19-0094. Epub 2019 Jun 13.
30. Gao, H., Priebe, W., Glod, J., & Banerjee, D. (2009). Activation of signal transducers and activators of transcription 3 and focal adhesion kinase by stromal cell-derived factor 1 is required for migration of human mesenchymal stem cells in response to tumor cell-conditioned medium. *Stem Cells, 27*(4), 857–865. https://doi.org/10.1002/stem.23
31. Hanahan, D., & Coussens, L. M. (2012). Accessories to the crime: Functions of cells recruited to the tumor microenvironment. *Cancer Cell, 21*(3), 309–322. https://doi.org/10.1016/j.ccr.2012.02.022
32. Hanahan, D., & Weinberg, R. A. (2011). Hallmarks of cancer: The next generation. *Cell, 144*(5), 646–674. https://doi.org/10.1016/j.cell.2011.02.013
33. Hanahan, D., & Weinberg, R. A. (2000, January 7). The hallmarks of cancer. *Cell, 100*(1), 57–70. https://doi.org/10.1016/s0092-8674(00)81683-9
34. Hirschey, M. D., DeBerardinis, R. J., Diehl, A. M. E., Drew, J. E., Frezza, C., Green, M. F., Jones, L. W., Ko, Y. H., Le, A., Lea, M. A., Locasale, J. W., Longo, V. D., Lyssiotis, C. A., McDonnell, E., Mehrmohamadi, M., Michelotti, G., Muralidhar, V., Murphy, M. P., Pedersen, P. L., … Target Validation Team. (2015, December). Dysregulated metabolism contributes to oncogenesis. *Seminars in Cancer Biology, 35*(Suppl), S129–S150. https://doi.org/10.1016/j.semcancer.2015.10.002
35. Jiang, L., Gonda, T. A., Gamble, M. V., Salas, M., Seshan, V., Tu, S., Twaddell, W. S., Hegyi, P., Lazar, G., Steele, I., Varro, A., Wang, T. C., & Tycko, B. (2008, December 1). Global hypomethylation of genomic DNA in cancer-associated myofibroblasts. *Cancer Research, 68*(23), 9900–9908. https://doi.org/10.1158/0008-5472.CAN-08-1319
36. Joyce, J. A. (2005). Therapeutic targeting of the tumor microenvironment. *Cancer Cell, 7*(6), 513–520. https://doi.org/10.1016/j.ccr.2005.05.024
37. Junttila, M. R., & de Sauvage, F. J. (2013). Influence of tumour micro-environment heterogeneity on therapeutic response. *Nature, 501*(7467), 346–354. https://doi.org/10.1038/nature12626
38. Kalluri, R., & Zeisberg, M. (2006). Fibroblasts in cancer. *Nature Reviews. Cancer, 6*(5), 392–401. https://doi.org/10.1038/nrc1877
39. Kalluri, R. (2016, August 23). The biology and function of fibroblasts in cancer. *Nature Reviews. Cancer, 16*(9), 582–598. https://doi.org/10.1038/nrc.2016.73
40. Kaps, L., & Schuppan, D. (2020, September 3). Targeting cancer associated fibroblasts in liver fibrosis and liver cancer using nanocarriers. *Cell, 9*(9), 2027. https://doi.org/10.3390/cells9092027
41. Katanov, C., Lerrer, S., Liubomirski, Y., Leider-Trejo, L., Meshel, T., Bar, J., Feniger-Barish, R., Kamer, I., Soria-Artzi, G., Kahani, H., Banerjee, D., & Ben-Baruch, A. (2015, May 1). Regulation of the inflammatory profile of stromal cells in human breast cancer: Prominent roles for TNF-α and the NF-κB pathway. *Stem Cell Research & Therapy, 6*(1), 87. https://doi.org/10.1186/s13287-015-0080-7
42. Kocher, H. M., Basu, B., Froeling, F. E. M., Sarker, D., Slater, S., Carlin, D., deSouza, N. M., De Paepe, K. N., Goulart, M. R., Hughes, C., Imrali, A., Roberts, R., Pawula, M., Houghton, R., Lawrence, C., Yogeswaran, Y., Mousa, K., Coetzee, C., Sasieni, P., … Propper, D. J. (2020, September 24). Phase I clinical trial repurposing all-trans retinoic acid as a stromal targeting agent for pancreatic cancer. *Nature Communications, 11*(1), 4841. https://doi.org/10.1038/s41467-020-18636-w
43. Kramer, N., Schmöllerl, J., Unger, C., Nivarthi, H., Rudisch, A., Unterleuthner, D., Scherzer, M., Riedl, A., Artaker, M., Crncec, I., Lenhardt, D., Schwarz, T., Prieler, B., Han, X., Hengstschläger, M., Schüler, J., Eferl, R., Moriggl, R., Sommergruber, W., & Dolznig, H. (2017, September 28). Autocrine WNT2 signaling in fibroblasts promotes colorectal cancer progression. *Oncogene, 36*(39), 5460–5472. https://doi.org/10.1038/onc.2017.144
44. LeBleu, V. S., & Kalluri, R. (2018, April 19). A peek into cancer-associated fibroblasts: Origins, functions and translational impact. *Disease Models & Mechanisms, 11*(4), dmm029447. https://doi.org/10.1242/dmm.029447
45. Ligorio, M., Sil, S., Malagon-Lopez, J., Nieman, L. T., Misale, S., Di Pilato, M., Ebright, R. Y., Karabacak, M. N., Kulkarni, A. S., Liu, A., Vincent Jordan, N., Franses, J. W., Philipp, J., Kreuzer, J., Desai, N., Arora, K. S., Rajurkar, M., Horwitz, E., Neyaz, A., … Ting, D. T. (2019, June 27). Stromal microenvironment shapes the intratumoral architecture of pancreatic cancer. *Cell, 178*(1), 160–175.e27. https://doi.org/10.1016/j.cell.2019.05.012
46. Lin, S. Y., Dolfi, S. C., Amiri, S., Li, J., Budak-Alpdogan, T., Lee, K. C., Derenzo, C., Banerjee, D., & Glod, J. (2013, December). P53 regulates the migration of mesenchymal stromal cells in response to the tumor microenvironment through both

CXCL12-dependent and -independent mechanisms. *International Journal of Oncology, 43*(6), 1817–1823. https://doi.org/10.3892/ijo.2013.2109

47. Lin, S. Y., Yang, J., Everett, A. D., Clevenger, C. V., Koneru, M., Mishra, P. J., Kamen, B., Banerjee, D., & Glod, J. (2008, October 15). The isolation of novel mesenchymal stromal cell chemotactic factors from the conditioned medium of tumor cells. *Experimental Cell Research, 314*(17), 3107–3117. https://doi.org/10.1016/j.yexcr.2008.07.028
48. Lisanti, M. P., Martinez-Outschoorn, U. E., & Sotgia, F. (2013, September 1). Oncogenes induce the cancer-associated fibroblast phenotype: Metabolic symbiosis and "fibroblast addiction" are new therapeutic targets for drug discovery. *Cell Cycle, 12*(17), 2723–2732. https://doi.org/10.4161/cc.25695
49. Ma, X. J., Dahiya, S., Richardson, E., Erlander, M., & Sgroi, D. C. (2009). Gene expression profiling of the tumor microenvironment during breast cancer progression. *Breast Cancer Research, 11*(1), R7. https://doi.org/10.1186/bcr2222
50. Martinez-Outschoorn, U. E., Goldberg, A., Lin, Z., Ko, Y. H., Flomenberg, N., Wang, C., Pavlides, S., Pestell, R. G., Howell, A., Sotgia, F., & Lisanti, M. P. (2011a, November 15). Anti-estrogen resistance in breast cancer is induced by the tumor microenvironment and can be overcome by inhibiting mitochondrial function in epithelial cancer cells. *Cancer Biology & Therapy, 12*(10), 924–938. https://doi.org/10.4161/cbt.12.10.17780
51. Martinez-Outschoorn, U. E., Pavlides, S., Whitaker-Menezes, D., Daumer, K. M., Milliman, J. N., Chiavarina, B., Migneco, G., Witkiewicz, A. K., Martinez-Cantarin, M. P., Flomenberg, N., Howell, A., Pestell, R. G., Lisanti, M. P., & Sotgia, F. (2010, June 15). Tumor cells induce the cancer associated fibroblast phenotype via caveolin-1 degradation: Implications for breast cancer and DCIS therapy with autophagy inhibitors. *Cell Cycle, 9*(12), 2423–2433. https://doi.org/10.4161/cc.9.12.12048
52. Martinez-Outschoorn, U. E., Prisco, M., Ertel, A., Tsirigos, A., Lin, Z., Pavlides, S., Wang, C., Flomenberg, N., Knudsen, E. S., Howell, A., Pestell, R. G., Sotgia, F., & Lisanti, M. P. (2011b, April 15). Ketones and lactate increase cancer cell "stemness," driving recurrence, metastasis and poor clinical outcome in breast cancer: Achieving personalized medicine via Metabolo-Genomics. *Cell Cycle, 10*(8), 1271–1286. https://doi.org/10.4161/cc.10.8.15330
53. Mathot, P., Grandin, M., Devailly, G., Souaze, F., Cahais, V., Moran, S., Campone, M., Herceg, Z., Esteller, M., Juin, P., Mehlen, P., & Dante, R. (2017, October 23). DNA methylation signal has a major role in the response of human breast cancer cells to the microenvironment. *Oncogenesis, 6*(10), e390. https://doi.org/10.1038/oncsis.2017.88
54. Menon, L. G., Picinich, S., Koneru, R., Gao, H., Lin, S. Y., Koneru, M., Mayer-Kuckuk, P., Glod, J., & Banerjee, D. (2007, February). Differential gene expression associated with migration of mesenchymal stem cells to conditioned medium from tumor cells or bone marrow cells. *Stem Cells, 25*(2), 520–528. https://doi.org/10.1634/stemcells.2006-0257
55. Micke, P., & Ostman, A. (2005, December). Exploring the tumour environment: Cancer-associated fibroblasts as targets in cancer therapy. *Expert Opinion on Therapeutic Targets, 9*(6), 1217–1233. https://doi.org/10.1517/14728222.9.6.1217
56. Mishra, D., & Banerjee, D. (2019). Lactate dehydrogenases as metabolic links between tumor and stroma in the tumor microenvironment. *Cancers (Basel), 11*(6), 750. Published 2019 May 29. https://doi.org/10.3390/cancers11060750
57. Mishra, P., Banerjee, D., & Ben-Baruch, A. (2011, January). Chemokines at the crossroads of tumor-fibroblast interactions that promote malignancy. *Journal of Leukocyte Biology, 89*(1), 31–39. https://doi.org/10.1189/jlb.0310182
58. Mishra, P. J., Mishra, P. J., Humeniuk, R., Medina, D. J., Alexe, G., Mesirov, J. P., Ganesan, S., Glod, J. W., & Banerjee, D. (2008, June 1). Carcinoma-associated fibroblast-like differentiation of human mesenchymal stem cells. *Cancer Research, 68*(11), 4331–4339. https://doi.org/10.1158/0008-5472.CAN-08-0943
59. Mishra, R., Haldar, S., Placencio, V., Madhav, A., Rohena-Rivera, K., Agarwal, P., Duong, F., Angara, B., Tripathi, M., Liu, Z., Gottlieb, R. A., Wagner, S., Posadas, E. M., & Bhowmick, N. A. (2018, October 1). Stromal epigenetic alterations drive metabolic and neuroendocrine prostate cancer reprogramming. *The Journal of Clinical Investigation, 128*(10), 4472–4484. https://doi.org/10.1172/JCI99397
60. Morais-Santos, F., Granja, S., Miranda-Gonçalves, V., Moreira, A. H., Queirós, S., Vilaça, J. L., Schmitt, F. C., Longatto-Filho, A., Paredes, J., Baltazar, F., & Pinheiro, C. (2015, August 7). Targeting lactate transport suppresses in vivo breast tumour growth. *Oncotarget, 6*(22), 19177–19189.
61. Orimo, A., Gupta, P. B., Sgroi, D. C., Arenzana-Seisdedos, F., Delaunay, T., Naeem, R., Carey, V. J., Richardson, A. L., & Weinberg, R. A. (2005, May 6). Stromal fibroblasts present in invasive human breast carcinomas promote tumor growth and angiogenesis through elevated SDF-1/CXCL12 secretion. *Cell, 121*(3), 335–348. https://doi.org/10.1016/j.cell.2005.02.034
62. Orimo, A., & Weinberg, R. A. (2006). Stromal fibroblasts in cancer: A novel tumor-promoting cell type. *Cell Cycle, 5*(15), 1597–1601. https://doi.org/10.4161/cc.5.15.3112
63. Palm, W., & Thompson, C. B. (2017). Nutrient acquisition strategies of mammalian cells. *Nature, 546*(7657), 234–242. https://doi.org/10.1038/nature22379
64. Patel, B. B., Ackerstaff, E., Serganova, I. S., Kerrigan, J. E., Blasberg, R. G., Koutcher, J. A., & Banerjee, D. (2017, March 1). Tumor stroma interaction is mediated by monocarboxylate metabolism. *Experimental Cell Research, 352*(1), 20–33. https://doi.org/10.1016/j.yexcr.2017.01.013

65. Pavlova, N. N., & Thompson, C. B. (2016). The emerging hallmarks of cancer metabolism. *Cell Metabolism, 23*(1), 27–47. https://doi.org/10.1016/j.cmet.2015.12.006
66. Picinich, S. C., Glod, J. W., & Banerjee, D. (2010). Protein kinase C zeta regulates interleukin-8-mediated stromal-derived factor-1 expression and migration of human mesenchymal stromal cells. *Experimental Cell Research, 316*(4), 593–602. https://doi.org/10.1016/j.yexcr.2009.11.011
67. Pietras, K., & Ostman, A. (2010, May 1). Hallmarks of cancer: Interactions with the tumor stroma. *Experimental Cell Research, 316*(8), 1324–1331. https://doi.org/10.1016/j.yexcr.2010.02.045
68. Pisarsky, L., Bill, R., Fagiani, E., Dimeloe, S., Goosen, R. W., Hagmann, J., Hess, C., & Christofori, G. (2016, May 10). Targeting metabolic symbiosis to overcome resistance to anti-angiogenic therapy. *Cell Reports, 15*(6), 1161–1174. https://doi.org/10.1016/j.celrep.2016.04.028
69. Raman, D., Baugher, P. J., Thu, Y. M., & Richmond, A. (2007, October 28). Role of chemokines in tumor growth. *Cancer Letters, 256*(2), 137–165. https://doi.org/10.1016/j.canlet.2007.05.013
70. Rattigan, Y., Hsu, J. M., Mishra, P. J., Glod, J., & Banerjee, D. (2010). Interleukin 6 mediated recruitment of mesenchymal stem cells to the hypoxic tumor milieu. *Experimental Cell Research, 316*(20), 3417–3424. https://doi.org/10.1016/j.yexcr.2010.07.002
71. Rattigan, Y. I., Patel, B. B., Ackerstaff, E., Sukenick, G., Koutcher, J. A., Glod, J. W., & Banerjee, D. (2012, February 15). Lactate is a mediator of metabolic cooperation between stromal carcinoma associated fibroblasts and glycolytic tumor cells in the tumor microenvironment. *Experimental Cell Research, 318*(4), 326–335. https://doi.org/10.1016/j.yexcr.2011.11.014
72. Rot, A., & von Andrian, U. H. (2004). Chemokines in innate and adaptive host defense: Basic chemokinese grammar for immune cells. *Annual Review of Immunology, 22*, 891–928. https://doi.org/10.1146/annurev.immunol.22.012703.104543
73. San-Millán, I., & Brooks, G. A. (2017 Feb 1). Reexamining cancer metabolism: Lactate production for carcinogenesis could be the purpose and explanation of the Warburg Effect. *Carcinogenesis, 38*(2), 119–133. https://doi.org/10.1093/carcin/bgw127
74. Sandri, B. J., Masvidal, L., Murie, C., Bartish, M., Avdulov, S., Higgins, L., Markowski, T., Peterson, M., Bergh, J., Yang, P., Rolny, C., Limper, A. H., Griffin, T. J., Bitterman, P. B., Wendt, C. H., & Larsson, O. (2019, August 1). Distinct cancer-promoting stromal gene expression depending on lung function. *American Journal of Respiratory and Critical Care Medicine, 200*(3), 348–358. https://doi.org/10.1164/rccm.201801-0080OC
75. Schwörer, S., Vardhana, S. A., & Thompson, C. B. (2019). Cancer metabolism drives a stromal regenerative response. *Cell Metabolism, 29*(3), 576–591. https://doi.org/10.1016/j.cmet.2019.01.015
76. Sherman, M. H., Yu, R. T., Tseng, T. W., Sousa, C. M., Liu, S., Truitt, M. L., He, N., Ding, N., Liddle, C., Atkins, A. R., Leblanc, M., Collisson, E. A., Asara, J. M., Kimmelman, A. C., Downes, M., & Evans, R. M. (2017, January 31). Stromal cues regulate the pancreatic cancer epigenome and metabolome. *Proceedings of the National Academy of Sciences of the United States of America, 114*(5), 1129–1134. https://doi.org/10.1073/pnas.1620164114
77. Sperb, N., Tsesmelis, M., & Wirth, T. (2020). Crosstalk between tumor and stromal cells in pancreatic ductal adenocarcinoma. *International Journal of Molecular Science, 21*(15), 5486. Published 2020 July 31. https://doi.org/10.3390/ijms21155486
78. Tennant, D. A., Durán, R. V., & Gottlieb, E. (2010). Targeting metabolic transformation for cancer therapy. *Nature Reviews. Cancer, 10*(4), 267–277. https://doi.org/10.1038/nrc2817
79. Tran, E., Chinnasamy, D., Yu, Z., Morgan, R. A., Lee, C. C., Restifo, N. P., & Rosenberg, S. A. (2013, June 3). Immune targeting of fibroblast activation protein triggers recognition of multipotent bone marrow stromal cells and cachexia. *The Journal of Experimental Medicine, 210*(6), 1125–1135. https://doi.org/10.1084/jem.20130110
80. Tripathi, M., Billet, S., & Bhowmick, N. A. (2012). Understanding the role of stromal fibroblasts in cancer progression. *Cell Adhesion & Migration, 6*(3), 231–235. https://doi.org/10.4161/cam.20419
81. Tyekucheva, S., Bowden, M., Bango, C., Giunchi, F., Huang, Y., Zhou, C., Bondi, A., Lis, R., Van Hemelrijck, M., Andrén, O., Andersson, S. O., Watson, R. W., Pennington, S., Finn, S. P., Martin, N. E., Stampfer, M. J., Parmigiani, G., Penney, K. L., Fiorentino, M., … Loda, M. (2017, September 4). Stromal and epithelial transcriptional map of initiation progression and metastatic potential of human prostate cancer. *Nature Communications, 8*(1), 420. https://doi.org/10.1038/s41467-017-00460-4
82. Valkenburg, K. C., de Groot, A. E., & Pienta, K. J. (2018, June). Targeting the tumour stroma to improve cancer therapy. *Nature Reviews. Clinical Oncology, 15*(6), 366–381. https://doi.org/10.1038/s41571-018-0007-1
83. Vander Heiden, M. G., Lunt, S. Y., Dayton, T. L., Fiske, B. P., Israelsen, W. J., Mattaini, K. R., Vokes, N. I., Stephanopoulos, G., Cantley, L. C., Metallo, C. M., & Locasale, J. W. (2011). Metabolic pathway alterations that support cell proliferation. *Cold Spring Harbor Symposia on Quantitative Biology, 76*, 325–334. https://doi.org/10.1101/sqb.2012.76.010900
84. Vander Heiden, M. G. (2011). Targeting cancer metabolism: A therapeutic window opens. *Nature Reviews Drug Discovery, 10*(9), 671–684. Published 2011 Aug 31. https://doi.org/10.1038/nrd3504
85. Warburg, O. (1956). On the origin of cancer cells. *Science, 123*(3191), 309–314. https://doi.org/10.1126/science.123.3191.309

86. Warburg, O. P., & Negelein, E. (1927). Uber den Stoffwechsel der Carcinomzelle. *Biochemische Zeitschrift, 152*, 309–344.
87. Ward, P. S., & Thompson, C. B. (2012). Metabolic reprogramming: A cancer hallmark even Warburg did not anticipate. *Cancer Cell, 21*(3), 297–308. https://doi.org/10.1016/j.ccr.2012.02.014
88. Weyandt, J. D., Thompson, C. B., Giaccia, A. J., & Rathmell, W. K. (2017). Metabolic alterations in cancer and their potential as therapeutic targets. *American Society of Clinical Oncology Educational Book, 37*, 825–832. https://doi.org/10.1200/EDBK_175561
89. Wingrove, E., Liu, Z. Z., Patel, K. D., Arnal-Estapé, A., Cai, W. L., Melnick, M. A., Politi, K., Monteiro, C., Zhu, L., Valiente, M., Kluger, H. M., Chiang, V. L., & Nguyen, D. X. (2019, April 23). Transcriptomic hallmarks of tumor plasticity and stromal interactions in brain metastasis. *Cell Reports, 27*(4), 1277–1292.e7. https://doi.org/10.1016/j.celrep.2019.03.085
90. Xiang, H., Ramil, C. P., Hai, J., Zhang, C., Wang, H., Watkins, A. A., Afshar, R., Georgiev, P., Sze, M. A., Song, X. S., Curran, P. J., Cheng, M., Miller, J. R., Sun, D., Loboda, A., Jia, Y., Moy, L. Y., Chi, A., & Brandish, P. E. (2020, April). Cancer-associated fibroblasts promote immunosuppression by inducing ROS-generating monocytic MDSCs in lung squamous cell carcinoma. *Cancer Immunology Research, 8*(4), 436–450. https://doi.org/10.1158/2326-6066.CIR-19-0507
91. Xiao, Q., Zhou, D., Rucki, A. A., Williams, J., Zhou, J., Mo, G., Murphy, A., Fujiwara, K., Kleponis, J., Salman, B., Wolfgang, C. L., Anders, R. A., Zheng, S., Jaffee, E. M., & Zheng, L. (2016, September 15). Cancer-associated fibroblasts in pancreatic cancer are reprogrammed by tumor-induced alterations in genomic DNA methylation. *Cancer Research, 76*(18), 5395–5404. https://doi.org/10.1158/0008-5472.CAN-15-3264
92. Yoshida, G. J. (2015). Metabolic reprogramming: The emerging concept and associated therapeutic strategies. *Journal of Experimental & Clinical Cancer Research, 34*, 111. Published 2015 Oct 6. https://doi.org/10.1186/s13046-015-0221-y
93. Zhu, Z., Achreja, A., Meurs, N., Animasahun, O., Owen, S., Mittal, A., Parikh, P., Lo, T. W., Franco-Barraza, J., Shi, J., Gunchick, V., Sherman, M. H., Cukierman, E., Pickering, A. M., Maitra, A., Sahai, V., Morgan, M. A., Nagrath, S., Lawrence, T. S., & Nagrath, D. (2020, August). Tumour-reprogrammed stromal BCAT1 fuels branched-chain ketoacid dependency in stromal-rich PDAC tumours. *Nature Metabolism, 2*(8), 775–792. https://doi.org/10.1038/s42255-020-0226-5
94. Zou, A., Lambert, D., Yeh, H., Yasukawa, K., Behbod, F., Fan, F., & Cheng, N. (2014, October 24). Elevated CXCL1 expression in breast cancer stroma predicts poor prognosis and is inversely associated with expression of TGF-β signaling proteins. *BMC Cancer, 14*, 781. https://doi.org/10.1186/1471-2407-14-781

Interacting Genetic Lesions of Melanoma in the Tumor Microenvironment: Defining a Viable Therapy

R. R. Maniyar, S. Chakraborty, T. Jarboe, R. Suriano, M. Wallack, J. Geliebter, and R. K. Tiwari

Melanoma results from the transformation of melanocytes as a consequence of genetic mutations, which leads to uninhibited growth and proliferation [1]. It is the least common, however the most aggressive, of skin cancers.

1 Types of Melanoma

There are primarily four types of cutaneous melanoma, i.e., occurring on the skin. It manifests most commonly as **superficial spreading melanoma** which accounts for about 70% of all cases in the age range of 30–50. Here, it presents as a lesion with irregular borders, color variegation, and a large diameter, usually 6–8 mm. *Nodular melanoma* occurs in patients above 50 years of age, and accounts for approximately 15% of all cases, making it the second most commonly occurring form of melanoma. It manifests as a raised dark brown-back papule or nodule and can appear independently from existing moles/skin lesions. It is often accompanied with bleeding and ulceration. Presenting with a thickness greater than superficial spreading melanoma, it is associated with worse outcomes and a poor response to therapies including BRAF targeted therapy [2]. *Lentigo maligna melanoma* accounts for approximately 10% of melanoma cases and is commonly found on the faces of elderly people whose skin has undergone sun damage. *Acral lentiginous melanoma* is the rarest form and occurs in only 5% of melanoma cases. It is often found in darker skinned individuals and can develop anywhere on the body including on nail beds [1, 2].

2 Therapeutic Options

Until 2011, when the first therapy targeting the BRAFV600E genetic lesion was approved, therapies for metastatic melanoma were extremely limited and mainly included *surgery, radiotherapy, and chemotherapy*.

R. R. Maniyar
Human Oncology and Pathogenesis Program, Ludwig Collaborative and Swim Across America Laboratory, Memorial Sloan Kettering Cancer Center, New York, NY, USA

S. Chakraborty
Department of Medicine, Division of Hematology and Medical Oncology, Weill Cornell Medicine, New York, NY, USA

T. Jarboe · J. Geliebter · R. K. Tiwari (✉)
Departments of Pathology, Microbiology and Immunology, New York Medical College, Valhalla, NY, USA
e-mail: Raj_Tiwari@nymc.edu

R. Suriano
Division of Natural Sciences, College of Mount Saint Vincent, Bronx, NY, USA

M. Wallack
Department Surgery, Metropolitan Hospital, New York, NY, USA

D. Banerjee, R. K. Tiwari (eds.), *Tumor Microenvironment: Cellular, Metabolic and Immunologic Interactions*, Advances in Experimental Medicine and Biology 1350,
https://doi.org/10.1007/978-3-030-83282-7_6

(a) **Surgery:** Primary melanoma tumors are surgically excised, wherein the tumor is resected along with a margin of surrounding healthy tissue to ensure complete removal of cancer cells [3]. In cases where it is deemed beneficial, resection is carried out for distant metastasis, slightly improving survival rates [4, 5].
(b) **Radiotherapy**: Melanoma has long been known as a radioresistant cancer, prior to fine-tuning and improvements in radiation therapy protocols [6]. Multiple cases of melanoma occur in elderly patients who are unfit for surgery. In such cases, definitive radiation therapy is administered. Radiation therapy as an adjuvant to surgery is administered to primary lesions in cases of cutaneous melanoma with a high risk of recurrence. In cases of metastatic melanoma, radiation therapy is administered to the lesions that are symptomatic. However, many lesions, particularly those in the bowel, are not treatable with radiation therapy, limiting its use [7].
(c) **Chemotherapy**: In advanced melanoma, with radiation therapy administered for targetable symptomatic lesions, chemotherapy remained a mainstay treatment until recently. Alkylating agents like dacarbazine, the only chemotherapeutic drug approved by the FDA for melanoma, is a standard chemotherapeutic drug used for metastatic melanoma, albeit is not the first line of treatment anymore. It acts by introducing alkyl groups to guanine bases, inducing DNA damage and eventually cell death by apoptosis. It has advantages in being able to cross the blood-brain barrier and target brain metastases; however, the response rate to dacarbazine is a meager 20% [8, 9]. Combination therapies with dacarbazine have been under investigation for several years but are yet to demonstrate significant improvements over single agent treatments, to gain the "standard of care" status. The Dartmouth regimen combines four chemotherapeutics in a treatment regimen against melanoma. These include dacarbazine, cisplatin (a platinum drug that cross-links with purine bases and causes DNA damage and interferes with DNA repair and consequently cellular apoptosis [10]), tamoxifen (a nonsteroidal selective estrogen receptor modulator that binds and inhibits the function of estrogen receptor), and carmustine (a nitrosourea alkylating agent with a similar mechanism of action to dacarbazine, but with a higher toxicity) [11]. In a trial that compared the Dartmouth regimen to single agent dacarbazine therapy in patients with malignant melanoma, there was no significant difference in the overall survival between the two treatment groups [12, 13]. With these poor treatment outcomes, there was a dire need for new therapeutics.

However, due to this seemingly untreatable disease, the focus on melanoma had considerably reduced until the discovery of the genetic lesion BRAFV600E in melanoma [14] which rekindled interest in melanoma research around the year 2002.

3 Genetic Lesions and Immunogenicity in Melanoma

Cancers are typically caused by an accumulation of somatic mutations resulting in either gain of function or loss of function in oncogenes and tumor suppressor genes, respectively. These mutations are associated with exposure to mutagens and/or carcinogenic environments. One of the hallmarks of melanoma is the exceptionally high somatic mutational rate (16.8 mutations/Mb) owing largely to UV exposure [15–17]. Mutations occur in several key driver pathways in melanoma [18, 19]. The Cancer Genome Atlas (TCGA) published a study with 331 melanoma patients and found 13 significant hot-spot mutations in key driver pathways. These included BRAF, N-RAS, CDKN2A, TP53, ARID2, IDH1, PPP6C, PTEN, DDX3X, RAC1, MAP 2 K1, NF1, and RB1 [20].

A pan-cancer analysis confirmed that owing to the high mutational rate in melanoma, and the high number of amino acid substitutions, melanoma also has the highest number of neoepitopes

[21]. This, theoretically, makes melanoma an extremely immunogenic cancer. Not all the melanoma-associated antigens are as strongly immunogenic in the context of an MHC-I peptide complex. Development of a strong immune response against differentiation antigens, like tyrosinase, is stunted owing to self-tolerance mechanisms. Even cancer testis-specific antigens like MAGE have demonstrated an extremely poor immunogenicity in patients [22]. However, there is still an immune response mounted against melanoma, evidenced by T cell infiltration, partial regression, and antibodies against melanoma-associated antigens like gp100 [23–26]. Despite this high mutational burden, large amount of neo-epitopes, and high immune infiltration into the tumor, melanoma manages to escape immune clearance and persists. This is in major part due to the immunosuppressive tumor microenvironment elicited by melanoma and its genetic lesions, particularly the BRAFV600E lesion, and in another part due to ligands for checkpoint molecules expressed on melanoma cells, e.g., PDL1.

4 The Melanoma Tumor Microenvironment

Melanoma develops as a cell autonomous event as a result of interactions with genetic factors, environmental factors, and host factors, e.g., the immune system, and metabolism. Melanoma cells do not exist in isolation in the tumor microenvironment. The importance of the tumor microenvironment was first thought about as the concept of the "seed and soil" theory coined by an English pathologist, Stephen Paget in 1889 based on his observations in breast cancer patients' metastases developing mainly in the bones and visceral organs. He proposed that metastasis was not a random occurrence; instead, tumor cells would only metastasize and grow in favorable organ microenvironments, like a seed will only germinate if the environment or "soil" is fertile and conducive to its germination [27]. This theory was proved correct almost a century later by a veterinary surgical oncologist, Isaiah Fidler. Fidler injected radiolabeled melanoma cells into mice and discovered that only 0.01% of the injected cells survived and only metastasized in the lung. He realized that some organs were more conducive to developing metastatic lesions than others and designed a defining experiment to prove this theory. He transplanted lung and kidney tissues into the muscle of mice. He then injected radiolabeled melanoma cells intravenously. He found that while the same number of melanoma cells populated the transplanted lung and kidney tissue in the muscle, only the lungs and the transplanted lung tissue developed metastatic lesions. This experiment conclusively proved that the organ microenvironment played a prominent role in the development and spread of cancer, proving the Paget "seed and soil" theory for metastasis correct [28].

In the decades that followed, research into the tumor microenvironment gathered steam. We now know that in addition to the malignant cells, a tumor comprises supporting stroma which includes immune cells, tumor-associated fibroblasts, endothelial cells, and soluble molecules in the extracellular matrix. There is a constant bidirectional interaction that is established between malignant cells and the rest of the components in the tumor microenvironment, which begins right from the time of initial tumor development with promotion of angiogenesis and continues as the tumor adapts mechanisms to evade the immune system and progress. These interactions are exploited by the tumor to promote its own survival and growth. They can be direct receptor/ligand interactions or driven by cytokines and chemokines secreted by tumor cells and the other cellular components of the microenvironment.

As malignant cells rapidly proliferate, they have a high nutrient and oxygen consumption, leading to a hypoxic and nutrient-depleted environment. However, in order to sustain growth, invasion, and metastasis, malignant cells need to replenish oxygen and nutrients and get rid of metabolic waste products that accumulate. To this end, one of the most crucial steps in tumor progression is the induction of angiogenesis. There exists evidence for the role of environmental factors like estrogen and ethanol playing a role in the induction and promotion of angiogenesis [29, 30]. Additionally, one of the primary drivers for induction of angiogenesis in the tumor microenvironment is hypoxia. Hypoxia leads to the stabilization of HIF-1α, which in turn leads to the expression of proangiogenic factors, from malignant cells and the surrounding endothelial cells, vascular endothelial growth factor (VEGF) and VEGF receptor (VEGFR), respectively [31]. Hypoxia also induces angiogenesis indirectly by stabilizing proangiogenic factors, e.g., via the induction of phosphoducin-like-3 that stabilizes VEGFR2 expression [32]. In microvascular endothelial cells, hypoxia has been shown to induce the expression of integrins including integrin β_3 to enhance tube formation [33]. These discoveries led to the development of antiangiogenic drugs like the anti-VEGF monoclonal antibody bevacizumab, which in case of melanoma demonstrated improved disease-free intervals, but did not provide an improved overall survival benefit [34].

One family of molecules that play a role in normal tissue remodeling and wound healing are matrix metalloproteinases. They lead to the degradation of extracellular matrix proteins and allow for cell migration and tissue replacement and remodeling [35]. Tumors co-opt this mechanism. The hypoxic environment in the tumor leads to tissue remodeling by way of upregulating matrix metalloproteinases like MMP2 and MMP9 either directly or indirectly via the induction of VEGF and other chemokines and growth factors [36]. Secretion of MMP2 and MMP9 by malignant cells enables their increased migration, invasion, and metastasis [37, 38]. Targeting MMPs has been an attractive therapeutic approach, however a largely unsuccessful one owing to multiple reasons, including large-scale systemic adverse effects [39].

While tissue remodeling, angiogenesis, invasion, and metastasis involve endothelial cells, stromal cells, fibroblasts, extracellular matrix proteins, and the malignant cells, one other major cellular component in the tumor microenvironment is the immune cell compartment. Owing to the high immunogenicity of melanoma due to the presence of high mutational burden, and melanoma antigen-specific T cells in the melanoma microenvironment, targeting melanoma with immunotherapeutic modalities has always been an attractive approach. The cellular components of the immune landscape in the tumor microenvironment include both innate and adaptive components of the immune system. Suppressive cells include pro-tumorigenic macrophages, FoxP3+ regulatory T cells, regulatory B cells, and myeloid-derived suppressor cells (MDSCs). Antitumor components include antigen-presenting dendritic cells and macrophages, CD8+ cytotoxic T cells, CD4+ effector T helper cells, B cells, natural killer (NK) cells, and NKT cells. Multiple studies have positively correlated the presence of tumor-infiltrating lymphocytes (TILs) in melanoma with an improved prognosis, a reduction in risk of recurrence, and improved clinicopathological features [40, 41]. However, these findings are not unanimous, as other studies have found that only an increase in TILs in primary melanomas did not necessarily correlate with better prognosis, but the sentinel lymph node should also be included for a better prediction [42]. Thus, a high TIL infiltration in the tumor does not always indicate a good clinical outcome. This underscores the importance of better understanding the immune cell make up in the tumor microenvironment. Defining immune cell heterogeneity, and ratios of cytotoxic T cells to T regulatory cells or activated effector T cells to exhausted T cells, provides stronger associations between clinical outcomes and tumor TIL infiltration [43].

The primary lymphocyte that plays a crucial and active role in an antitumor immune response is the CD8+ cytotoxic T cell. It specifically recognizes tumor cells via MHCI-peptide complex/T cell receptor interaction and kills them using cytotoxic granules like perforin and granzyme or via the interaction of FasL with Fas receptors on target cells. T cell activation is a complex process involving cellular interactions via their cell surface molecules, and secreted cytokines. The first signal for T cell activation is the T cell receptor recognizing the MHC-peptide complex on its interacting cell (either an antigen-presenting cell or a virus-infected/tumor cell). However, this alone is insufficient, and there is a second signal involving CD28 on the T cell binding CD80/86 on the antigen-presenting cell, in order to fulfill the two-signal criteria for T cell activation. Then came the discovery of the inhibitory CTLA-4 molecule that competitively binds CD80/86 and renders effector T cells inactive, and in a state of exhaustion (PMID: 8596936). The binding of CTLA-4 to CD80/86 is a naturally occurring process that prevents an overactive immune response and hence autoimmunity. The discovery of additional costimulatory and co-inhibitory molecules led to the understanding that T cell activation/inactivation was a way more complex and finely balanced process than was once thought, evolving the two-step hypothesis [44]. The interaction between PD-1 on the T cell and PD-L1 on the APC or the tumor cell was another major discovery involved in T cell inactivation and subsequent exhaustion [45]. As the state of T cell exhaustion was further examined, it was discovered that T cell exhaustion is a state of dysfunction. This dysfunctional state is present in settings of persistent antigen-driven TCR signaling like in chronic infections, and in cancer. Thus, tonic signaling plays a key role in inducing T cell exhaustion [46]. Exhausted T cells are transcriptionally, phenotypically, and functionally distinct from effector T cells. The transcription factor TOX has been recently shown to be the driver of T cell exhaustion [47, 48]. TOX expression is driven via NFAT activation through TCR signaling. Deletion of TOX led to the abrogation of exhaustion in T cells. A phenotypic characteristic of this dysfunctional T cells is the upregulation of multiple inhibitory receptors like TIM3, LAG3, PD-1, CTLA-4, CD38, and CD69. They also lose their ability to secrete IFN-γ and TNF [49].

Another key lymphocyte in determining a pro vs antitumor immune response is the FoxP3 + CD4+ T regulatory cell. Ligation of CTLA-4, constitutively expressed as a result of FoxP3, on T regulatory cells leads to an enhanced immunosuppressive environment by way of increased IL-10 and TGFβ secretion [50, 51]. With these discoveries of inhibitory molecules driving, in part, the dysfunctional T cell phenotype came the two current mainstay therapies that have effectively replaced chemotherapy and radiation as first-line standard of care in melanoma. Ipilimumab is a monoclonal antibody that binds CTLA-4, neutralizing it and thus preventing it from inactivating a T cell, and also abrogating T regulatory cell activation, serving as a dual pronged approach in alleviating some of the immunosuppressive effects observed within the tumor microenvironment [52, 53]. Preclinical studies in a B16 melanoma mouse model demonstrated that a combination of GMCSF and CTLA4 blockade has an effect on the tumor-infiltrating T regulatory cell population, altering the intratumoral T regulatory cell to T effector cell ratio to favor tumor clearance [54]. Preclinical studies using CTLA-4 blockade along with PD-1 blockade demonstrated antitumor activity in murine colorectal tumor models, along with enhanced T cell infiltration. Additionally, it led to a favorable T regulatory cell to T effector cell ratio, increasing the secretion of pro-inflammatory cytokine and activation of tumor-specific effector T cells [55].

MDSCs also play a key role in promoting an immune suppressive environment in melanoma. They have been demonstrated to have a predictive value; their presence negatively correlated with a patient's response to ipilimumab therapy [56]. MDSCs are activated by a sleuth of soluble factors in the tumor microenvironment, including IL-6, GM-CSF, IL-10, and VEGF [57–59]. Once activated, MDSCs produce nitric oxide and upregulate arginase-1 which leads to further nutrient deprivation in the tumor microenvironment leading to a cell cycle arrest in effector T cells. It also leads to a reduction in expression of ζ-chain in the T cell receptor, destabilizing effector T cells and suppressing their functions [60]. In B16 melanoma mouse models, a combination of CTLA-4 and PD-1 blockade led to a depletion of T regulatory and myeloid suppressor cells, and an effective increase in the T effector/MDSC and T effector/T regulatory cell ratio [53]. The reduction of T regulatory cells on treatment with CTLA-4 blockade was mainly attributed to the presence of FcγR expressing macrophages that infiltrated the tumor microenvironment [61]. The preclinical studies and the enhancement of immune activation as a result of CTLA4 and PD1 blockade led to clinical trials targeting these two molecules.

Trials with ipilimumab showed an increase in overall survival compared to a control arm of gp100 peptide vaccine [62]. However, coupled with an improved overall survival were immune-related adverse effects [63]. Nivolumab targets PD-1, binding it and preventing its ligands from binding and inactivating T cells. Initial trials with nivolumab showed a higher response rate of about 41%, with, comparatively, a more acceptable safety profile [64–66]. A trial combining ipilimumab and nivolumab demonstrated a much higher response rate of 57.6% in untreated melanoma cases and in advanced melanoma with a 2-year overall survival of 53% [67–70].

While we have two effective therapies as our first-line standard of care in metastatic melanoma, there is still significant room for improvement in terms of response rates and therapeutic efficiency. To this end, explorations into alternative immune stimulators and checkpoint molecules have begun. T cell activation is an extremely intricate and well-balanced process involving not only signal 1 and 2 as previously described but multiple other molecules. In addition to CTLA4 and PD1, there are numerous other receptors that interact with their respective ligands to fine-tune T cell activation and prevent overactive T cells. These molecules belong to various superfamilies of receptors, the primary families being the tumor necrosis factor receptor superfamily (TNFRSF) and the immunoglobulin superfamily (IGSF) which includes the CD28 and B7 molecule family along with the TIM family of proteins [44].

4.1 Immunoglobulin Superfamily

The immunoglobulin superfamily includes multiple subfamilies of molecules. The B7 family and the CD28 family are two members of the immunoglobulin superfamily, among many others including cell adhesion molecules and growth factor receptors, and are the most well studied [71]. This family is characterized by the presence of a conserved fold structure comprised of two β pleated sheets with multiple strands [71, 72]. The members of the IgSF primarily bind to ligands that also belong to the same family [44]. CD226, a member of the immunoglobulin superfamily, is a costimulatory molecule on the T cell, which on binding CD155 (poliovirus receptor) or CD112 (nectin-1) leads to T cell activation [44, 73]. It competes with TIGIT for the same epitope on CD155. TIGIT binds CD155 with an affinity 100X greater than CD226 [74]. CD226 also serves as an activating receptor for natural killer (NK) cells. The binding of CD226 with its ligands leads to the activation/inactivation balance tipping toward activating the NK cell. ICOS, another costimulatory molecule in this superfamily, present on the T cell leads to T cell activation when bound by its ligand ICOSL [75]. Among the checkpoint molecules exists CTLA4 which, as previously elaborated, binding B71/2 also called CD80/86, PDL1 binding to PD1, and LAG3 binding to MHCII all leading to a dampened T cell activation. A subfamily of the immunoglobulin superfamily is the TIM (T cell immunoglobulin and mucin domain) family of genes which includes TIM3 binding to galectin-9 which leads to a dampened T cell response. Among the TIM family of proteins, TIM1 is a costimulatory molecule present on T cells. When bound to TIM4, it is said to play a role in allergic responses leading to Th2 cell hyper-proliferation [76]. With the discovery of these multiple immunomodulatory molecules, and the clinical success observed with ipilimumab and nivolumab in melanoma, multiple targets and diseases started to be investigated in clinic.

4.2 Tumor Necrosis Factor Receptor Superfamily

The TNFRSF proteins are structurally diverse. However, they all contain extracellular cysteine-rich domains. They can be stimulatory or inhibitory in nature, their function not correlated with their structure [77]. The costimulatory molecules of this TNFRSF include herpesvirus entry mediatory (HVEM) when it binds LIGHT; death receptor-3 (DR3) when it binds TL1A; CD40 interacting with CD40L, and GITR interacting

GITRL. OX-40, also belonging to the TNFRSF, is a costimulatory molecule on T cells which when bound with its ligand OX40L leads to T cell activation [44]. Usually members of the TNFRSF interact with ligands that belong to the tumor necrosis factor superfamily (TNFSF). However, one extremely intriguing exception to this rule is HVEM. Belonging to the tumor necrosis factor superfamily, it not only interacts with LIGHT, a TNFSF member, but also with BTLA and CD160, both belonging to the immunoglobulin superfamily. The ligand bound by HVEM dictates its effect on T cell activation. When HVEM on the T cell binds LIGHT on an antigen-presenting cell, or in its soluble form, it leads to T cell activation. In contrast when HVEM on an antigen-presenting cell binds CD160 or BTLA on a T cell, both belonging to the immunoglobulin superfamily, it leads to dampening of T cell activation.

The role of these immunomodulatory targets, while well-defined in the vacuum of the immune synapse, is yet to be defined in the context of the malignant cell as there is increasing evidence that these molecules do not exist in isolation. In addition to their presence on cells involved in immune activation, co-stimulatory and co-inhibitory molecules are also expressed by a third player, the tumor cells themselves, and have been demonstrated to have a prognostic significance [78–86].

In gastric cancer, the presence of BTLA and HVEM, in the cytoplasm of cancer cells detected by immunohistochemistry, was associated with progression and poor prognosis [82]. HVEM interacts with BTLA and CD160 on the T cell, to render the T cell inactive [44]. In some melanoma cases, BTLA remains highly expressed on CD8+ T cells, leaving them susceptible to HVEM-mediated inactivation [87]. BTLA on effector T cells has been demonstrated to bind HVEM on T regulatory cells and increase their immunosuppressive activity [88]. Thus, the presence of BTLA on cancer cells might play a similar role in binding HVEM on T regulatory cells and enhancing their immunosuppressive functions. These interactions make the HVEM/BTLA/CD160 axis tempting targets to add to the existing repertoire of checkpoint inhibitors.

5 Expression of Immune Targets on Melanoma Cells

We characterized five patient-derived melanoma cell lines, MEL2, MELV, 3MM, KFM, and GLM2, and three established melanoma cell lines, SKMEL-28, SKMEL-37, and SKMEL-103, for the expression of 23 immunomodulatory molecules by RT-PCR and compared them to adult normal melanocytes (Fig. 1). Additionally, we explored this expression based on the BRAFV600E status of these cells. Checkpoint molecules are differentially expressed in melanoma cell lines and adult normal melanocytes. Individual patient-derived melanoma cells have a distinct expression profile of immune checkpoint molecules. The presence of BRAFV600E promotes constitutive expression of ICOS, CTLA4, and HVEM (Fig. 2).

Among the checkpoint molecules, HVEM was significantly downregulated in the melanoma cells compared to normal melanocytes, independent of BRAFV600E status. HVEM is an intriguing molecule since it functions as a bidirectional switch. When HVEM binds to BTLA or CD160, it leads to dampening of T cell activation. When HVEM binds to LIGHT, it leads to T cell activation (Fig. 1). Additionally, HVEM ligand BTLA demonstrated a similar difference in the overall survival of patients with higher expression. Patients positive for the BRAFV600E lesion demonstrated a better overall survival with higher expression of BTLA. This was reversed in patients without the BRAFV600E lesion who demonstrated a poorer overall survival in case of higher BTLA expression. CD160, the other ligand of HVEM, though showing no difference in overall survival, demonstrated a statistically significant downregulation in BRAFV600E-positive cell lines compared to normal melanocytes. Moreover, HVEM belongs to the tumor necrosis factor receptor superfamily, and its ability to bind to proteins of the immunoglobulin

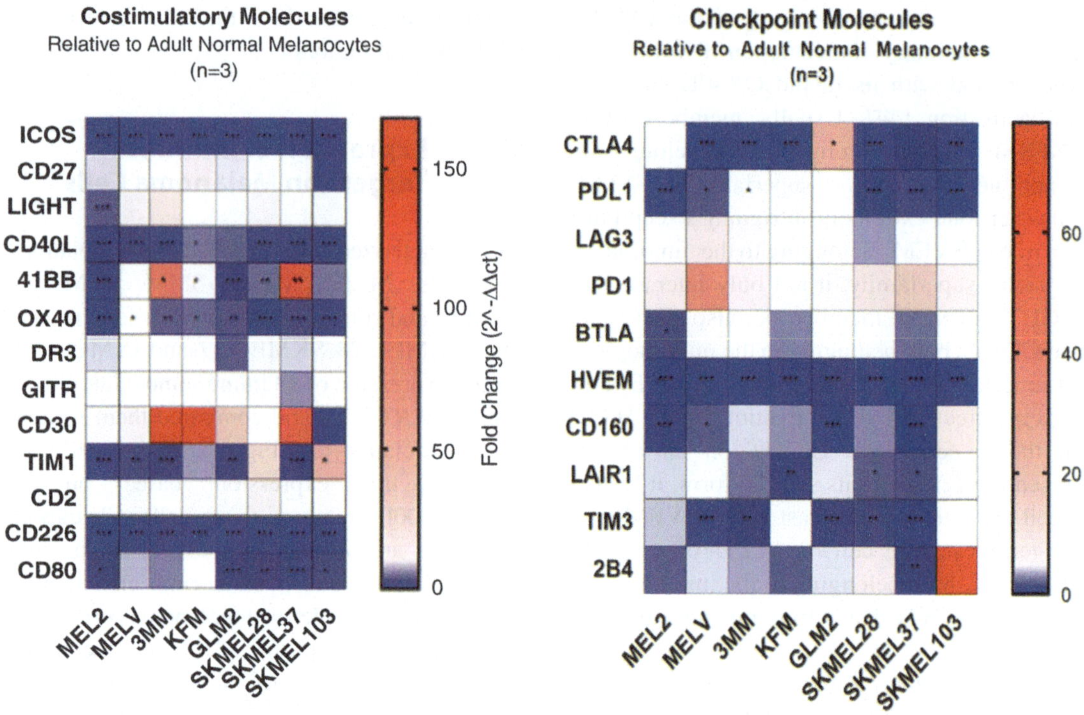

Fig. 1 Immunomodulatory molecule expression in patient-derived melanoma cells. RT-PCR for mRNA expression of costimulatory molecules in melanoma cells relative to adult normal melanocytes. Mean fold change of N = 3 independent experiments. Multiple Student's t-tests were used to compare mean fold change between normal melanocytes and melanoma cells. *p < 0.05 **p < 0.01 ***p < 0.001

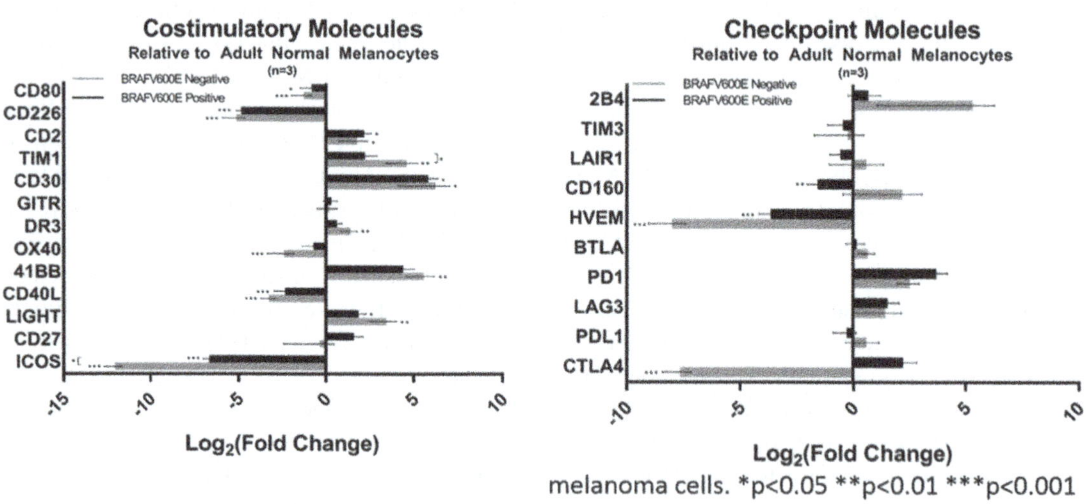

Fig. 2 Immunomodulatory molecule expression in patient-derived BRAFV600E-positive and BRAFV600E-negative melanoma cells. RT-PCR determining log2 fold change of checkpoint molecules in BRAFV600E-positive (n = 6) and BRAFV600E-negative melanoma cells (n = 2) relative to adult normal melanocytes. Mean ± SEM of N = 3 independent experiments was calculated. One-way ANOVA followed by a Tukey's post-test was used to compare fold changes between normal melanocytes and BRAFV600E-positive and BRAFV600E-negative melanoma cells. *p < 0.05 **p < 0.01 ***p < 0.001

superfamily (CD160 and BTLA) makes this trio of molecules an interesting set to explore.

Since these molecules are usually expressed on cells involved in an immune response, e.g., T cells and antigen-presenting cells, this observation opens up a new area for potential exploration of the role of these molecules on the third major player in the antitumor response: the tumor cells. While much is known about the roles of these positive and negative regulators in the immunological synapse, there remains to be seen the role played by these molecules in the context of the tumor cell with respect to manipulating an immune response. Molecules that have shown a poor prognosis when present in tumor samples include HVEM, BTLA, and CD160 [79, 82].

In an effort to visualize the location of the immunomodulatory molecules in melanoma cells, immunofluorescence was performed in all our cell lines. We observed that HVEM, BTLA, and CD160 are present on the membranes as well as in the cytoplasm of the melanoma cells. Some cells were brightly stained and some dimly stained within a field of view, this time pointing out the intra-cell line heterogeneity (Fig. 3). Checkpoint molecules HVEM, BTLA, and CD160 are present in the cytoplasm as well as on the membrane of melanoma cells, determined by flow cytometry surface staining (Fig. 4). There is a heterogeneity in the expression level of these molecules in each cell line. Moreover, the presence of the BRAFV600E genetic lesion correlates with a higher surface expression of immunomodulatory molecules in melanoma cells (Fig. 5).

The hot-spot somatic mutation for BRAF results in a valine residue at the 600th position being replaced by a glutamic acid (V600E) or lysine (V600K) residue. As seen with the mutations in RAS, different mutations in BRAF also lead to different outcomes. The presence of BRAFV600K in cutaneous melanoma has been linked with highly aggressive tumors that metastasize faster than BRAFV600E tumors [89]. However, the most frequently found BRAF genetic lesion is BRAFV600E [90]. The presence of BRAFV600E is associated with poor prognosis in cancers, including skin cutaneous melanoma [91, 92].

The presence of the BRAFV600E genetic lesion in melanoma aids in immune escape. It was observed that inhibiting BRAFV600E with a small molecule inhibitor led to an upregulation of MHC-I molecules on melanoma cells [93]. Additionally, inhibiting mutated BRAF with interfering RNA reduced the production of immunosuppressive cytokines like IL-10 and VEGF [94]. Various studies, including our group, have observed that treatment with a BRAFV600E inhibitor leads to an increased expression of melanoma-associated antigens and consequently better immune activation via T cell recognition [95, 96]. The efficacy of adoptive T cell transfer was also enhanced on treatment of melanoma cells with BRAFV600E and MEK inhibitors [97]. BRAFV600E-positive melanoma cell lines demonstrated an increased IL-1 expression. IL-1 was shown to enhance the immunosuppressive activity of tumor-associated fibroblasts. Treatment of tumor-associated fibroblasts with IL-1 led to reduced proliferation and function of melanoma-specific cytotoxic T cells [98]. BRAFV600E was also shown to govern T regulatory cell infiltration during tumorigenesis. The induction of BRAFV600E oncogene led to a localized accumulation of FoxP3+ T regulatory cells within 1 week of increases in melanoma-associated antigen expression [99]. With this discovery, a new class of drugs was added to the then existing, extremely limited treatment palate for melanoma.

(a) Small Molecule Inhibitors.

With profound impacts on melanoma progression and survival, as well as immune escape, it was reasonable to assume that inhibition of BRAFV600E, in addition to causing melanoma regression, would also alleviate metastasis and the immunosuppressive environment. To that end, the therapeutic landscape of melanoma became vastly different with the discovery of small molecule inhibitors of BRAFV600E, like vemurafenib, that gained FDA approval in August 2011 and quickly

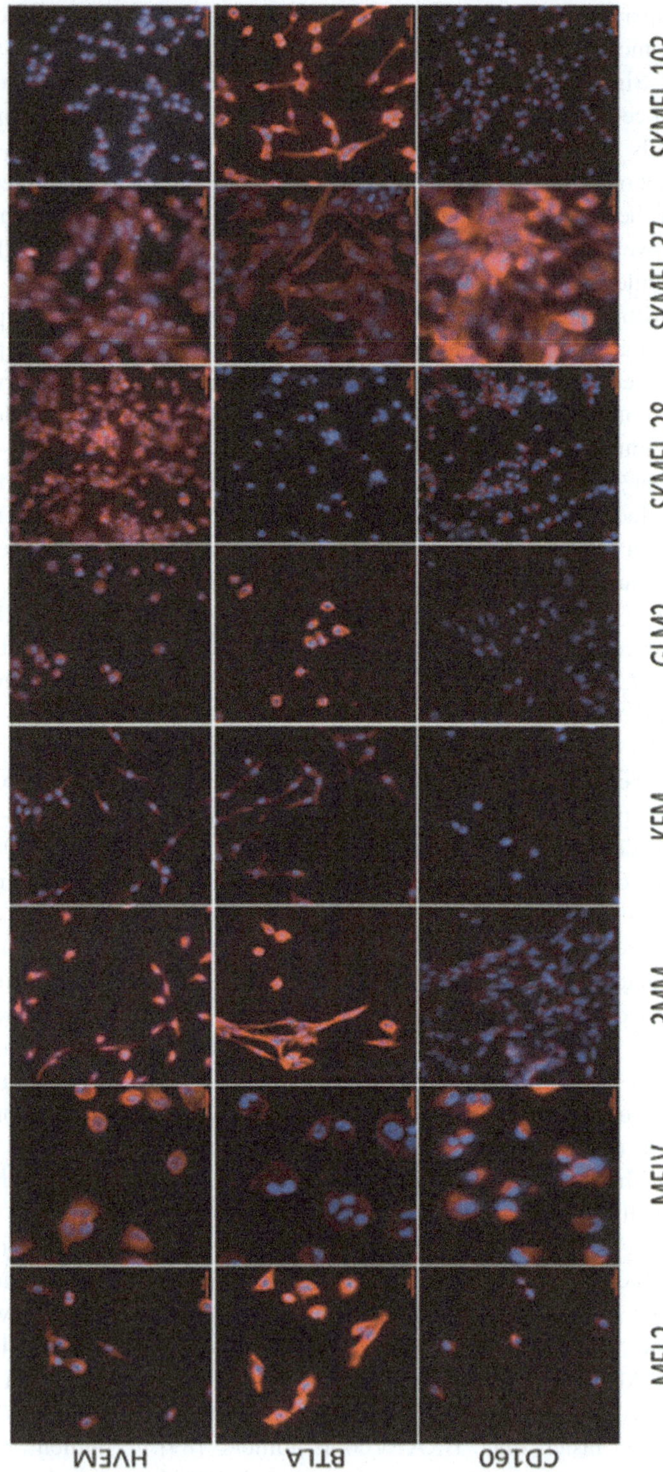

Fig. 3 Localization of immunomodulatory molecules in cytoplasm of melanoma cells. Immunofluorescence was carried out for HVEM, BTLA, and CD160 on melanoma cells. Blue, nucleus; red, immunomodulatory molecule. Images are 400X magnified

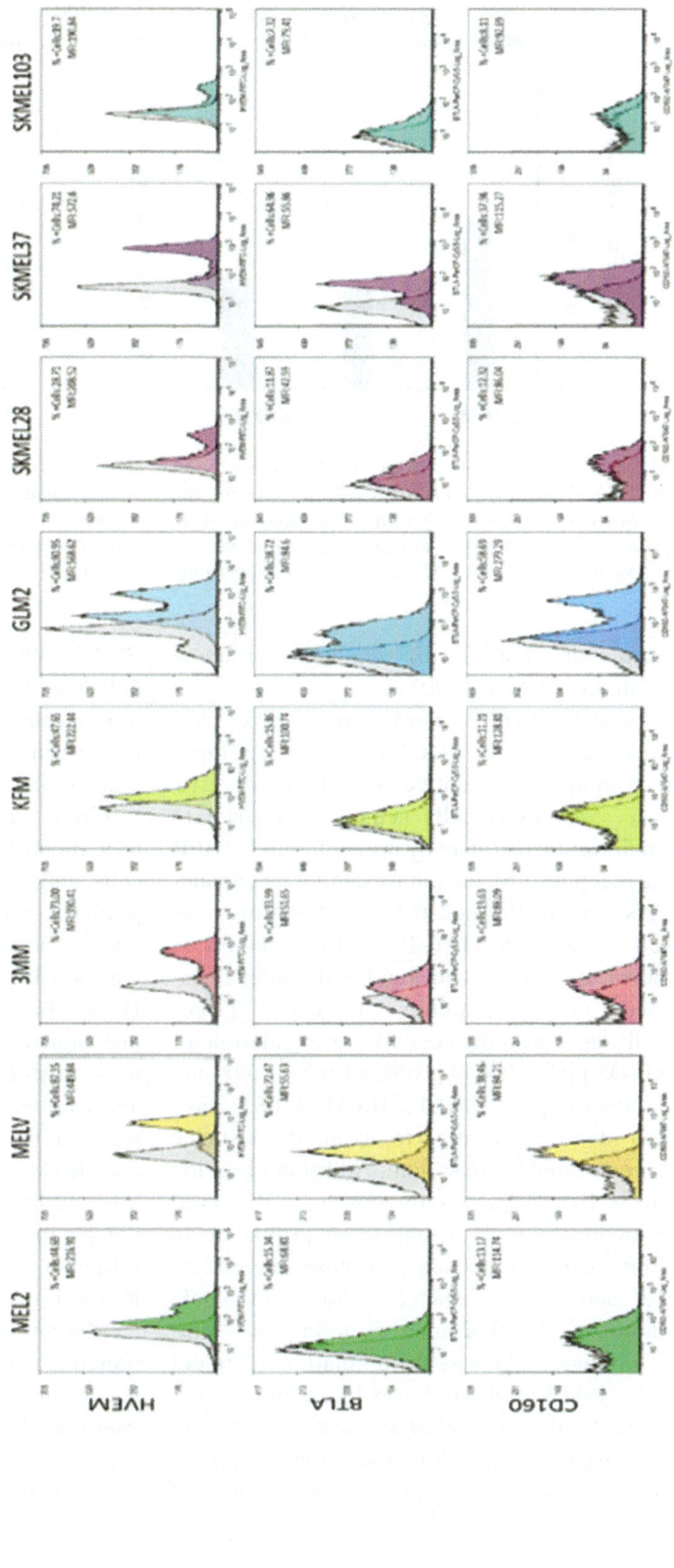

Fig. 4 **Immunomodulatory molecule surface expression on melanoma cells**. Flow cytometry was carried out for HVEM, BTLA, and CD160, on melanoma cells. Gray, unstained control; colored histogram, stained cells. Top right corner shows the percentage of positive cells and mean fluorescence intensity from one representative of n = 3 independent experiments

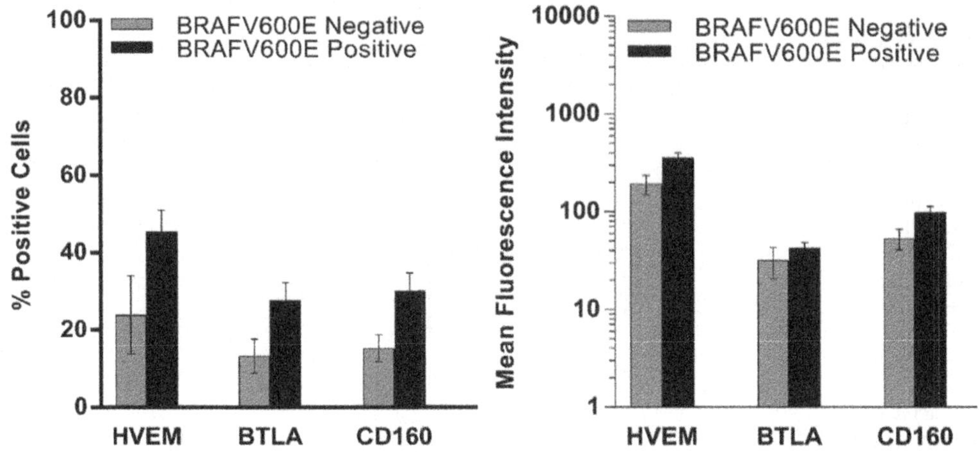

Fig. 5 Percentage of BRAFV600E-positive and BRAFV600E-negative melanoma cells positive for the expression of immunomodulatory molecules on their surface. Five-color flow cytometry was carried out for HVEM, BTLA, CD160, TIM1, and CD226 on melanoma cells. Gates were drawn on the cells positive for expression and percentage of positive cells determined. Bars represent mean ± SEM percent positive cells from n = 3 independent experiments. One-way ANOVA with Tukey's post hoc test was carried out to determine statistical significance

became the first line of treatment for many melanoma patients [100].

Treatment with vemurafenib, however, was accompanied with side effects and a rapid development of adaptive and acquired resistance. Melanoma cells acquire resistance to vemurafenib treatment by upregulating PDGFR like receptor tyrosine kinases and thus enhancing signaling through the pAKT pathway, as well as N-RAS [101–103]. Beta-catenin is known to interact with Stat3 and confer resistance to vemurafenib treatment [104]. Additional mechanisms, like upregulation of FOXD3 [105], BAG3 [106], AEBP1 [107], and the fusion gene AGAP3-BRAF [108], have been identified, leading to acquired resistance to vemurafenib treatment. Additionally, side effects like keratoacanthomas were observed on treatment with vemurafenib [109]. In an effort to circumvent some of these side effects and acquired resistances, small molecule inhibitors of MEK like trametinib or cobimetinib were added as a combination treatment with BRAFV600E inhibitors like dabrafenib or vemurafenib and showed an improved survival and safety [110]. While the phenomenon of small molecule-mediated inhibition of BRAFV600E was yet unfolding, owing to the enhanced immunogenicity as well as unwanted immunosuppressive microenvironment, the interest in immunotherapeutic intervention for melanoma persisted.

Given our observations of immune modulatory molecules being expressed on melanoma cells, and the small molecule inhibitors working primarily on tumor cells, it was important to understand the effect of treating malignant cells with small molecules on the expression of the HVEM/BTLA/CD160 axis which remains as yet unexplored and can bear a crucial significance in the ability of tumor cells to escape immune clearance, as well as in designing a combinatorial regimen combining small molecule inhibitors and checkpoint inhibitors. We observed that inhibition of BRAFV600E with PLX4032 leads to an upregulation of HVEM, BTLA, and CD160 transcripts in melanoma cells that harbor the genetic lesion (Fig. 6).

Moreover, the treatment does not diminish the protein expression of these molecules, nor change localization of these molecules in the cell. Additionally, HVEM, BTLA, and CD160 are expressed in melanoma patient tissues as observed via IHC (Figs. 7 and 8).

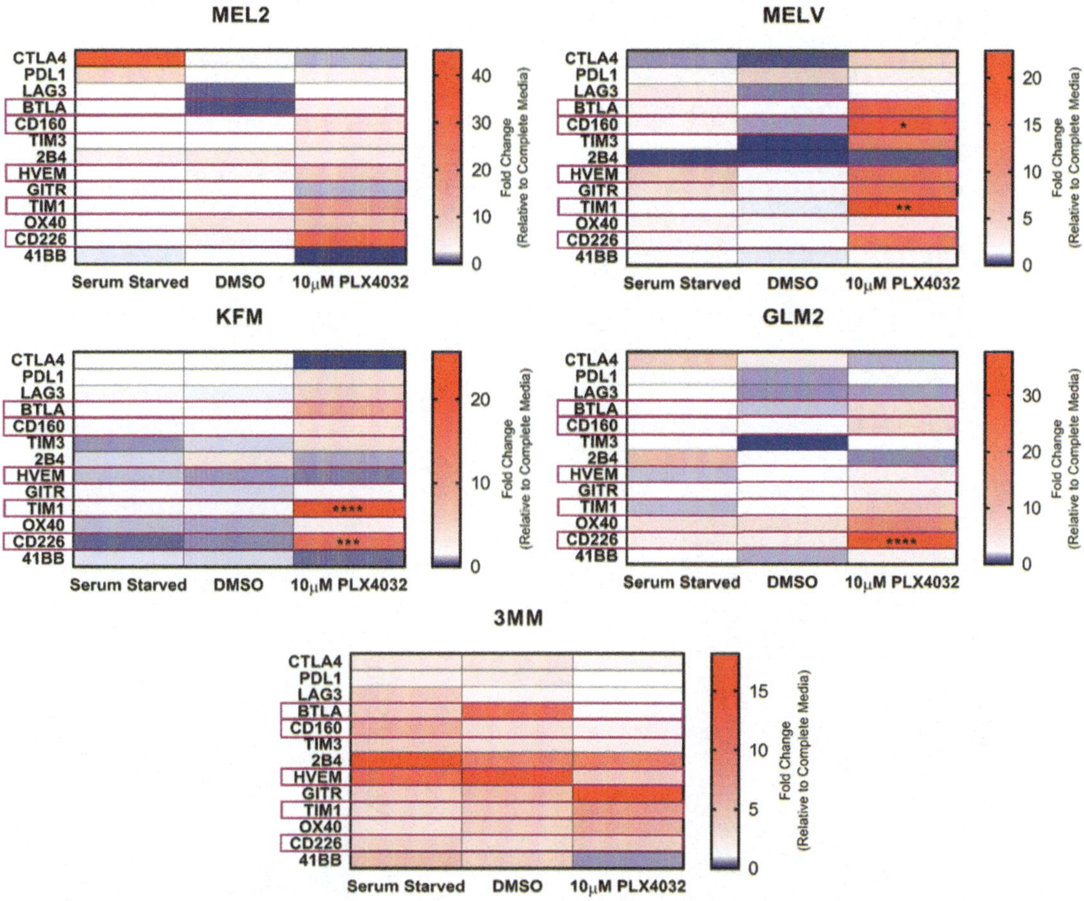

Fig. 6 Expression of immunomodulatory molecules on inhibition of BRAFV600E in patient-derived melanoma cells. Patient-derived melanoma cells were serum starved (5% charcoal stripped FBS containing RPMI), treated with DMSO (1:1000 vehicle control), or BRAFV600E inhibitor, 10 μM PLX4032. RT-PCR was carried out and fold change relative to complete RPMI was calculated. Heat maps represent mean fold change relative to complete media control of n = 3 independent experiments. Two-way ANOVA followed by a Tukey's multiple comparisons test was carried out to determine statistical significance. *$p < 0.05$ **$p < 0.01$ ***$p < 0.001$ ****$p < 0.0001$

6 Perspectives

Cancer growth and progression can be attributed to two major drivers: accumulation of genetic mutations in key driver pathways that give cancer cells a survival advantage and the ability of cancer cells to evade the immune system. We attempted to dissect the relationship between the most frequently found genetic lesion, BRAFV600E, and the expression of novel immunomodulatory molecules in melanoma, identifying BTLA as a potential immunotherapeutic target, amenable to a combinatorial therapeutic regimen with small molecule inhibitors of the MAPK pathway.

Melanoma has the highest mutational rate among all cancers. These somatic mutations can occur in molecules of key driver pathways leading to the activation of oncogenes and subsequently cellular proliferation and cancer progression. High somatic mutations also lead to an increase in neo-epitopes that subsequently lead to melanoma having an increased immunogenicity. However, melanoma is notorious for immune evasion, negating the effect of immu-

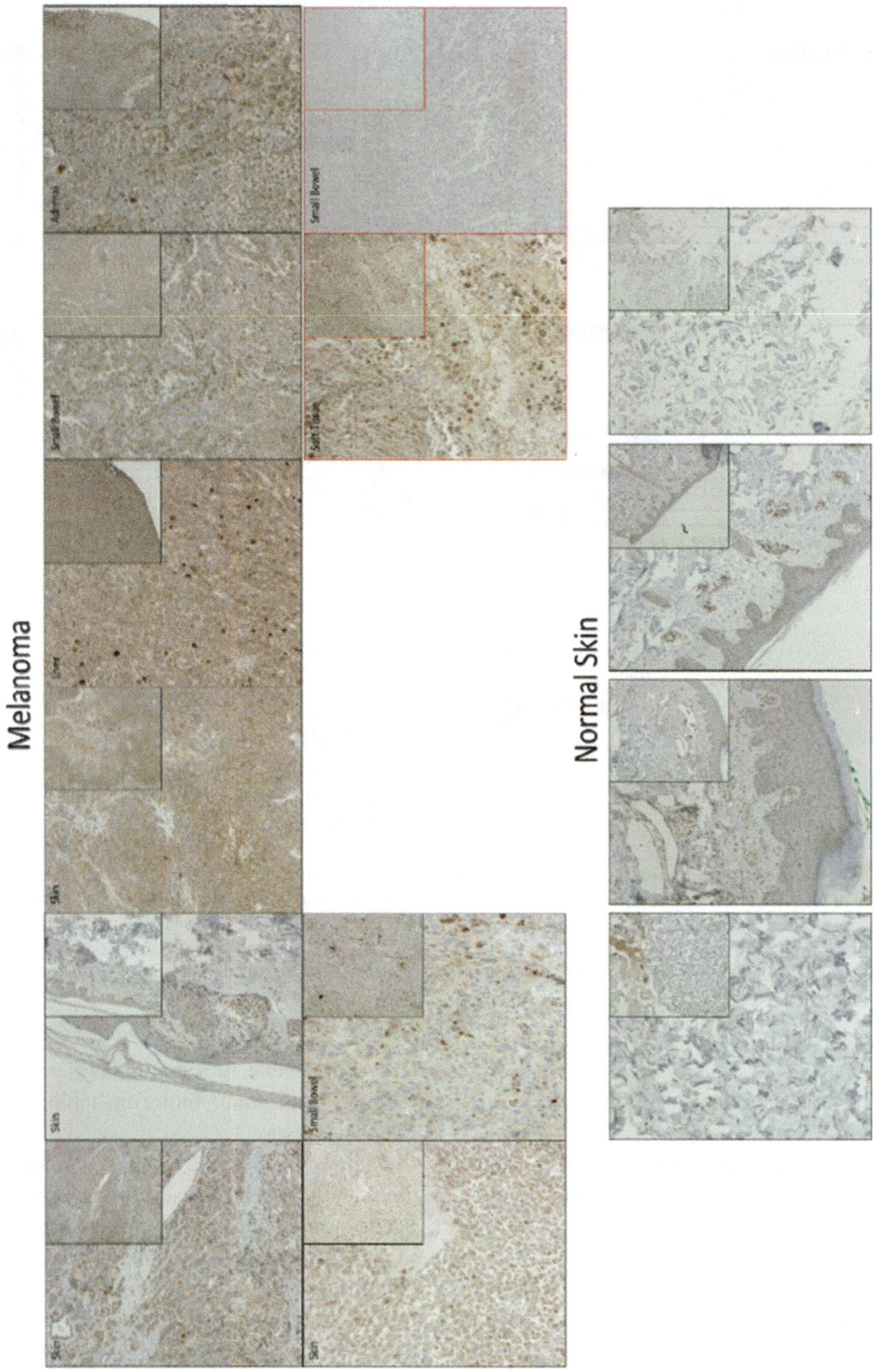

Fig. 7 Protein expression of immunomodulatory molecules in human melanoma and normal skin tissues. Immunohistochemistry staining for (A) HVEM, (B) BTLA, and (C) CD160 was evaluated in BRAFV600E-negative (n = 8) and BRAFV600E-positive (n = 2; red border) melanoma tissues and melanocytes in normal skin tissues (n = 4). The top left corner indicates the site of surgical excision. Pictures are 200X magnified. Insets are 100X magnified

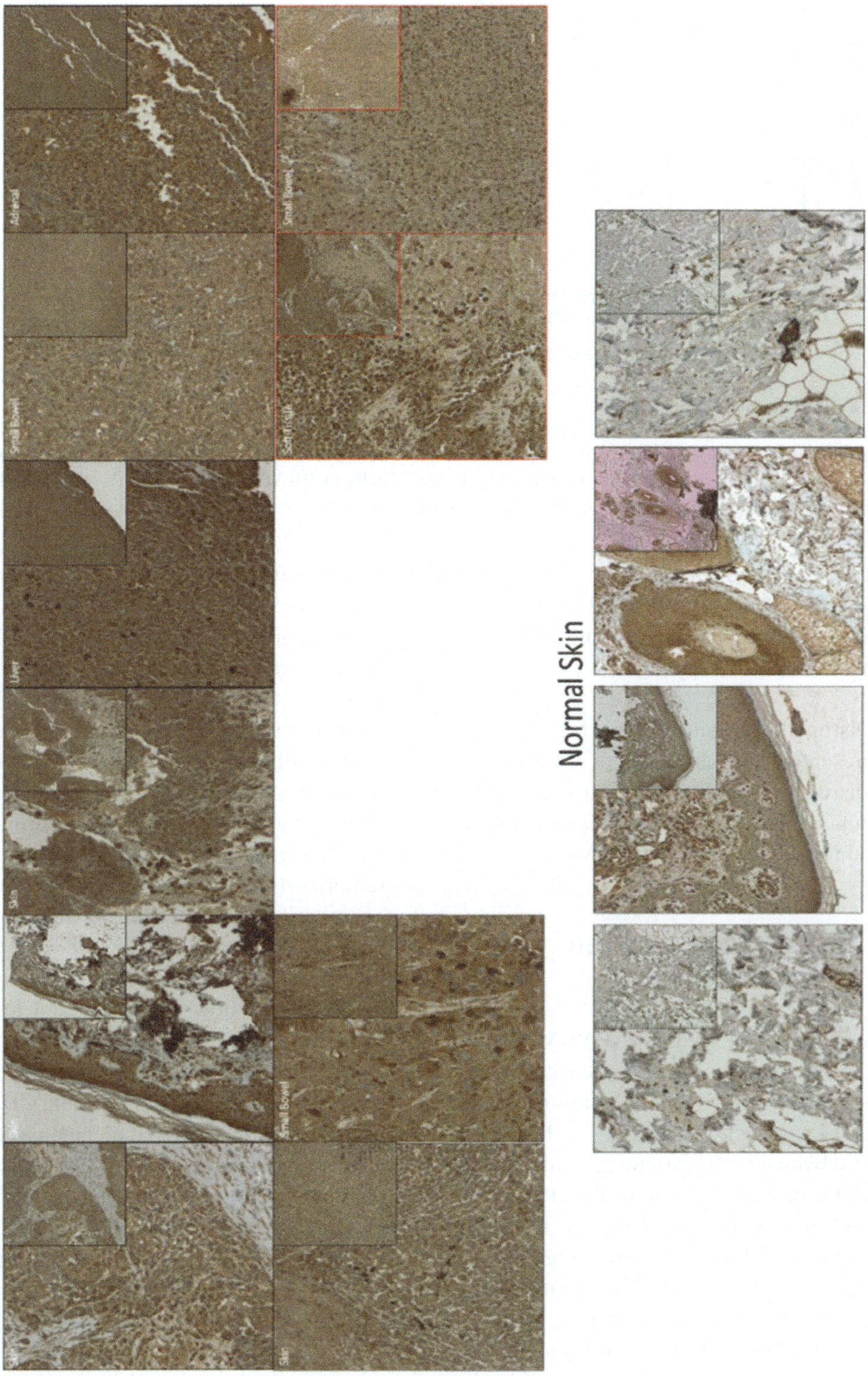

Fig. 7 (continued)

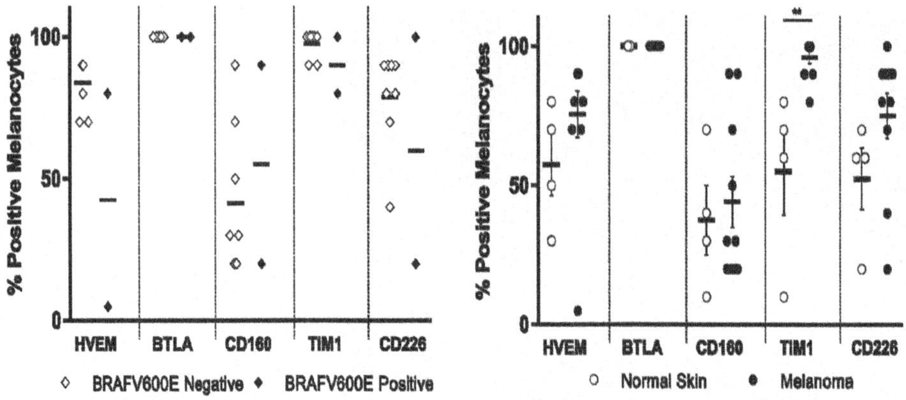

Fig. 8 Immunomodulatory molecule expression in human melanoma and normal skin tissue melanocytes by immunohistochemistry. Melanoma (n = 10) and normal skin (n = 4) tissues were stained for HVEM, BTLA, and CD160. (**a**) Percent positive melanocytes in normal skin and melanoma tissues. Line and bars represent mean ± SEM. Student's t-test was used to determine statistical significance $**p < 0.01$. (**b**) Percent positive melanoma cells in BRAFV600E-positive (n = 2) and BRAFV600E-negative (n = 8) melanoma tissues. Line represents the mean

nogenicity. Thus, a rational therapy would involve targeting melanoma at both drivers, activation of oncogenes and immune evasion.

An effective therapy should:

1. Disrupt the inhibitory signal between antigen-presenting cells and effector T cells.
2. Disrupt the inhibitory signal imposed by the tumor cell on an activated effector T cell.
3. Inhibit T regulatory cell activation.

7 HVEM/BTLA/CD160 Interactome

Herpesvirus entry mediator (HVEM) belongs to the TNFR superfamily. It is a checkpoint molecule when it binds B and T lymphocyte attenuator (BTLA) or CD160 on the T cell. BTLA and CD160 belong to the immunoglobulin superfamily and play a critical role in the HVEM/BTLA/CD160 axis interaction. They are unique molecules in that despite being a member of the immunoglobulin superfamily, they interact with a member of the TNFR superfamily, HVEM [44]. BTLA or CD160 on the T cell interacting with HVEM on the antigen-presenting cell leads to T cell inactivation [111].

While the role of BTLA in immune cell interactions is fairly well elucidated, its role in cancer cells remains to be explored. The presence of a high expression of BTLA is associated with a poor prognosis in gastric cancer patients [82]. Here we report, by immunohistochemistry, that BTLA is also expressed in tumor cells in melanoma tissues. The expression of BTLA in melanocytes of normal skin and melanoma patient tissues was the same. However, the frequency of melanocytes within the subepidermal layer of normal skin is very low compared to a melanoma tumor, 5–10%. We believe that this gives BTLA a quantitative advantage in the tumor microenvironment. Moreover, the presence of BTLA on the membrane of patient-derived melanoma cells, as evidenced by flow cytometry and immunofluorescence, makes BTLA an easy molecule to target with a therapeutic blocking antibody. We also report the presence of HVEM, and CD160, on the surface of patient-derived melanoma cells in vitro and in melanoma tissue sections by immunohistochemistry. Increased expression of HVEM is also associated with poor prognosis in gastric cancer [82]. HVEM on a T regulatory cell being engaged by BTLA leads to an increased T regulatory cell effector function [88]. We speculate that BTLA on the tumor cell may engage HVEM on the T regulatory cell and lead to an enhanced T regulatory cell effector function. HVEM silenced ovarian cancer cells were more susceptible to T cell-mediated killing compared to ovarian cancer cells expressing HVEM [112]. Thus, HVEM on the tumor cell could bind to BTLA and CD160 on T effector cells, rendering them inactive.

Thus, targeting BTLA meets all the criteria defined in this study:

1. It disrupts the T cell inactivating signal between HVEM on an antigen-presenting cell and BTLA on the T effector cell.
2. It disrupts the negative signal between HVEM on the tumor cell and BTLA on the T effector cell.
3. It would lead to an inhibition of T regulatory cell activity by disrupting the interaction of BTLA on the tumor cell with HVEM on the T regulatory cell.

Additionally, singularly targeting BTLA might not lead to as robust a clinical response as combining it with FDA-approved small molecule inhibitors of the MAPK pathway: BTLA and MAPK inhibitors.

We report that treatment of BRAFV600E-positive patient-derived melanoma cell lines leads to an upregulation of BTLA, HVEM, as well as CD160. Moreover, there is a persistent protein expression on the surface of melanoma cells on inhibition of the MAPK pathway, thus BTLA and HVEM on tumor cells can potentially interact with immune cells, aiding in immune suppression and immune escape. Combining small molecule inhibitors of the MAPK pathway with an antibody blocking BTLA interactions might lead to an enhanced tumor clearance by way of reduced T regulatory cell activation, and enhanced T effector cell function leading to a better overall survival in melanoma patients. Thus, a combination of BTLA blockade and MAPK pathway inhibition with small molecule inhibitors should be tested in preclinical models.

References

1. Liu, Y., & Sheikh, M. S. (2014). Melanoma: Molecular pathogenesis and therapeutic management. *Molecular and Cellular Pharmacology, 6*, 228–228.
2. Lattanzi, M., et al. (2019). Primary melanoma histologic subtype: Impact on survival and response to therapy. *Journal of the National Cancer Institute, 111*, 180–188. https://doi.org/10.1093/jnci/djy086
3. Corrie, P., Hategan, M., Fife, K., & Parkinson, C. (2014). Management of melanoma. *British Medical Bulletin, 111*, 149–162. https://doi.org/10.1093/bmb/ldu019
4. Wong, J. H., Fau, S. K., Kim, K. A., Fau, K. K., Foshag, L. J., Fau, F. L., Morton, D. L., & Morton, D. L. (1993). The role of surgery in the treatment of nonregionally recurrent melanoma. *Surgery, 113*, 389–394.
5. Leung, A. M., Hari, D. M., & Morton, D. L. (2012). Surgery for distant melanoma metastasis. *Cancer Journal, 18*, 176–184. https://doi.org/10.1097/PPO.0b013e31824bc981
6. Shi, W. (2015). Role for radiation therapy in melanoma. *Surgical Oncology Clinics of North America, 24*, 323–335. https://doi.org/10.1016/j.soc.2014.12.009
7. Fogarty, G. B., & Hong, A. (2014). Radiation therapy for advanced and metastatic melanoma. *Journal of Surgical Oncology, 109*, 370–375. https://doi.org/10.1002/jso.23509
8. Eggermont, A. M. M., & Kirkwood, J. M. (2004). Re-evaluating the role of dacarbazine in metastatic melanoma: What have we learned in 30 years? *European Journal of Cancer, 40*, 1825–1836. https://doi.org/10.1016/j.ejca.2004.04.030
9. Jiang, G., Li, R.-H., Sun, C., Liu, Y.-Q., & Zheng, J.-N. (2014). Dacarbazine combined targeted therapy versus dacarbazine alone in patients with malignant melanoma: A meta-analysis. *PLoS One, 9*, e111920. https://doi.org/10.1371/journal.pone.0111920
10. Dasari, S., & Tchounwou, P. B. (2014). Cisplatin in cancer therapy: Molecular mechanisms of action. *European Journal of Pharmacology, 740*, 364–378. https://doi.org/10.1016/j.ejphar.2014.07.025
11. Johnston, S. R., et al. (1998). Randomized phase II trial of BCDT [carmustine (BCNU), cisplatin, dacarbazine (DTIC) and tamoxifen] with or without interferon alpha (IFN-alpha) and interleukin (IL-2) in patients with metastatic melanoma. *British Journal of Cancer, 77*, 1280–1286. https://doi.org/10.1038/bjc.1998.214
12. Propper, D. J., et al. (2000). Phase II study of second-line therapy with DTIC, BCNU, cisplatin and tamoxifen (Dartmouth regimen) chemotherapy in patients with malignant melanoma previously treated with dacarbazine. *British Journal of Cancer, 82*, 1759–1763. https://doi.org/10.1054/bjoc.2000.1141
13. Chapman, P. B. et al. Phase III multicenter randomized trial of the Dartmouth regimen versus dacarbazine in patients with metastatic melanoma.
14. Davies, H., et al. (2002). Mutations of the BRAF gene in human cancer. *Nature, 417*, 949–954. https://doi.org/10.1038/nature00766

15. Alexandrov, L. B., et al. (2013). Signatures of mutational processes in human cancer. *Nature, 500*, 415–421. https://doi.org/10.1038/nature12477
16. Hocker, T., & Tsao, H. (2007). Ultraviolet radiation and melanoma: A systematic review and analysis of reported sequence variants. *Human Mutation, 28*, 578–588. https://doi.org/10.1002/humu.20481
17. Pleasance, E. D., et al. (2010). A comprehensive catalogue of somatic mutations from a human cancer genome. *Nature, 463*, 191–196. https://doi.org/10.1038/nature08658
18. Hodis, E., et al. (2012). A landscape of driver mutations in melanoma. *Cell, 150*, 251–263. https://doi.org/10.1016/j.cell.2012.06.024
19. Zhang, T., Dutton-Regester, K., Brown, K. M., & Hayward, N. K. (2016). The genomic landscape of cutaneous melanoma. *Pigment Cell & Melanoma Research, 29*, 266–283. https://doi.org/10.1111/pcmr.12459
20. Cancer Genome Atlas. (2015). N. Genomic classification of cutaneous melanoma. *Cell, 161*, 1681–1696. https://doi.org/10.1016/j.cell.2015.05.044
21. Teku, G. N., & Vihinen, M. (2018). Pan-cancer analysis of neoepitopes. *Scientific Reports, 8*, 12735. https://doi.org/10.1038/s41598-018-30724-y
22. Kirkin, A. F., Fau, D. K., Zeuthen, J., & Zeuthen, J. (1998). The immunogenic properties of melanoma-associated antigens recognized by cytotoxic T lymphocytes. *Experimental and Clinical Immunogenetics, 15*, 19–32. https://doi.org/10.1159/000019050
23. Zörnig, I., et al. (2015). Prognostic significance of spontaneous antibody responses against tumor-associated antigens in malignant melanoma patients. *International Journal of Cancer, 136*, 138–151. https://doi.org/10.1002/ijc.28980
24. Mihm, M. C., Jr., & Mulé, J. J. (2015). Reflections on the histopathology of tumor-infiltrating lymphocytes in melanoma and the host immune response. *Cancer Immunology Research, 3*, 827–835. https://doi.org/10.1158/2326-6066.CIR-15-0143
25. Fortes, C., et al. (2015). Tumor-infiltrating lymphocytes predict cutaneous melanoma survival. *Melanoma Research, 25*.
26. Obeid, J. M., Hu, Y., Erdag, G., Leick, K. M., & Slingluff, C. L., Jr. (2017). The heterogeneity of tumor-infiltrating CD8+ T cells in metastatic melanoma distorts their quantification: How to manage heterogeneity? *Melanoma Research,* **27**.
27. Paget, S. (1889). The distribution of secondary growths in cancer of the breast. *The Lancet, 133*, 571–573. https://doi.org/10.1016/S0140-6736(00)49915-0
28. Hart, I. R., & Fidler, I. J. (1980). Role of organ selectivity in the determination of metastatic patterns of B16 melanoma. *Cancer Research, 40*, 2281.
29. Maniyar, R., Chakraborty, S., & Suriano, R. (2018). Ethanol enhances estrogen mediated angiogenesis in breast cancer. *Journal of Cancer, 9*, 3874–3885. https://doi.org/10.7150/jca.25581
30. Rajoria, S., et al. (2011). Estradiol-mediated tumor neo-vascularization. *Oncology Letters, 2*, 453–457. https://doi.org/10.3892/ol.2011.283
31. Ramakrishnan, S., Anand, V., & Roy, S. (2014). Vascular endothelial growth factor signaling in hypoxia and inflammation. *Journal of Neuroimmune Pharmacology, 9*, 142–160. https://doi.org/10.1007/s11481-014-9531-7
32. Srinivasan, S., et al. (2015). Hypoxia-induced expression of phosducin-like 3 regulates expression of VEGFR-2 and promotes angiogenesis. *Angiogenesis, 18*, 449–462. https://doi.org/10.1007/s10456-015-9468-3
33. Befani, C., & Liakos, P. (2017). Hypoxia upregulates integrin gene expression in microvascular endothelial cells and promotes their migration and capillary-like tube formation. *Cell Biology International, 41*, 769–778. https://doi.org/10.1002/cbin.10777
34. Corrie, P. G., et al. (2018). Adjuvant bevacizumab for melanoma patients at high risk of recurrence: Survival analysis of the AVAST-M trial. *Annals of Oncology, 29*, 1843–1852. https://doi.org/10.1093/annonc/mdy229
35. Caley, M. P., Martins, V. L. C., & O'Toole, E. A. (2015). Metalloproteinases and Wound Healing. *Advances in Wound Care (New Rochelle), 4*, 225–234. https://doi.org/10.1089/wound.2014.0581
36. Yan, C., & Boyd, D. D. (2007). Regulation of matrix metalloproteinase gene expression. *Journal of Cellular Physiology, 211*, 19–26. https://doi.org/10.1002/jcp.20948
37. Hofmann, U. B., Eggert, A. A. O., Blass, K., Bröcker, E.-B., & Becker, J. C. (2003). Expression of matrix metalloproteinases in the microenvironment of spontaneous and experimental melanoma metastases reflects the requirements for tumor formation. *Cancer Research, 63*, 8221.
38. Hofmann, U. B., et al. (1999). Matrix metalloproteinases in human melanoma cell lines and xenografts: Increased expression of activated matrix metalloproteinase-2 (MMP-2) correlates with melanoma progression. *British Journal of Cancer, 81*, 774–782. https://doi.org/10.1038/sj.bjc.6690763
39. Cathcart, J., Pulkoski-Gross, A. & Cao, J. Targeting matrix metalloproteinases in cancer: Bringing new life to old ideas.
40. Azimi, F., et al. (2012). Tumor-infiltrating lymphocyte grade is an independent predictor of sentinel lymph node status and survival in patients with cutaneous melanoma. *Journal of Clinical Oncology, 30*, 2678–2683. https://doi.org/10.1200/JCO.2011.37.8539
41. Erdag, G., et al. (2012). Immunotype and immunohistologic characteristics of tumor-infiltrating immune cells are associated with clinical outcome in metastatic melanoma. *Cancer Research, 72*, 1070–1080. https://doi.org/10.1158/0008-5472.CAN-11-3218

42. Murali, R., Desilva, C., Thompson, J. F., & Scolyer, R. A. (2011). Factors predicting recurrence and survival in sentinel lymph node-positive melanoma patients. *Annals of Surgery, 253*.
43. Saleh, R., & Elkord, E. (2020). FoxP3+ T regulatory cells in cancer: Prognostic biomarkers and therapeutic targets. *Cancer Letters, 490*, 174–185. https://doi.org/10.1016/j.canlet.2020.07.022
44. Chen, L., & Flies, D. B. (2013). Molecular mechanisms of T cell co-stimulation and co-inhibition. *Nature Reviews Immunology, 13*, 227–242. https://doi.org/10.1038/nri3405
45. Ishida, Y., Agata, Y., Shibahara, K., & Honjo, T. (1992). Induced expression of PD-1, a novel member of the immunoglobulin gene superfamily, upon programmed cell death. *The EMBO Journal, 11*, 3887–3895.
46. Wherry, E. J., & Kurachi, M. (2015). Molecular and cellular insights into T cell exhaustion. *Nature Reviews Immunology, 15*, 486–499. https://doi.org/10.1038/nri3862
47. Khan, O., et al. (2019). TOX transcriptionally and epigenetically programs CD8+ T cell exhaustion. *Nature, 571*, 211–218. https://doi.org/10.1038/s41586-019-1325-x
48. Mann, T. H., & Kaech, S. M. (2019). Tick-TOX, it's time for T cell exhaustion. *Nature Immunology, 20*, 1092–1094. https://doi.org/10.1038/s41590-019-0478-y
49. Scott, A. C., et al. (2019). TOX is a critical regulator of tumour-specific T cell differentiation. *Nature, 571*, 270–274. https://doi.org/10.1038/s41586-019-1324-y
50. Takahashi, T., et al. (2000). Immunologic self-tolerance maintained by CD25(+)CD4(+) regulatory T cells constitutively expressing cytotoxic T lymphocyte-associated antigen 4. *The Journal of Experimental Medicine, 192*, 303–310. https://doi.org/10.1084/jem.192.2.303
51. Jain, N., Nguyen, H., Chambers, C., & Kang, J. (2010). Dual function of CTLA-4 in regulatory T cells and conventional T cells to prevent multiorgan autoimmunity. *Proceedings of the National Academy of Sciences of the United States of America, 107*, 1524–1528. https://doi.org/10.1073/pnas.0910341107
52. Peggs, K. S., Quezada, S. A., Chambers, C. A., Korman, A. J., & Allison, J. P. (2009). Blockade of CTLA-4 on both effector and regulatory T cell compartments contributes to the antitumor activity of anti-CTLA-4 antibodies. *The Journal of Experimental Medicine, 206*, 1717–1725. https://doi.org/10.1084/jem.20082492
53. Curran, M. A., Montalvo, W., Yagita, H., & Allison, J. P. (2010). PD-1 and CTLA-4 combination blockade expands infiltrating T cells and reduces regulatory T and myeloid cells within B16 melanoma tumors. *Proceedings of the National Academy of Sciences, 107*, 4275. https://doi.org/10.1073/pnas.0915174107
54. Quezada, S. A., Peggs, K. S., Curran, M. A., & Allison, J. P. (2006). CTLA4 blockade and GM-CSF combination immunotherapy alters the intratumor balance of effector and regulatory T cells. *The Journal of Clinical Investigation, 116*, 1935–1945. https://doi.org/10.1172/JCI27745
55. Selby, M. J., et al. (2016). Preclinical development of Ipilimumab and Nivolumab combination immunotherapy: Mouse tumor models, in vitro functional studies, and Cynomolgus macaque toxicology. *PLoS One, 11*, e0161779–e0161779. https://doi.org/10.1371/journal.pone.0161779
56. Meyer, C., et al. (2014). Frequencies of circulating MDSC correlate with clinical outcome of melanoma patients treated with ipilimumab. *Cancer immunology. Immunotherapy, 63*, 247–257. https://doi.org/10.1007/s00262-013-1508-5
57. Bah, I., Kumbhare, A., Nguyen, L., McCall, C. E., & El Gazzar, M. (2018). IL-10 induces an immune repressor pathway in sepsis by promoting S100A9 nuclear localization and MDSC development. *Cellular Immunology, 332*, 32–38. https://doi.org/10.1016/j.cellimm.2018.07.003
58. Hutchison, S., et al. (2019). Characterization of myeloid-derived suppressor cells and cytokines GM-CSF, IL-10 and MCP-1 in dogs with malignant melanoma receiving a GD3-based immunotherapy. *Veterinary Immunology and Immunopathology, 216*, 109912. https://doi.org/10.1016/j.vetimm.2019.109912
59. Tobin, R. P., et al. (2019). IL-6 and IL-8 are linked with myeloid-derived suppressor cell accumulation and correlate with poor clinical outcomes in melanoma patients. *Frontiers in Oncology, 9*, 1223–1223. https://doi.org/10.3389/fonc.2019.01223
60. Baniyash, M. (2004). TCR ζ-chain downregulation: Curtailing an excessive inflammatory immune response. *Nature Reviews Immunology, 4*, 675–687. https://doi.org/10.1038/nri1434
61. Simpson, T. R., et al. (2013). Fc-dependent depletion of tumor-infiltrating regulatory T cells co-defines the efficacy of anti-CTLA-4 therapy against melanoma. *The Journal of Experimental Medicine, 210*, 1695–1710. https://doi.org/10.1084/jem.20130579
62. Hodi, F. S., et al. (2010). Improved survival with Ipilimumab in patients with metastatic melanoma. *New England Journal of Medicine, 363*, 711–723. https://doi.org/10.1056/NEJMoa1003466
63. Verschuren, E. C., et al. (2016). Clinical, endoscopic, and histologic characteristics of Ipilimumab-associated colitis. *Clinical Gastroenterology and Hepatology, 14*, 836–842. https://doi.org/10.1016/j.cgh.2015.12.028
64. Topalian, S. L., Drake, C. G., & Pardoll, D. M. (2015). Immune checkpoint blockade: A common denominator approach to cancer therapy. *Cancer Cell, 27*, 450–461. https://doi.org/10.1016/j.ccell.2015.03.001
65. Topalian, S. L., et al. (2012). Safety, activity, and immune correlates of anti-PD-1 antibody in cancer.

The New England Journal of Medicine, 366, 2443–2454. https://doi.org/10.1056/NEJMoa1200690
66. Topalian, S. L., et al. (2014). Survival, durable tumor remission, and long-term safety in patients with advanced melanoma receiving Nivolumab. *Journal of Clinical Oncology, 32*, 1020–1030. https://doi.org/10.1200/JCO.2013.53.0105
67. Hodi, F. S., et al. (2016). Combined nivolumab and ipilimumab versus ipilimumab alone in patients with advanced melanoma: 2-year overall survival outcomes in a multicentre, randomised, controlled, phase 2 trial. *The Lancet Oncology, 17*, 1558–1568. https://doi.org/10.1016/S1470-2045(16)30366-7
68. Larkin, J., et al. (2015). Combined Nivolumab and Ipilimumab or monotherapy in untreated melanoma. *New England Journal of Medicine, 373*, 23–34. https://doi.org/10.1056/NEJMoa1504030
69. Wolchok, J. D., et al. (2017). Overall survival with combined nivolumab and Ipilimumab in advanced melanoma. *The New England Journal of Medicine, 377*, 1345–1356. https://doi.org/10.1056/NEJMoa1709684
70. Wolchok, J. D., et al. (2013). Nivolumab plus Ipilimumab in advanced melanoma. *New England Journal of Medicine, 369*, 122–133. https://doi.org/10.1056/NEJMoa1302369
71. Halaby, D. M., & Mornon, J. P. E. (1998). The immunoglobulin superfamily: An insight on its tissular, species, and functional diversity. *Journal of Molecular Evolution, 46*, 389–400. https://doi.org/10.1007/PL00006318
72. Halaby, D. M., Poupon, A., & Mornon, J. P. (1999). The immunoglobulin fold family: Sequence analysis and 3D structure comparisons. *Protein Engineering, Design and Selection, 12*, 563–571. https://doi.org/10.1093/protein/12.7.563
73. Gilfillan, S., et al. (2008). DNAM-1 promotes activation of cytotoxic lymphocytes by nonprofessional antigen-presenting cells and tumors. *The Journal of Experimental Medicine, 205*, 2965–2973. https://doi.org/10.1084/jem.20081752
74. Lozano, E., Dominguez-Villar, M., Kuchroo, V., & Hafler, D. A. (2012). The TIGIT/CD226 axis regulates human T cell function. *Journal of Immunology, 188*, 3869–3875. https://doi.org/10.4049/jimmunol.1103627
75. Wang, S., & Chen, L. (2004). Co-signaling molecules of the B7-CD28 family in positive and negative regulation of T lymphocyte responses. *Microbes and Infection, 6*, 759–766. https://doi.org/10.1016/j.micinf.2004.03.007
76. Meyers, J. H., et al. (2005). TIM-4 is the ligand for TIM-1, and the TIM-1-TIM-4 interaction regulates T cell proliferation. *Nature Immunology, 6*, 455–464. https://doi.org/10.1038/ni1185
77. Chattopadhyay, K., et al. (2009). Sequence, structure, function, immunity: Structural genomics of costimulation. *Immunological Reviews, 229*, 356–386. https://doi.org/10.1111/j.1600-065X.2009.00778.x
78. Kishimoto, W., et al. (2016). Expression of Tim-1 in primary CNS lymphoma. *Cancer Medicine, 5*, 3235–3245. https://doi.org/10.1002/cam4.930
79. Inoue, T., et al. (2015). HVEM expression contributes to tumor progression and prognosis in human colorectal cancer. *Anticancer Research, 35*, 1361.
80. Gadiot, J., et al. (2011). Overall survival and PD-L1 expression in metastasized malignant melanoma. *Cancer, 117*, 2192–2201. https://doi.org/10.1002/cncr.25747
81. Wang, H., et al. (2016). Activation of TIM1 induces colon cancer cell apoptosis via modulating Fas ligand expression. *Biochemical and Biophysical Research Communications, 473*, 377–381. https://doi.org/10.1016/j.bbrc.2016.02.085
82. Lan, X., et al. (2017). Increased BTLA and HVEM in gastric cancer are associated with progression and poor prognosis. *OncoTargets and Therapy, 10*, 919–926. https://doi.org/10.2147/OTT.S128825
83. Bertucci, F., et al. (2017). PDL1 expression is a poor-prognosis factor in soft-tissue sarcomas. *Oncoimmunology, 6*, e1278100-e1278100. https://doi.org/10.1080/2162402X.2016.1278100
84. Cuadros, T., et al. (2014). HAVCR/KIM-1 activates the IL-6/STAT-3 pathway in clear cell renal cell carcinoma and determines tumor progression and patient outcome. *Cancer Research, 74*, 1416. https://doi.org/10.1158/0008-5472.CAN-13-1671
85. Wu, J., et al. (2017). Low TIM3 expression indicates poor prognosis of metastatic prostate cancer and acts as an independent predictor of castration resistant status. *Scientific Reports, 7*, 8869. https://doi.org/10.1038/s41598-017-09484-8
86. Laurent, S., et al. (2013). The engagement of CTLA-4 on primary melanoma cell lines induces antibody-dependent cellular cytotoxicity and TNF-α production. *Journal of Translational Medicine, 11*, 108. https://doi.org/10.1186/1479-5876-11-108
87. Haymaker, C. L., et al. (2015). BTLA marks a less-differentiated tumor-infiltrating lymphocyte subset in melanoma with enhanced survival properties. *Oncoimmunology, 4*, e1014246-e1014246. https://doi.org/10.1080/2162402X.2015.1014246
88. Tao, R., Wang, L., Murphy, K. M., Fraser, C. C., & Hancock, W. W. (2008). Regulatory T cell expression of herpesvirus entry mediator suppresses the function of B and T lymphocyte attenuator-positive effector T cells. *The Journal of Immunology, 180*, 6649. https://doi.org/10.4049/jimmunol.180.10.6649
89. Li, Y., Umbach, D. M., & Li, L. (2017). Putative genomic characteristics of BRAF V600K versus V600E cutaneous melanoma. *Melanoma Research, 27*, 527–535. https://doi.org/10.1097/CMR.0000000000000388
90. Greaves, W. O., et al. (2013). Frequency and Spectrum of BRAF mutations in a retrospective, single-institution study of 1112 cases of melanoma. *The Journal of Molecular Diagnostics, 15*, 220–226. https://doi.org/10.1016/j.jmoldx.2012.10.002

91. Roth, A. D., et al. (2009). Prognostic role of KRAS and BRAF in stage II and III resected colon cancer: Results of the translational study on the PETACC-3, EORTC 40993, SAKK 60-00 trial. *Journal of Clinical Oncology, 28*, 466–474. https://doi.org/10.1200/JCO.2009.23.3452
92. Moreau, S., et al. (2012). Prognostic value of BRAFV600 mutations in melanoma patients after resection of metastatic lymph nodes. *Annals of Surgical Oncology, 19*, 4314–4321. https://doi.org/10.1245/s10434-012-2457-5
93. Sapkota, B., Hill, C. E., & Pollack, B. P. (2013). Vemurafenib enhances MHC induction in BRAF(V600E) homozygous melanoma cells. *Oncoimmunology, 2*, e22890. https://doi.org/10.4161/onci.22890
94. Sumimoto, H., Imabayashi, F., Iwata, T., & Kawakami, Y. (2006). The BRAF-MAPK signaling pathway is essential for cancer-immune evasion in human melanoma cells. *The Journal of Experimental Medicine, 203*, 1651–1656. https://doi.org/10.1084/jem.20051848
95. Frederick, D. T., et al. (2013). BRAF inhibition is associated with enhanced melanoma antigen expression and a more favorable tumor microenvironment in patients with metastatic melanoma. *Clinical Cancer Research, 19*, 1225–1231. https://doi.org/10.1158/1078-0432.CCR-12-1630
96. George, A. L., et al. (2015). PLX4032 mediated melanoma associated antigen potentiation in patient derived primary melanoma cells. *Journal of Cancer, 6*, 1320–1330. https://doi.org/10.7150/jca.11126
97. Hu-Lieskovan, S., et al. (2015). Improved antitumor activity of immunotherapy with BRAF and MEK inhibitors in BRAF(V600E) melanoma. *Science Translational Medicine, 7*, 279ra241-279ra241. https://doi.org/10.1126/scitranslmed.aaa4691
98. Khalili, J. S., et al. (2012). Oncogenic BRAF(V600E) promotes stromal cell-mediated immunosuppression via induction of interleukin-1 in melanoma. *Clinical Cancer Research, 18*, 5329–5340. https://doi.org/10.1158/1078-0432.CCR-12-1632
99. Shabaneh, T. B., et al. (2018). Oncogenic BRAF(V600E) governs regulatory T-cell recruitment during melanoma tumorigenesis. *Cancer Research, 78*, 5038–5049. https://doi.org/10.1158/0008-5472.CAN-18-0365
100. Kim, G., et al. (2014). FDA approval summary: Vemurafenib for treatment of unresectable or metastatic melanoma with the BRAFV600E mutation. *Clinical Cancer Research, 20*, 4994. https://doi.org/10.1158/1078-0432.CCR-14-0776
101. Nazarian, R., et al. (2010). Melanomas acquire resistance to B-RAF(V600E) inhibition by RTK or N-RAS upregulation. *Nature, 468*, 973–977. https://doi.org/10.1038/nature09626
102. Shi, H., et al. (2014). Acquired resistance and clonal evolution in melanoma during BRAF inhibitor therapy. *Cancer Discovery, 4*, 80. https://doi.org/10.1158/2159-8290.CD-13-0642
103. Gerlinger, M., et al. (2014). Cancer: Evolution within a lifetime. *Annual Review of Genetics, 48*, 215–236. https://doi.org/10.1146/annurev-genet-120213-092314
104. Sinnberg, T., et al. (2016). A nexus consisting of Beta-catenin and Stat3 attenuates BRAF inhibitor efficacy and mediates acquired resistance to Vemurafenib. *eBioMedicine, 8*, 132–149. https://doi.org/10.1016/j.ebiom.2016.04.037
105. Basile, K. J., Abel, E. V., & Aplin, A. E. (2012). Adaptive upregulation of FOXD3 and resistance to PLX4032/4720-induced cell death in mutant B-RAF melanoma cells. *Oncogene, 31*, 2471–2479. https://doi.org/10.1038/onc.2011.424
106. Guerriero, L., et al. (2017). The anti-apoptotic BAG3 protein is involved in BRAF inhibitor resistance in melanoma cells. *Oncotarget, 8*, 80393–80404. https://doi.org/10.18632/oncotarget.18902
107. Hu, W., et al. (2013). AEBP1 upregulation confers acquired resistance to BRAF (V600E) inhibition in melanoma. *Cell Death & Disease, 4*, e914–e914. https://doi.org/10.1038/cddis.2013.441
108. Kulkarni, A., et al. (2017). BRAF Fusion as a Novel Mechanism of Acquired Resistance to Vemurafenib in BRAFV600E mutant melanoma. *Clinical Cancer Research, 23*, 5631. https://doi.org/10.1158/1078-0432.CCR-16-0758
109. Chu, E. Y., et al. (2012). Diverse cutaneous side effects associated with BRAF inhibitor therapy: A clinicopathologic study. *Journal of the American Academy of Dermatology, 67*, 1265–1272. https://doi.org/10.1016/j.jaad.2012.04.008
110. Long, G. V., et al. (2017). Dabrafenib plus trametinib versus dabrafenib monotherapy in patients with metastatic BRAF V600E/K-mutant melanoma: Long-term survival and safety analysis of a phase 3 study. *Annals of Oncology, 28*, 1631–1639. https://doi.org/10.1093/annonc/mdx176
111. Jones, A., et al. (2016). Immunomodulatory functions of BTLA and HVEM govern induction of extrathymic regulatory T cells and tolerance by dendritic cells. *Immunity, 45*, 1066–1077. https://doi.org/10.1016/j.immuni.2016.10.008
112. Zhang, T., Ye, L., Han, L., He, Q., & Zhu, J. (2016). Knockdown of HVEM, a lymphocyte regulator gene, in ovarian cancer cells increases sensitivity to activated T cells. *Oncology Research, 24*, 189–196. https://doi.org/10.3727/096504016X14641336229602

Noncoding RNAs in Papillary Thyroid Cancer: Interaction with Cancer-Associated Fibroblasts (CAFs) in the Tumor Microenvironment (TME) and Regulators of Differentiation and Lymph Node Metastasis

Sina Dadafarin, Michelle Carnazza, Humayun K. Islam, Augustine Moscatello, Raj K. Tiwari, and Jan Geliebter

1 Introduction

1.1 Overview of the Thyroid Gland

1.1.1 Normal Thyroid Differentiation and Thyroid Hormone Synthesis

The thyroid is a butterfly-shaped organ that is situated anterior to the trachea at the level of the C5 to T1 vertebrae. The gland is endodermal in origin, derived from the foramen cecum positioned at the base of the tongue and descends the midline of the neck [1]. At its native position, the thyroid gland has symmetrical lateral lobes and a centrally located isthmus. Dual blood supply, from the superior and inferior thyroid arteries, provides a disproportionate share of cardiac output relative to its size. This rich blood supply allows the endocrine organ to detect and secrete circulating hormones as well as offset the cellular energetic demands [1].

Histologically, the thyroid is enclosed by a fibrous capsule and organized into follicles, a circular structure composed of a single layer of follicular cells and a central collection of the colloid. The colloid is acellular and eosinophilic and contains a reservoir of thyroglobulin (Tg). Follicular thyroid epithelial cells are responsible for the synthesis and secretion of the thyroid hormones T4 and T3 which are derived from the precursor Tg. Normally differentiated follicular cells express transcription factors paired box gene 8 (PAX8) and NK2 homeobox 1 (NKX2-1). Key features of the basolateral membrane include thyrotropin receptors (TSHR) and the sodium-iodide transporter (SLC5A5). The apical membrane contains a chloride-iodide exchanger (SLC26A4) and thyroperoxidase (TPO). In between follicles is a second cell type known as parafollicular cells, or C cells, that are responsible for the production of calcitonin. A third, rarer cell type is oncocytic cells called Hürthle cells that are rich

S. Dadafarin · M. Carnazza · H. K. Islam · R. K. Tiwari · J. Geliebter (✉)
Department of Pathology, Microbiology, and Immunology, New York Medical College, Valhalla, NY, USA
e-mail: Jan_Geliebter@nymc.edu

A. Moscatello
Department of Otolaryngology, New York Medical College, Westchester Medical Center, Valhalla, NY, USA

D. Banerjee, R. K. Tiwari (eds.), *Tumor Microenvironment: Cellular, Metabolic and Immunologic Interactions*, Advances in Experimental Medicine and Biology 1350,
https://doi.org/10.1007/978-3-030-83282-7_7

in mitochondria and are of unknown function. These cells are often found in chronic autoimmune thyroid diseases, such as Graves' disease and Hashimoto's thyroiditis [2].

1.1.2 Thyroid Hormone Production and Regulation

Thyrotropin-releasing hormone (TRH) is secreted by the hypothalamus and stimulates release of thyrotropin thyroid-stimulating hormone (TSH) from basophil cells in the anterior pituitary. TSH is a glycoprotein hormone that binds to TSHR on the surface of follicular epithelial cells in the thyroid gland to stimulate thyroid hormone production. This initiates the import of iodide from the basolateral membrane of follicular cells via SLC5A5 and expression of Tg. Iodide then is transported across the apical membrane via SLC26A4 and organified and incorporated onto Tg by TPO. Iodination occurs on tyrosine residues of Tg and coupling of these iodinated residues to form iodothyronine residues. The predominant form of iodothyronine contains four iodine atoms and acts as a precursor to T4. Iodinated Tg from the colloid is then endocytosed and processed in an endovesicle, where free T4 and T3 are produced and released into circulation. T4 is converted into the more active T3 hormone at target tissues via the deiodinase DIO1, upregulating cellular metabolism, protein synthesis, neuronal maturation, and the response to catecholamines. Regulation of thyroid hormone exists along the hypothalamic-pituitary axis, whereby circulating T4 or products of peripheral deiodination (T3 and rT3) inhibit TSH and TRH release [3].

1.2 Papillary Thyroid Carcinoma

1.2.1 Classification of Thyroid Cancers

Thyroid malignancies were formerly classified based on their histopathological characteristics and cell type the cancer is derived from. All thyroid malignancies, with the exception of medullary carcinoma, are derived from follicular cells [4]. A large majority (>80%) of all thyroid cancers are papillary thyroid carcinomas (PTC), named for the specific papillary architecture observed histologically. Follicular thyroid cancer (FTC) is the second most common subtype and retains features of normal thyroid architecture, including a ring of follicular cells surrounding a central colloid [5]. Either of these cancers can progress to more dedifferentiated and aggressive variants, such as poorly differentiated papillary thyroid cancer (PDPTC) and anaplastic thyroid cancer (ATC) [6]. Recent molecular classification by The Cancer Genome Atlas [4] and other groups [7] have stratified the subtypes of PTC and FTC along a spectrum, whereby BRAF-mutant, papillary cancers are more dedifferentiated and likely to metastasize, while RAS-mutant and RAS and BRAF-nonmutant tumors are better differentiated and less aggressive.

1.3 Diagnostic and Therapeutic Approach to Thyroid Nodules

1.3.1 Initial Evaluation of a Thyroid Nodule

The first sign of a thyroid malignancy typically begins with a physical exam finding of a neck nodule or as an incidental finding on imaging. The initial test following identification of a thyroid nodule is a TSH measurement to determine if the nodule is autonomously producing thyroid hormone (also known as a functional or "hot" nodule). A low TSH indicates elevated levels of thyroid hormone, and the next diagnostic step is scintigraphy with either technetium (99mTc), 123I, or 131I [8]. A focal uptake of radioactive material in the nodule with reduced uptake in the remainder of the thyroid is diagnostic for a functional adenoma, which bears a very low risk of malignancy, and the patient is subsequently evaluated and treated for thyrotoxicosis. In the setting of normal or elevated TSH levels, ultrasound-guided fine needle aspiration (FNA) biopsy is recommended in the next step as cytologic assessment is critical for determining good candidates for surgical intervention [9].

1.3.2 FNA and Current Molecular Classifiers

The interpretation of FNA biopsy is made using the Bethesda class II classification schema [10]. Classes I and II are considered benign and only require nodule surveillance with serial ultrasound, while classes V and VI warrant primary treatment for malignancy. Classes III and IV are considered indeterminate and the clinical decision at this point is more complex. FNA can be repeated in an attempt to obtain a more definitive cytological finding. Recently, molecular classifiers such as the Afirma Gene Expression Classifier [11] or the ThyroSeq sequencing classifier [12] use mutational status and expression levels from FNA samples to guide therapeutic decisions. Finally, patients with indeterminate FNA biopsies who also have radiologic or sonographic findings suggestive of malignancy may be directed to definitive treatment with lobectomy or total thyroidectomy.

1.3.3 Treatment Modalities

For patients with PTC or suspected PTC, thyroid and neck imaging with ultrasound or CT/MRI is performed to identify tumor-bearing lymph nodes and possible extension of the primary into nearby structures. Results from imaging also guide the surgical approach, including the decision to perform total thyroidectomy or lobectomy and removal of cervical lymph nodes. Lobectomy can successfully treat a patient with small PTC tumors and without extrathyroidal extension while preserving thyroid function and minimizes risk of complications (e.g., hypocalcemia) [13]. Specific indications for total thyroidectomy include tumor diameter >4 cm, evidence of nodal or distant metastasis, extrathyroidal extension, or bilateral, multifocal disease.

For patients with residual disease that is unresectable in the neck, postsurgical management involves serial TSH and Tg monitoring to detect recurrence and 123I or 131I total body imaging to determine if remaining cancer cells are responsive to radioactive iodine (RAI). Responsive tumors are then treated with whole body 131I, also called RAI ablation. This combination of surgical removal of primary disease followed by RAI therapy has led to an overall 5-year survival rate of >95%, making PTC among the most effectively treated human malignancies [14].

1.3.4 Potential Role of Novel Biomarkers

Despite the high rate of success with modern diagnostic and therapeutic algorithms, there are significant areas where the management of PTC can be improved. Aggressive PTC subtypes that are refractory to RAI therapy carry a much worse prognosis and account for the majority of PTC-related deaths [15]. Thus, methods that could accurately classify RAI avidity could better tailor the therapeutic approach by identifying patients with resistant subtypes of the disease earlier. To date methods for determining the response to RAI carry significant drawbacks. Low-dose 131I imaging may cause a phenomenon known as "thyroid stunning" whereby the use of 131I for imaging reduces the efficacy of subsequent high-dose therapeutic 131I use, resulting in incomplete ablation of remaining disease [16]. An alternative isotope, 123I, does not cause this stunning phenomenon but is more expensive and not as widely available. Serum Tg level may act as an indicator of thyroid differentiation and, therefore, avidity to RAI; however, endogenous TSH levels and the presence of anti-Tg antibodies, such as in autoimmune thyroiditis, can confound Tg measurements. Recent evidence suggests that thyroid differentiation characterized by gene expression signatures is directly associated with RAI avidity [17]. These metrics are inelastic to TSH levels or endogenous thyroglobulin (TG) antibodies. Additionally, gene markers bypass adverse effects of 131I imaging such as radiation exposure and thyroid stunning [18].

When trying to detect tumor-positive lymph nodes in the neck, current imaging methods have low sensitivity [19, 20]. With low specificity, these tests allow too many false negative results to be presented to patients, thus not allowing them to receive the treatment that they need. As lymph node metastasis is present in roughly 40% of all adult PTC cases, higher specificity in these tests is a clinical need, especially since lymph node metastases are associated with reduced survival and higher recurrence rates [21–23]. Using molecular markers as adjuvants with ultrasound imaging has been shown to improve the detection of lymph node metastasis [24]. Additionally, development of more sensitive and specific detection methods that allow unnecessary surgeries to be avoided is of the utmost importance. For example, routine practice shies away from the use of prophylactic cervical lymph node dissections guided by single-gene mutation profiles (e.g., BRAF) [25–27]. The discovery of novel biomarkers better suited toward predicting lymph node metastases could identify the PTC patient subset most likely to benefit from lymph node dissection.

1.4 lncRNAs in Papillary Thyroid Cancer

1.4.1 Structure and Function of lncRNAs

The body of large-scale, unbiased gene expression analysis in PTC has focused on the coding transcriptome, specifically mRNAs and microRNAs [4, 28]. However, protein-coding genes constitute only 2% of the entire genome, and recent genome-wide investigations have uncovered long noncoding transcripts of 200 nucleotides or greater that are transcribed in unique genomic positions [29, 30]. These long noncoding RNAs (lncRNAs) have diverse regulatory potential in gene expression, alternative splicing, posttranscriptional mRNA modification, and epigenomic alterations [31–33]. Many lncRNAs have tissue-specific expression [34, 35]. Furthermore, there are lncRNAs that have been demonstrated to play key roles in cancer progression and prognosis [35–37]. However, lncRNAs are not being exploited as biomarkers or therapeutic targets currently, despite their elucidated effects on oncogenesis [32, 38, 39]. For example, in thyroid cancer, dysregulation of lncRNAs has been correlated with a more aggressive phenotypes; however, this has yet to be exploited therapeutically [40, 41]. Hence, the identification of differentially expressed lncRNAs could fill the gap in knowledge and applications in PTC diagnosis, prognosis, and treatment.

1.4.2 lncRNA Investigation in Papillary Thyroid Cancer

There have been implications for the potential use of lncRNAs in PTC diagnosis, prognosis, and treatment via the utilization of genome-wide studies of patient samples. Most of the transcriptomic data is from microarray and quantitative reverse transcription polymerase chain reaction (qRT-PCR) with this data analysis uncovering the dysregulation of lncRNAs in cancerous tissue [42–45]. Unfortunately, this methodology only probes for a fraction of the noncoding transcriptome [46, 47]. Whole-exome RNA sequencing of a small number of patient samples has revealed an association of certain lncRNAs with molecular and clinical characteristics of PTC [48, 49]. The Cancer Genome Atlas Thyroid Carcinoma (TCGA THCA) study further demonstrated this with larger patient sample sizes [41, 50, 51]. However, it should be noted that RNA sequencing by the TCGA may not have captured all lncRNAs, specifically those lacking polyadenylated tails, due to the sequencing on polyA-purified RNA [52, 53]. In order to circumvent that caveat, the J. Geliebter lab performed RNA sequencing on 45 matched-paired PTC tumors with more diverse staging than those previously described, and normal adjacent tissue samples utilizing rRNA-depleted total RNA. The goal was to supplement existing analyses while maximizing detection of differentially expressed (DE) lncRNAs in PTC that associated with clinical characteristics including thyroid differentiation and lymph node metastasis. The identification of these lncRNAs was done via the examination of their co-expression with mRNAs.

Relative to protein-coding genes, lncRNAs are underutilized as biomarkers and underrepresented and not fully enriched in the existing datasets. This work saw that relative to the TCGA, there was a greater detection of antisense, sense intronic, sense overlapping, and 3′ overlapping lncRNAs. It was speculated the decrease in long intergenic RNA (lincRNA) detection was due to poly-adenylation of intergenic transcripts that facilitates higher enrichment by the poly-A RNA isolation methods mentioned above [53].

2 lncRNAs Highly Associated with Thyroid Differentiation and Tissue-Specific Expression

For a particular tissue, cells are differentiated; they have gone from pluripotent to unipotent with the capability of doing the one function of this tissue. As cells differentiate, they are restricted to how many of them can then be produced. Differentiation is a regulated process of gene expression and via accumulation of mutations, cancer can form. Cancer is a disease of proliferation due to the loss of normal controls on cell growth as well as dedifferentiation resulting typically in cells that are undifferentiated or partially differentiated. Anaplastic cells are those that are undifferentiated or poorly differentiated, as they cannot be identified as a specific tissue cell due to the loss of the defining characteristics such as markers or morphology. Thyroid cancer has enormous heterogeneity regarding morphology and prognosis. Anaplastic thyroid cancer (ATC) is the most advanced and aggressive form of thyroid cancer. It is one of the fastest growing and these cells do not look or behave at all like thyroid cells. Poorly differentiated thyroid cancer (PDTC) is another rare and aggressive form of thyroid cancer. The cause is unknown; however, it has been seen to arise from differentiated thyroid cancers such as PTC or follicular thyroid cancer (FTC). While most types of thyroid cancer are associated with a relatively good prognosis, ATC and PDTC are associated with an increased risk of recurrence and death. These more aggressive forms are difficult to treat due to their ease of spreading and metastasis.

Dedifferentiation can clinically manifest as unresponsiveness to RAI therapy and, therefore, impairs the ability to treat unresectable or metastatic malignancies [4]. The BRAFV600E mutation is present in the vast majority of dedifferentiated tumors; however, not all BRAF-mutant patients have poorly differentiated PTC [4]. This indicates that the BRAFV600E mutation is necessary but not sufficient for the development of RAI-resistant cancer [4]. Thus, additional markers/variables are needed to better stratify patients based on the differentiation status of their disease. Furthermore, this line of investigation may also reveal molecular targets to rescuing differentiation of thyroid cancer cells and make previously RAI-refractory disease amenable to RAI therapy.

A recent clinical trial of the BRAF inhibitor vemurafenib in RAI-refractory thyroid cancer used an expanded thyroid differentiation score (eTDS) as a proxy for differentiation status and showed RAI responsiveness was associated with an increase in eTDS scores [17]; thus, the authors concluded that the eTDS as a molecular marker may better predict RAI responsiveness compared to existing serum biomarkers such as Tg or TSH levels.

Long noncoding RNAs are increasingly investigated for their role in a variety of cancer-related processes, yet underutilized as biomarkers relative to protein-coding genes [32, 54, 55]. Furthermore, many lncRNAs are exquisitely tissue-specific and stable enough to be detected in serum [56], making them excellent candidate biomarkers and potential therapeutic targets. In PTC, lncRNAs have been identified as key regulatory elements in mediating proliferation, apoptosis, angiogenesis, invasion, metastasis, and differentiation [57–61], and as such, the use of these tissue- and stage-specific lncRNAs could be a potential treatment option to induce differentiation or suppress dedifferentiation.

The Geliebter lab used the TDS score first described by the TCGA Thyroid Carcinoma (THCA) project and correlated the TDS to every annotated and expressed lncRNA to identify noncoding transcripts that showed strong positive and negative associations with thyroid differentiation. These include FAM95C and AC004603, respectively (Spearman = 0.842 and

Spearman = −0.571). This strong positive correlation of FAM95C led to the investigation of this previously uncharacterized long intergenic RNA (lincRNA). A lincRNA is distinguished from the broader transcript class of lncRNA as they are located between protein-coding genes and are transcribed independently [62]. They do not overlap with protein-coding genes and will usually have their own promoters and regulatory elements. FAM95C is located on the short arm of chromosome 9 and is downstream to the 3′end of the ANKRD18A gene, a potential epigenetic regulator that is commonly downregulated in thyroid cancer [63, 64]. FAM95C is also co-expressed with ANKRD18A, suggesting possible cis-regulatory activity.

Intriguingly, FAM95C outperformed the TDS constituent genes in predictivity of TDS with the exception of TPO. Notably, TPO expression can be influenced by TSH levels and inflammatory cytokines, making its use as a molecular marker limited in thyroid cancer patients with concomitant hypothyroidism or thyroiditis [65, 66]. Next, patient tumors were subdivided into four groups based on high or low FAM95C expression and *BRAF* mutational status. Tumors that were BRAFV600E positive with low FAM95C expression showed significantly lower TDS scores compared to the other groups and detected 88% of tumors with a TDS < −2 (denoting a fourfold mean reduction in thyroid differentiation genes). This provided preliminary evidence of the possibility that these two metrics of BRAF status and FAM95C expression could characterize differentiation status.

Additionally, the expression of FAM95C in TCGA normal tissues was examined to determine if FAM95C is expressed in a tissue-specific manner. This analysis revealed that the first and second highest transcript levels of FAM95C were in the testis and thyroid, respectively. The GTEx data were also examined and indicated the top five tissues with highest transcript levels of FAM95C were endocrine organs, including the testis, thyroid, pituitary gland, pancreas, and prostate. This indicates it may be detected reliably in a tissue-specific manner, especially in females.

3 lncRNAs Expressed in Primary Tumors that Predict LNM

Detection of lymph node metastasis (LNM) in the preoperative setting can guide the surgical approach as well as postoperative decision-making regarding the use of RAI. Furthermore, patients with LNM have higher rates of recurrence and reduced overall survival [21–23]. Consistent with the advantages sought when identifying molecular markers for thyroid differentiation, the large-scale regulatory function [31], tissue-specific expression [34, 62], and dysregulation in cancer [57] make lncRNAs potential mediators of LNM and good candidate biomarkers as well as therapeutic targets. However, there was not a gene expression marker, such as the TDS for thyroid differentiation, that can be used as a proxy for identifying lncRNAs that are significantly associated with LNM. Furthermore, since the vast majority of the noncoding transcriptome is poorly characterized, there is no currently available functional annotation method for lncRNAs as there is for protein-coding genes (e.g., KEGG pathway and GO enrichment analyses).

A common method for identifying the functional role of lncRNAs in large-scale transcriptomics experiments is by constructing co-expression networks of mRNAs and lncRNAs [67]. This method allows one to infer the biological role of noncoding transcripts by functionally annotating the mRNAs co-expressed within the same gene network. A popular method for creating co-expression networks from transcriptomics data is by using weighted gene coexpression analysis (WGCNA) first developed by the Horvath lab [68]. WGCNA not only allows gene networks to be formed from a global analysis but also provides a method to associate co-expression networks to clinical, demographic, and genomic features via linear regression for continuous variables (e.g., age, tumor size) or logistic regression for categorical variables (e.g., lymph node status, stage, gender). Thus, gene networks derived from WGCNA identify sets of genes, including noncoding ones, tightly associated with disease states and potential therapeutic targets [69].

To identify lncRNAs associated with LNM in PTC, WGCNA was used to identify a gene co-expression module that was significantly correlated with LNM. This module contained approximately 730 genes, 74 of which were lncRNAs. Functional annotation of protein-coding genes in this module revealed enrichment of biological processes including epithelial-mesenchymal transition, hypoxia, and TNFa activation, all of which have been implicated in cancer metastasis [70, 71]. Given this module's statistical and biologic association with LNM, we next examined lncRNAs within the module. Ranked by module membership (MM) score denoting the importance of a gene within a module, the lncRNA MEG3 was most predictive of LNM. Transcriptomic analysis showed that MEG3 is expressed higher in tumors with LNM compared to those without LNM and high MEG3 expression is associated with lower overall survival, particularly among patients with BRAF-mutant tumors.

Interestingly, these findings regarding MEG3 contrast much in the current cancer literature [72–75]. Wang and colleagues specifically showed in PTC that MEG3 may prevent invasion and metastasis by inhibiting GTPases, such as RAC1, that promote cell motility and cytoskeletal rearrangement [76–78]. As many studies of MEG3 in the cancer biology literature have focused on the role in tumor cells, we hypothesized that our seemingly contrasting findings may be due to the expression of MEG3 within the tumor microenvironment from nonmalignant cell types. Cancer cells engage in complex interactions with infiltrating immune cells, vasculature, extracellular matrix, and stromal cells [79]. Using deconvolution methods for bulk RNA sequencing data to predict cell types in PTC tumors, we found MEG3 expression was highly correlated with infiltration of cancer-associated fibroblasts (CAF). CAFs have been shown to be key mediators of tumor invasion and metastasis via the role in extracellular matrix remodeling [80]. Furthermore, recent findings from the cardiovascular literature have shown that MEG3 expression in cardiac fibroblasts is associated with cardiac remodeling post-coronary infarction via increased expression of ECM processing genes such as MMP-2 [81]. We also found MEG3 expression to be highly correlated with MMP-2 expression in PTC tumors. These findings may indicate that, while MEG3 may typically function as a tumor suppressor in cancer cells, the expression of MEG3 in CAFs may indicate propensity for LNM via higher rates of ECM processing.

4 lncRNas as Regulators of Molecular Phenotype and Interaction with Components of TME

Papillary thyroid cancer generally bears a favorable prognosis, oftentimes curable, as tumors are most often slow-growing and surgically resectable. However, PTC can transition into aggressive subtypes and metastasize in certain patients that nullifies the otherwise high survival rate [21]. Extended longevity has been achieved via a combination of pharmaceutical, surgical, and radiation-based therapies; however, it is difficult to predict which of these patients will benefit from these interventions [18, 25]. With the increased accessibility and decreased cost of high-throughput sequencing, novel biomarkers in PTC could be identified to fill the gap in knowledge and indicate which clinical approach would be best [82].

A common thread through these lines of investigation is the role key regulators, namely, the actions of lncRNAs, play in the development and progression of thyroid cancer. Using transcriptome-wide and genome-wide sequencing methods as well as a suite of computational tools, the aims were to identify specific regulatory actions of molecules that mediate the onset and progression of PTC that can be exploited for diagnostic and therapeutic purposes.

It is known that lncRNAs are involved in transcriptional regulation of protein-coding genes; oftentimes, however, this complexity is not easily integrated into clinical phenotypes.

Since RAI is a mainstay of metastatic PTC treatment, it was pertinent to explore lncRNAs associated with iodine handling and thyroid differentiation, key factors that lead to RAI resistance and increased mortality in this normally well-managed disease [18, 23]. Overall, the work in the J. Geliebter lab demonstrates a simpler metric for differentiation looking at just FAM95C expression and BRAF mutation status, as opposed to the arguably more complex parallel quantification of 16 genes that could pose more issues rather than not [17]. This two-factor metric could yield a cost-effective, simpler, but more precise assessment of differentiation compared to obtaining the TDS or eTDS in patient samples.

There are other studies utilizing TCGA, Genotype-Tissue Expression (GTEx) and Gene Expression Omnibus (GEO) datasets, to identify and investigate differentially expressed lncRNAs in thyroid cancer. Interestingly, there are few studies that investigate the role of lncRNAs in ATC. As mentioned, lncRNAs have implicated roles at essentially all steps of tumorigenesis. A July 2020 systematic review of studies of lncRNAs in ATC, there were only 30 lncRNAs that were identified for their role in ATC as oncogenes or tumor suppressors [83]. These potent biomarkers would be revolutionary in detection at early stages as this significantly increases the chances of survival. Their aberrant expression in cancer and correlation with steps in tumorigenesis as well as their role in differentiation would allow for a promising role as a prognostic and diagnostic biomarker in thyroid cancer. This would help prevent the more aggressive ATC that derives from dedifferentiation of the less aggressive PTC and FTC. Therefore, in the case of catching PTC or FTC early, one can hopefully prevent the progression to the more lethal ATC. Furthermore, targeting of the specific lncRNAs could also pose as a valuable treatment option via preventing or reversing this dedifferentiation process and making this usually refractory form of thyroid cancer more responsive to standard treatment options.

References

1. Allen, E., & Fingeret, A. (2019). Anatomy, head and neck, thyroid. In *StatPearls*. StatPearls Publishing.
2. Cannon, J. (2011). The significance of hurthle cells in thyroid disease. *The Oncologist, 16*(10), 1380–1387.
3. Zoeller, R. T., Tan, S. W., & Tyl, R. W. (2007). General background on the hypothalamic-pituitary-thyroid (HPT) axis. *Critical Reviews in Toxicology, 37*(1-2), 11–53.
4. Cancer Genome Atlas Research Network. (2014). Integrated genomic characterization of papillary thyroid carcinoma. *Cell, 159*(3), 676–690.
5. Grebe, S. K., & Hay, I. D. (1995). Follicular thyroid cancer. *Endocrinology and Metabolism Clinics of North America, 24*(4), 761–801.
6. Xing, M. (2013). Molecular pathogenesis and mechanisms of thyroid cancer. *Nature Reviews. Cancer, 13*(3), 184–199.
7. Yoo, S.-K., Lee, S., Kim, S.-J., et al. (2016). Comprehensive analysis of the transcriptional and mutational landscape of follicular and papillary thyroid cancers. *PLoS Genetics, 12*(8), e1006239.
8. Bomeli, S. R., LeBeau, S. O., & Ferris, R. L. (2010). Evaluation of a thyroid nodule. *Otolaryngologic Clinics of North America, 43*(2), 229–238. vii.
9. Sidawy, M. K., Vecchio, D. M. D., & Knoll, S. M. (1997). Fine-needle aspiration of thyroid nodules: Correlation between cytology and histology and evaluation of discrepant cases. *Cancer Cytopathology: Interdisciplinary International Journal of the American Cancer Society, 81*(4), 253–259.
10. Cibas, E. S., & Ali, S. Z. (2017). The 2017 Bethesda system for reporting thyroid cytopathology. *Thyroid, 27*(11), 1341–1346.
11. Alexander, E. K., Schorr, M., Klopper, J., et al. (2014). Multicenter clinical experience with the Afirma gene expression classifier. *The Journal of Clinical Endocrinology and Metabolism, 99*(1), 119–125.
12. Nikiforov, Y. E., Carty, S. E., Chiosea, S. I., et al. (2015). Impact of the multi-gene ThyroSeq next-generation sequencing assay on cancer diagnosis in thyroid nodules with atypia of undetermined significance/follicular lesion of undetermined significance cytology. *Thyroid, 25*(11), 1217–1223.
13. Vargas-Pinto, S., & Romero Arenas, M. A. (2018). Thyroid lobectomy vs total thyroidectomy for low risk papillary thyroid cancer: A systematic review. *Journal of the American College of Surgeons, 227*(4), e123.
14. Hay, I. D., Thompson, G. B., Grant, C. S., et al. (2002). Papillary thyroid carcinoma managed at the Mayo Clinic during six decades (1940–1999): Temporal trends in initial therapy and long-term outcome in 2444 consecutively treated patients. *World Journal of Surgery, 26*(8), 879–885. https://doi.org/10.1007/s00268-002-6612-1
15. Gruber, J. J., & Colevas, A. D. (2015). Differentiated thyroid cancer: Focus on emerging treatments for

radioactive iodine-refractory patients. *The Oncologist, 20*(2), 113–126.
16. Park, H.-M., & Gerard, S. K. (2006). Stunning: Untoward effect of 131I thyroid imaging prior to radioablation therapy. In L. Wartofsky & D. Van Nostrand (Eds.), *Thyroid cancer: A comprehensive guide to clinical management* (pp. 337–345). Humana Press.
17. Dunn, L. A., Sherman, E. J., Baxi, S. S., et al. (2019). Vemurafenib redifferentiation of BRAF mutant, RAI-refractory thyroid cancers. *The Journal of Clinical Endocrinology and Metabolism, 104*(5), 1417–1428.
18. Robbins, R. J., & Schlumberger, M. J. (2005). The evolving role of (^{131}I) for the treatment of differentiated thyroid carcinoma. *The Journal of Nuclear Medicine and Allied Sciences, 46*, 28S.
19. Ahn, J. E., Lee, J. H., Yi, J. S., et al. (2008). Diagnostic accuracy of CT and ultrasonography for evaluating metastatic cervical lymph nodes in patients with thyroid cancer. *World Journal of Surgery, 32*(7), 1552–1558.
20. Jeong, H.-S., Baek, C.-H., Son, Y.-I., et al. (2006). Integrated 18F-FDG PET/CT for the initial evaluation of cervical node level of patients with papillary thyroid carcinoma: Comparison with ultrasound and contrast-enhanced CT. *Clinical Endocrinology, 65*(3), 402–407.
21. Podnos, Y. D., Smith, D., Wagman, L. D., & Ellenhorn, J. D. I. (2005). The implication of lymph node metastasis on survival in patients with well-differentiated thyroid cancer. *The American Surgeon, 71*(9), 731–734.
22. Mazzaferri, E. L., & Jhiang, S. M. (1994). Long-term impact of initial surgical and medical therapy on papillary and follicular thyroid cancer. *The American Journal of Medicine, 97*(5), 418–428.
23. Mazzaferri, E. L. (1993). Management of a solitary thyroid nodule. *The New England Journal of Medicine, 328*(8), 553–559.
24. Xia, S., Wang, C., Ni, X., Ni, Z., Dong, Y., & Zhan, W. (2017). NONHSAT076754 aids ultrasonography in predicting lymph node metastasis and promotes migration and invasion of papillary thyroid cancer cells. *Oncotarget, 8*(2), 2293–2306.
25. Haugen, B. R., Alexander, E. K., Bible, K. C., et al. (2016). 2015 American Thyroid Association Management guidelines for adult patients with thyroid nodules and differentiated thyroid cancer: The American Thyroid Association Guidelines Task Force on thyroid nodules and differentiated thyroid cancer. *Thyroid, 26*(1), 1–133.
26. Aragon Han, P., Kim, H.-S., Cho, S., et al. (2016). Association of BRAFV600E mutation and MicroRNA expression with central lymph node metastases in papillary thyroid cancer: A prospective study from four endocrine surgery centers. *Thyroid, 26*(4), 532–542.
27. Dutenhefner, S. E., Marui, S., Santos, A. B. O., et al. (2013). BRAF: A tool in the decision to perform elective neck dissection? *Thyroid, 23*(12), 1541–1546.
28. Aragon Han, P., Weng, C.-H., Khawaja, H. T., et al. (2015). MicroRNA expression and association with clinicopathologic features in papillary thyroid cancer: A systematic review. *Thyroid, 25*(12), 1322–1329.
29. Pennisi, E. (2012). Genomics. ENCODE project writes eulogy for junk DNA. *Science, 337*(6099), 1159–1161.
30. ENCODE Project Consortium, Moore, J. E., Purcaro, M. J., et al. (2020). Expanded encyclopaedias of DNA elements in the human and mouse genomes. *Nature, 583*(7818), 699–710.
31. Lee, J. T. (2012). Epigenetic regulation by long noncoding RNAs. *Science, 338*(6113), 1435–1439.
32. Huarte, M. (2015). The emerging role of lncRNAs in cancer. *Nature Medicine, 21*(11), 1253–1261.
33. Tripathi, V., Ellis, J. D., Shen, Z., et al. (2010). The nuclear-retained noncoding RNA MALAT1 regulates alternative splicing by modulating SR splicing factor phosphorylation. *Molecular Cell, 39*(6), 925–938.
34. Gupta, R. A., Shah, N., Wang, K. C., et al. (2010). Long non-coding RNA HOTAIR reprograms chromatin state to promote cancer metastasis. *Nature, 464*(7291), 1071–1076.
35. Zhang, Y., Yu, S., Jiang, L., Wang, X., & Song, X. (2017). HOTAIR is a promising novel biomarker in patients with thyroid cancer. *Experimental and Therapeutic Medicine, 13*(5), 2274–2278.
36. Rinn, J. L., Kertesz, M., Wang, J. K., et al. (2007). Functional demarcation of active and silent chromatin domains in human HOX loci by noncoding RNAs. *Cell, 129*(7), 1311–1323.
37. Ji, P., Diederichs, S., Wang, W., et al. (2003). MALAT-1, a novel noncoding RNA, and thymosin beta4 predict metastasis and survival in early-stage non-small cell lung cancer. *Oncogene, 22*(39), 8031–8041.
38. Mercer, T. R., Dinger, M. E., & Mattick, J. S. (2009). Long non-coding RNAs: Insights into functions. *Nature Reviews. Genetics, 10*(3), 155–159.
39. Ponting, C. P., Oliver, P. L., & Reik, W. (2009). Evolution and functions of long noncoding RNAs. *Cell, 136*(4), 629–641.
40. Cui, M., Chang, Y., Du, W., et al. (2018). Upregulation of lncRNA-ATB by transforming growth factor β1 (TGF-β1) promotes migration and invasion of papillary thyroid carcinoma cells. *Medical Science Monitor, 24*, 5152–5158.
41. Goedert, L., Plaça, J. R., Fuziwara, C. S., et al. (2017). Identification of long noncoding RNAs deregulated in papillary thyroid cancer and correlated with BRAF V600E mutation by bioinformatics integrative analysis. *Scientific Reports, 7*(1), 1–11.
42. Lan, X., Zhang, H., Wang, Z., et al. (2015). Genome-wide analysis of long noncoding RNA expression profile in papillary thyroid carcinoma. *Gene, 569*(1), 109–117.
43. Yang, M., Tian, J., Guo, X., et al. (2016). Long noncoding RNA are aberrantly expressed in human papillary thyroid carcinoma. *Oncology Letters, 12*(1), 544–552.

44. Xu, B., Shao, Q., Xie, K., et al. (2016). The long non-coding RNA ENST00000537266 and ENST00000426615 influence papillary thyroid cancer cell proliferation and motility. *Cellular Physiology and Biochemistry, 38*(1), 368–378.
45. Li, T., Yang, X.-D., Ye, C.-X., et al. (2017). Long noncoding RNA HIT000218960 promotes papillary thyroid cancer oncogenesis and tumor progression by upregulating the expression of high mobility group AT-hook 2 (HMGA2) gene. *Cell Cycle, 16*(2), 224–231.
46. Vickers, K. C., Roteta, L. A., Hucheson-Dilks, H., Han, L., & Guo, Y. (2015). Mining diverse small RNA species in the deep transcriptome. *Trends in Biochemical Sciences, 40*(1), 4–7.
47. Han, L., Vickers, K. C., Samuels, D. C., & Guo, Y. (2015). Alternative applications for distinct RNA sequencing strategies. *Briefings in Bioinformatics, 16*(4), 629–639.
48. Liyanarachchi, S., Li, W., Yan, P., et al. (2016). Genome-wide expression screening discloses long noncoding RNAs involved in thyroid carcinogenesis. *The Journal of Clinical Endocrinology and Metabolism, 101*(11), 4005–4013.
49. Wang, Q., Yang, H., Wu, L., et al. (2016). Identification of specific long non-coding RNA expression: Profile and analysis of association with clinicopathologic characteristics and BRAF mutation in papillary thyroid cancer. *Thyroid, 26*(12), 1719–1732.
50. Ma, B., Liao, T., Wen, D., et al. (2017). Corrigendum: Long intergenic non-coding RNA 271 is predictive of a poorer prognosis of papillary thyroid cancer. *Scientific Reports, 7*, 42321.
51. Luo, Y.-H., Liang, L., He, R.-Q., et al. (2017). RNA-sequencing investigation identifies an effective risk score generated by three novel lncRNAs for the survival of papillary thyroid cancer patients. *Oncotarget, 8*(43), 74139–74158. https://doi.org/10.18632/oncotarget.18274
52. Zhao, W., He, X., Hoadley, K. A., Parker, J. S., Hayes, D. N., & Perou, C. M. (2014). Comparison of RNA-Seq by poly (A) capture, ribosomal RNA depletion, and DNA microarray for expression profiling. *BMC Genomics, 15*, 419.
53. Guo, Y., Zhao, S., Sheng, Q., et al. (2015). RNAseq by total RNA library identifies additional RNAs compared to Poly(A) RNA library. *BioMed Research International, 2015*, 1–9. https://doi.org/10.1155/2015/862130
54. Prensner, J. R., Iyer, M. K., Sahu, A., et al. (2013). The long noncoding RNA SChLAP1 promotes aggressive prostate cancer and antagonizes the SWI/SNF complex. *Nature Genetics, 45*(11), 1392–1398. https://doi.org/10.1038/ng.2771
55. Gutschner, T., & Diederichs, S. (2012). The hallmarks of cancer: A long non-coding RNA point of view. *RNA Biology, 9*(6), 703–719.
56. Qi, P., Zhou, X.-Y., & Du, X. (2016). Circulating long non-coding RNAs in cancer: Current status and future perspectives. *Molecular Cancer, 15*(1), 39.
57. Sedaghati, M., & Kebebew, E. (2019). Long non-coding RNAs in thyroid cancer. *Current Opinion in Endocrinology, Diabetes, and Obesity, 26*(5), 275–281.
58. Cao, J., Zhang, M., Zhang, L., Lou, J., Zhou, F., & Fang, M. (2021). Non-coding RNA in thyroid cancer- functions and mechanisms. *Cancer Letters, 496*, 117–126.
59. Javed, Z., Shah, F. A., Rajabi, S., Raza, Q., Iqbal, Z., Ullah, M., et al. (2020). LncRNAs as potential therapeutic targets in thyroid cancer. *Asian Pacific Journal of Cancer Prevention, 21*(2), 281–287.
60. Kung, J., Colognori, D., & Lee, J. T. (2013). Long noncoding RNAs: Past, present, and future. *Genetics, 193*(3), 651–669.
61. Murugan, A. K., Munirajan, A. K., & Alzahrani, A. S. (2018). Long noncoding RNAs: Emerging players in thyroid cancer pathogenesis. *Endocrine-Related Cancer, 25*, R59–R82.
62. Ransohoff, J. D., Wei, Y., & Khavari, P. A. (2018). The functions and unique features of long intergenic non-coding RNA. *Nature Reviews Molecular Cell Biology, 19*(3), 143–157.
63. Liu, W.-B., Han, F., Jiang, X., et al. (2012). ANKRD18A as a novel epigenetic regulation gene in lung cancer. *Biochemical and Biophysical Research Communications, 429*(3-4), 180–185.
64. Shen, Y., Dong, S., Liu, J., et al. (2020). Identification of potential biomarkers for thyroid cancer using bioinformatics strategy: A study based on GEO datasets. *BioMed Research International, 2020*, 9710421.
65. Ashizawa, K., Yamashita, S., Nagayama, Y., et al. (1989). INTERFERON- y INHIBITS THYROTROPIN-INDUCED THYROIDAL PEROXIDASE GENE EXPRESSION IN CULTURED HUMAN THYROCYTES. *The Journal of Clinical Endocrinology and Metabolism, 69*(2), 475–477.
66. Tominaga, T., Yamashita, S., Nagayama, Y., et al. (1991). Interleukin 6 inhibits human thyroid peroxidase gene expression. *Acta Endocrinologica, 124*(3), 290–294.
67. Wang, Q., Roy, B., & Dwivedi, Y. (2019). Co-expression network modeling identifies key long non-coding RNA and mRNA modules in altering molecular phenotype to develop stress-induced depression in rats. *Translational Psychiatry, 9*(1), 125.
68. Zhao, W., Langfelder, P., Fuller, T., Dong, J., Li, A., & Hovarth, S. (2010). Weighted gene coexpression network analysis: State of the art. *Journal of Biopharmaceutical Statistics, 20*(2), 281–300.
69. Chen, Y., Zhu, J., Lum, P. Y., et al. (2008). Variations in DNA elucidate molecular networks that cause disease. *Nature, 452*(7186), 429–435.
70. Martin, T. A., Ye, L., Sanders, A. J., Lane, J., & Jiang, W. G. (2013). Cancer invasion and metastasis: Molecular and cellular perspective. *Metastatic Cancer: Clinical and Biological Perspectives*.
71. Ham, B., Fernandez, M. C., D'Costa, Z., & Brodt, P. (2016). The diverse roles of the TNF axis in can-

cer progression and metastasis. *Trends Cancer Res, 11*(1), 1–27.
72. Gong, X., & Huang, M. (2020). Tumor-suppressive function of lncRNA-MEG3 in glioma cells by regulating miR-6088/SMARCB1 axis. *BioMed Research International*, 1–15.
73. Zhang, S., & Guo, W. (2019). Long non-coding RNA MEG3 suppresses the growth of glioma cells by regulating the miR-96-5p/MTSS1 signaling pathway. *Molecular Medicine Reports, 20*(5), 4215–4225.
74. Liu, Z., Chen, J. Y., Zhong, Y., Xie, L., & Li, J. S. (2019). lncRNA MEG3 inhibits the growth of hepatocellular carcinoma cells by sponging miR-9-5p to upregulate SOX11. *Brazilian Journal of Medical and Biological Research, 52*(10).
75. Ghafouri-Fard, S., & Taheri, M. (2019). Maternally expressed gene 3(MEG3): A tumor suppressor long non coding RNA. *Biomedicine & Pharmacotherapy, 118*, 109–120.
76. Wang, C., Yan, G., Zhang, Y., Jia, X., & Bu, P. (2015). Long non-coding RNA MEG3 suppresses migration and invasion of thyroid carcinoma by targeting of Rac1. *Neoplasma, 62*(4), 541–549.
77. Parri, M., & Chiarugi, P. (2010). Rac and Rho GTPases in cancer cell motility control. *Cell Communication and Signaling: CCS, 8*, 23.
78. Bauer, N. N., Chen, Y.-W., Samant, R. S., Shevde, L. A., & Fodstad, O. (2007). Rac1 activity regulates proliferation of aggressive metastatic melanoma. *Exp Cell Res, 313*(18), 3832–3839.
79. Jason Morton, J., Bird, G., Refaeli, Y., & Jimeno, A. (2016). Humanized mouse xenograft models: Narrowing the tumor–microenvironment gap. *Cancer Research, 76*(21), 6153–6158.
80. Chen, X., & Song, E. (2019). Turning foes to friends: Targeting cancer-associated fibroblasts. *Nature Reviews. Drug Discovery, 18*(2), 99–115.
81. Piccoli, M., Gupta, S. K., Viereck, J., Foinquinos, A., Samolovac, S., Kramer, F. L., Garg, A., Remke, J., Zimmer, K., Batkai, S., & Thum, T. (2017). Inhibition of the cardiac fibroblast–enriched lncRNA Meg3 prevents cardiac fibrosis and diastolic dysfunction. *Circulation Research, 121*(5), 575–583.
82. Marti, J. L., Avadhani, V., Donatelli, L. A., et al. (2015). Wide inter-institutional variation in performance of a molecular classifier for indeterminate thyroid nodules. *Annals of Surgical Oncology, 22*(12), 3996–4001.
83. Samimi, H., Sajjadi-Jazi, S. M., Seifirad, S., Atlasi, R., Mahmoozadeh, H., Faghihi, M. A., & Haghpanah, V. (2020). Molecular mechanisms of long non-coding RNAs in anaplastic thyroid cancer: A systematic review. *Cancer Cell International, 20*, 352.

Index

D. Banerjee, R. K. Tiwari (eds.), *Tumor Microenvironment: Cellular, Metabolic and Immunologic Interactions*, Advances in Experimental Medicine and Biology 1350,
https://doi.org/10.1007/978-3-030-83282-7

D

The manufacturer's authorised representative in the EU is Springer Nature Customer Service Centre GmbH, Europaplatz 3, 69115 Heidelberg, Germany. If you have any concerns regarding our products, please contact ProductSafety@springernature.com

Printed and bound by CPI Group (UK) Ltd, Croydon, CR0 4YY

30/09/2026

02225465-0020